VOLUME
7
Phobias

WPA Series
Evidence and Experience in Psychiatry

Other Titles in the *WPA Series* Evidence and Experience in Psychiatry

Volume 1—Depressive Disorders 1999
Mario Maj and Norman Sartorius

Depressive Disorders, Second Edition 2003
Mario Maj and Norman Sartorius

Volume 2—Schizophrenia 1999
Mario Maj and Norman Sartorius

Schizophrenia, Second Edition 2003
Mario Maj and Norman Sartorius

Volume 3—Dementia 1999
Mario Maj and Norman Sartorius

Dementia, Second Edition 2003
Mario Maj and Norman Sartorius

Volume 4—Obsessive–Compulsive Disorder 1999
*Mario Maj, Norman Sartorius,
Ahmed Okasha and Joseph Zohar*

Obsessive–Compulsive Disorder, Second Edition 2003
*Mario Maj, Norman Sartorius,
Ahmed Okasha and Joseph Zohar*

Volume 5—Bipolar Disorder
*Mario Maj, Hagop S. Akiskal,
Juan José López-Ibor and Norman Sartorius*

Volume 6—Eating Disorders
*Mario Maj, Katherine Halmi, Juan José López-Ibor
and Norman Sartorius*

VOLUME

7

Phobias

Editors

Mario Maj
University of Naples, Italy

Hagop S. Akiskal
University of California, San Diego, USA

Juan José López-Ibor
Complutense University of Madrid, Spain

Ahmed Okasha
Ain Shams University, Cairo, Egypt

WPA Series
Evidence and Experience in Psychiatry

John Wiley & Sons, Ltd

Copyright © 2004   John Wiley & Sons Ltd, The Atrium, Southern Gate, Chichester,
West Sussex PO19 8SQ, England

Telephone (+44) 1243 779777

E-mail (for orders and customer service enquiries): cs-books@wiley.co.uk
Visit our Home Page on www.wileyeurope.com or www.wiley.com

All Rights Reserved. No part of this publication may be reproduced, stored in a retrieval system or transmitted in any form or by any means, electronic, mechanical, photocopying, recording, scanning or otherwise, except under the terms of the Copyright, Designs and Patents Act 1988 or under the terms of a licence issued by the Copyright Licensing Agency Ltd, 90 Tottenham Court Road, London W1T 4LP, UK, without the permission in writing of the Publisher. Requests to the Publisher should be addressed to the Permissions Department, John Wiley & Sons Ltd, The Atrium, Southern Gate, Chichester, West Sussex PO19 8SQ, England, or E-mailed to permreq@wiley.co.uk, or faxed to (+44) 1243 770620.

This publication is designed to provide accurate and authoritative information in regard to the subject matter covered. It is sold on the understanding that the Publisher is not engaged in rendering professional services. If professional advice or other expert assistance is required, the services of a competent professional should be sought.

Other Wiley Editorial Offices

John Wiley & Sons Inc., 111 River Street, Hoboken, NJ 07030, USA

Jossey-Bass, 989 Market Street, San Francisco, CA 94103-1741, USA

Wiley-VCH Verlag GmbH, Boschstr. 12, D-69469 Weinheim, Germany

John Wiley & Sons Australia Ltd, 33 Park Road, Milton, Queensland 4064, Australia

John Wiley & Sons (Asia) Pte Ltd, 2 Clementi Loop #02-01, Jin Xing Distripark, Singapore 129809

John Wiley & Sons (Canada) Ltd, 22 Worcester Road, Etobicoke, Ontario, Canada M9W 1L1

Wiley also publishes its books in a variety of electronic formats. Some content that appears in print may not be available in electronic books.

Library of Congress Cataloging-in-Publication Data

Phobias / edited by Mario Maj ... [et al.].
    p. ; cm. – (WPA series, evidence and experience in psychiatry ; v. 7)
Includes bibliographical references and index.
    ISBN 0-470-85833-8 (cloth : alk. paper)
1. Phobias. 2. Phobias - - Treatment.
    [DNLM: 1. Phobic Disorders. WM 178 P5743 2004]   I. Maj, Mario, 1953-
II. Series.
RC535 .P466 2004

British Library Cataloguing in Publication Data

A catalogue record for this book is available from the British Library

ISBN 0-470-85833-8

Typeset in 10/12pt Palatino by Dobbie Typesetting Ltd, Tavistock, Devon
Printed and bound in Great Britain by T.J. International Ltd, Padstow, Cornwall
This book is printed on acid-free paper responsibly manufactured from sustainable forestry in which at least two trees are planted for each one used for paper production.

Contents

List of Review Contributors		xi
Preface		xiii

CHAPTER 1 DIAGNOSIS AND CLASSIFICATION OF PHOBIAS   1

Diagnosis and Classification of Phobias:
A Review   1
Isaac Marks and David Mataix-Cols

COMMENTARIES

1.1 Two Procrustean or One King-Size Bed for Comorbid Agoraphobia and Panic?   33
Heinz Katschnig

1.2 Politics and Pathophysiology in the Classification of Phobias   36
Franklin R. Schneier

1.3 A Critical Evaluation of the Classification of Phobias   38
David V. Sheehan

1.4 The Role of Spontaneous, Unexpected Panic Attacks in the Diagnosis and Classification of Phobic Disorders   40
Giulio Perugi and Cristina Toni

1.5 Anxiety and Phobia: Issues in Classification   43
George C. Curtis

1.6 Nosology of the Phobias: Clues from the Genome   46
Raymond R. Crowe

1.7 Clusters, Comorbidity and Context in Classification of Phobic Disorders   47
Joshua D. Lipsitz

1.8 Comorbidity in Social Phobia: Nosological Implications   50
Constantin R. Soldatos and Thomas J. Paparrigopoulos

1.9 Giving Credit to "Neglected" or "Minor" Disorders   52
Charles Pull and Caroline Pull

1.10	A Cognitive Approach to Phobias *Jean-Pierre Lépine and Catherine Musa*	55
1.11	Diagnosis and Classification of Phobias and Other Anxiety Disorders: Quite Different Categories or Just One Dimension? *Miguel R. Jorge*	59

CHAPTER 2 EPIDEMIOLOGY OF PHOBIAS 61

Epidemiology of Phobias: A Review 61
Gavin Andrews

COMMENTARIES

2.1	Risk-Factor and Genetic Epidemiology of Phobic Disorders: A Promising Approach *Assen Jablensky*	81
2.2	Defining a Case for Psychiatric Epidemiology: Threshold, Non-Criterion Symptoms, and Category versus Spectrum *Jack D. Maser and Jonathan M. Meyer*	85
2.3	Phobias: A Difficult Challenge for Epidemiology *Carlo Faravelli*	89
2.4	Phobias: Handy or Handicapping Conditions *Peter Tyrer*	91
2.5	Phobic Disorders: Can We Integrate Empirical Findings with Clinical Theories? *Marco Battaglia and Anna Ogliari*	94
2.6	Social Phobia and Bipolar Disorder: The Significance of a Counterintuitive and Neglected Comorbidity *Hagop S. Akiskal and Giulio Perugi*	98
2.7	Comorbidity between Phobias and Mood Disorders: Diagnostic and Treatment Implications *Zoltán Rihmer*	103
2.8	Epidemiology of Phobias: Old Terminology, New Relevance *Laszlo A. Papp*	105
2.9	Phobias: Reflections on Definitions *Elie G. Karam and Nay G. Khatcherian*	108
2.10	Phobias: Facts or Fiction? *Rudy Bowen and Murray B. Stein*	110

2.11	Epidemiology of Phobias: The Pathway to Early Intervention in Anxiety Disorders *Michael Van Ameringen, Beth Pipe and Catherine Mancini*	113

CHAPTER 3 PHARMACOTHERAPY OF PHOBIAS 117

Pharmacotherapy of Phobias: A Review 117
Dan J. Stein, Bavanisha Vythilingum and Soraya Seedat

COMMENTARIES

3.1	Placing the Pharmacotherapy of Phobic Disorders in a New Neuroscience Context *Jack M. Gorman*	143
3.2	Psychobiology and Pharmacotherapy of Phobias *Rudolf Hoehn-Saric*	146
3.3	The Neuropsychology of Defence: Implications for Syndromes and Pharmacotherapy *Neil McNaughton*	148
3.4	Social Phobia: Not Neglected, Just Misunderstood *David S. Baldwin*	152
3.5	Research in Pharmacotherapy of Social Anxiety Disorder *Siegfried Kasper and Dietmar Winkler*	154
3.6	Pharmacotherapy for Phobic Disorders: Where Do We Go from Here? *Mark H. Pollack*	156
3.7	Progress in Pharmacotherapy for Social Anxiety Disorder and Agoraphobia *Bruce Lydiard*	158
3.8	Psychopharmacology Treatment of Phobias and Avoidance Reactions *Carl Salzman*	160
3.9	Crowning Achievement: The Rise of Anti-phobic Pharmacotherapy *Murray B. Stein*	163
3.10	Comorbidity and Phobias: Diagnostic and Therapeutic Challenges *Joseph Zohar*	165
3.11	Comments on the Pharmacotherapy of Agoraphobia *Matig R. Mavissakalian*	167

3.12	Pharmacotherapy of Phobias: A Long-Term Endeavour *Marcio Versiani*	170
3.13	Behavioural Toxicity of Pharmacotherapeutic Agents Used in Social Phobia *Ian Hindmarch and Leanne Trick*	172
3.14	Medication Treatment of Phobias: Theories Hide Effectiveness *James C. Ballenger*	175

CHAPTER 4 PSYCHOTHERAPEUTIC INTERVENTIONS FOR PHOBIAS 179

Psychotherapeutic Interventions for Phobias: A Review   179
David H. Barlow, David A. Moscovitch and Jamie A. Micco

COMMENTARIES

4.1	Phobias: A Suitable Case for Treatment *Anthony D. Roth*	211
4.2	Cognitive-Behavioural Interventions for Phobias: What Works for Whom and When *Richard G. Heimberg and James P. Hambrick*	215
4.3	Practical Comments on Exposure Therapy *Matig R. Mavissakalian*	217
4.4	The Treatment of Phobic Disorders: Is Exposure Still the Treatment of Choice? *Paul M.G. Emmelkamp*	220
4.5	"Behavioural Experimentation" and the Treatment of Phobias *Yiannis G. Papakostas, Vasilios G. Masdrakis and George N. Christodoulou*	223
4.6	Evaluating the Durability of Cognitive-Behavioural Therapy *Eberhard H. Uhlenhuth, Deepa Nadiga and Paula Hensley*	226
4.7	Some Comments on Psychological Treatment of Phobias *Lars-Göran Öst*	228
4.8	Pushing the Envelope on Treatments for Phobia *Michael J. Telch*	232

4.9	Treatment of Phobic Disorders from a Public Health Perspective *Ronald M. Rapee*	235
4.10	Psychotherapeutic Interventions for Phobia: A Psychoanalytic-Attachment Perspective *Jeremy Holmes*	237
4.11	Psychotherapy in the Treatment of Phobias: A Perspective from Latin America *Flávio Kapczinski*	242

CHAPTER 5   PHOBIAS IN CHILDREN AND ADOLESCENTS   245

Phobias in Children and Adolescents: A Review   245
Thomas H. Ollendick, Neville J. King and Peter Muris

COMMENTARIES

5.1	Childhood Phobias: More Questions than Answers *Michael Rutter*	280
5.2	Fear, Anxieties and Treatment Efficacy in Children and Adolescents *Rachel G. Klein*	283
5.3	Where Are All the Fearful Children? *Gabrielle A. Carlson and Deborah M. Weisbrot*	285
5.4	Etiology and Treatment of Childhood Phobias *Deborah C. Beidel and Autumn Paulson*	288
5.5	From Development Fears to Phobias *Sam Tyano and Miri Keren*	290
5.6	Assessment and Treatment of Phobic Disorders in Youth *John S. March*	292
5.7	Phobias: From Little Hans to a Bigger Picture *Gordon Parker*	295
5.8	Phobias in Childhood and Adolescence: Implications for Public Policy *E. Jane Costello*	297
5.9	Phobias in Children and Adolescents: Data from Brazil *Heloisa H.A. Brasil and Isabel A.S. Bordin*	299

	5.10	Phobias: A View from the South Seas *John Scott Werry*	301
CHAPTER 6		**SOCIAL AND ECONOMIC BURDEN OF PHOBIAS**	303
		Social and Economic Burden of Phobias: A Review *Koen Demyttenaere, Ronny Bruffaerts and Andy De Witte*	303
		COMMENTARIES	
	6.1	Burden of Phobias: Focus on Health-Related Quality of Life *Mark H. Rapaport, Katia K. Delrahim and Rachel E. Maddux*	329
	6.2	Reducing the Burden of Phobias: Patient Factors, System Issues *Naomi M. Simon and Julia Oppenheimer*	332
	6.3	Health-Related Quality of Life: Disease-Specific and Generic Dimensions in Social Phobia *Per Bech*	335
	6.4	What's So Different about Anxiety Disorders (Such as Phobias)? *Paul E. Greenberg, Howard G. Birnbaum and Tamar Sisitsky*	337
	6.5	Why Take Social Phobia Seriously? *Fiona Judd*	339
	6.6	Phobias in Primary Care and in Young Children *Myrna M. Weissman*	342
	6.7	Treatments Are Needed to Reduce the Burden of Phobic Illness *Peter P. Roy-Byrne and Wayne Katon*	344
	6.8	Early Diagnosis Can Reduce the Social and Economic Burden of Phobias *Antonio E. Nardi*	348
	6.9	The High Cost of Underrecognition of Phobic Disorders *Julio Bobes*	350
	6.10	Unanswered Questions on Phobias: What Can We Do to Meet the Need? *T. Bedirhan Üstün*	352
Index			355

Review Contributors

Gavin Andrews Clinical Research Unit for Anxiety and Depression, School of Psychiatry, University of New South Wales at St. Vincent's Hospital, 299 Forbes St., Darlinghurst, NSW 2010, Australia

David H. Barlow Center for Anxiety and Related Disorders at Boston University, 648 Beacon Street, Boston, MA 02215-2002, USA

Ronny Bruffaerts Department of Psychiatry, University Hospital Gasthuisberg, Herestraat 49, B-3000 Leuven, Belgium

Koen Demyttenaere Department of Psychiatry, University Hospital Gasthuisberg, Herestraat 49, B-3000 Leuven, Belgium

Andy De Witte Department of Psychiatry, University Hospital Gasthuisberg, Herestraat 49, B-3000 Leuven, Belgium

Neville J. King Faculty of Education, Monash University, Melbourne, Australia

Isaac Marks Institute of Psychiatry, King's College, London SE5 8AF, UK

David Mataix-Cols Institute of Psychiatry, King's College, London SE5 8AF, UK

Jamie A. Micco Center for Anxiety and Related Disorders at Boston University, 648 Beacon Street, Boston, MA 02215-2002, USA

David A. Moscovitch Center for Anxiety and Related Disorders at Boston University, 648 Beacon Street, Boston, MA 02215-2002, USA

Peter Muris Department of Medical, Clinical and Experimental Psychology, Maastricht University, The Netherlands

Thomas H. Ollendick Department of Psychology, Child Study Center, Virginia Polytechnic Institute and State University, 3110 Prices Fork Road, Blacksburg, VA 24061, USA

Soraya Seedat MRC Unit on Anxiety Disorders, University of Stellenbosch, Cape Town, South Africa

Dan J. Stein MRC Unit on Anxiety Disorders, University of Stellenbosch, Cape Town, South Africa

Bavanisha Vythilingum MRC Unit on Anxiety Disorders, University of Stellenbosch, Cape Town, South Africa

CHAPTER 1

Diagnosis and Classification of Phobias: A Review

Isaac Marks and David Mataix-Cols

Institute of Psychiatry, King's College, London SE5 8AF, UK

HISTORY OF THE CONCEPT OF PHOBIA

From Hippocrates to the 18th century, phobic problems were described occasionally but not distinguished clearly as disorders in their own right. "Phobia" began to be used as a term early in the 19th century, after which it gradually gained acceptance in its current sense: an intense fear that is out of proportion to the apparent stimulus, cannot be explained or reasoned away, and leads to avoidance of the feared stimulus.

In the later 19th century, many careful descriptions of phobic disorders appeared, starting with Westphal's classic account of agoraphobia in 1871. In 1895 Freud separated common phobias of things most people fear to some extent (death, illness, snakes etc.) from phobias of things or situations that inspire no fear in the average person, e.g. agoraphobia. That same year Henry Maudsley in his *Pathology of Mind* approved Westphal's agoraphobia as a separate syndrome; in his 1895 edition, however, Maudsley included all phobias under melancholia and derided the big-sounding names given to each type of phobic situation, since many phobias were often found together or successively in the same case. In 1913 Kraepelin included in his textbook a brief description of irresistible fears and irrepressible ideas, but did not separate phobic from obsessive–compulsive phenomena.

Phobias achieved a separate diagnostic label in the International Classification of Diseases (ICD) in 1947, and in the American Psychiatric Association classification (now called DSM, for Diagnostic and Statistical Manual) in 1952. By 1959 just three out of nine classifications used in various countries listed phobic disorder as a diagnosis on its own [1]. In the first two editions of the DSM all phobias were grouped together [2,3]. In the

---

Phobias. Edited by Mario Maj, Hagop S. Akiskal, Juan José López-Ibor and Ahmed Okasha.
©2004 John Wiley & Sons Ltd: ISBN 0-470-85833-8

1960s Marks and colleagues observed that the various phobias had different ages of onset and gender distribution [4,5] and this provided the initial impetus for the split of phobias into agoraphobia, social and specific phobia; this was later adopted by the 3rd edition of the DSM [6] and continued until the current DSM-IV [7] and DSM-IV-TR [8]. Anxiety and related disorders appeared in the ICD for the first time in its 7th revision [9] and came under 18 rubrics in its 9th revision [10]. This constituted the basis of the current classification of phobias in the ICD-10 [11].

PURPOSES OF DIAGNOSTIC AND OTHER CLASSIFICATIONS

Classification is the arrangement of phenomena into classes with common features. Classes can be categories that are mutually exclusive, like most animal species, even though we cannot say exactly when the apes that preceded hominids became hominid on gradually evolving dimensions of change. Classes may overlap, like human physical types. Classes may shade into one another along continuous dimensions like age. We cannot say exactly when an infant becomes a toddler, a toddler a child, a child an adolescent, an adolescent an adult, but we can reliably tell an infant from an adult (except regarding behaviour sometimes!) and so carve out two mutually exclusive categories from the opposite ends of a continuous dimension. Even a continuous dimension like age has relative discontinuities, with more rapid change during pubertal than preceding years. Thus certain quantitative changes along dimensions can also mean qualitative categorical changes. Dimensional and categorical classes need not be mutually exclusive. Any category of disorder may be mild, moderate or severe (dimensional), and a category of disorder can overlap with some but not other categories (e.g. agoraphobia overlaps with social phobia but not with hypomania). There is an argument for adopting a mixed categorical and dimensional classification of mental disorders [12].

Classifications are fictions imposed on a complex world to understand and manage it. We can classify any set of features in endless ways, the value of which depends on the purpose of our classification. Health care planners and funders find certain administrative classifications useful (e.g. problems needing intensive inpatient care versus just outpatient or day-patient care, psychosis versus neurosis, serious versus minor mental illness, child versus adult psychiatry, forensic versus other mental health problems). Some medical specialists practise with an anatomical label (e.g. ear, nose and throat diseases versus genito-urinary diseases). Other specialists use an etiological taxonomy (e.g. auto-immune versus infectious diseases or even substance abuse disorders have lower treatment rates). In the Epidemiologic Catchment Area study, only about 17% of respondents with a phobic disorder reported a mental health outpatient visit in the last year, and about 70% of phobic individuals who sought professional help did so for physical health reasons only. In only 5–6% of social phobics without comorbid depression, psychological problems were the main reason for seeking help.

There are certainly patient-related barriers to seeking treatment: many phobic individuals do not interpret their problems in mental health terms, or are afraid of what others might think, or prefer to handle the situation on their own, or are not aware of available treatment options. However, physician-related barriers also exist: the recognition rate of phobic disorders by general practitioners is very low and, unfortunately, even some psychiatrists are not familiar with all the treatment modalities for phobic disorders whose efficacy is now proven by research. Indeed, these treatment modalities are not available in many clinical contexts worldwide, whereas a variety of interventions whose efficacy is not demonstrated are widely applied.

With the only exception of pharmacotherapy for social phobia, the management of phobic disorders is usually not a very visible topic in psychiatric congresses, and the literature on these disorders is mostly perused by a small circle of clinicians and researchers. This book focusing on phobias within a series reaching general psychiatrists of all regions of the world may contribute to disseminate information on currently available evidence and experience in the management of these disorders and probably to reduce the current significant gap between research advances and clinical practice.

Finally, pursuing the other main objective of the series "Evidence and Experience in Psychiatry", this book may increase the visibility of some controversies that do exist in the area of phobic disorders, and that require the clinicians' attention, discretion and judgment in their own particular treatment setting. These controversies include those on the relationship between agoraphobia and panic disorder (so differently addressed in ICD-10 and DSM-IV), the usefulness of psychodynamic psychotherapies in phobic disorders, and the role of pharmacotherapy vs. psychotherapies in the management of the various types of phobias.

Mario Maj
Hagop S. Akiskal
Juan José López-Ibor
Ahmed Okasha

Preface

This book focusing on phobias is the seventh of the WPA series "Evidence and Experience in Psychiatry". Initiated in 1999, this series of books has involved up to now as contributors more than 700 experts from more than 60 countries, and has reached many thousands of readers in all regions of the world. All the books of the series have been translated into various languages, and a second edition of four of them have already been published.

Since the beginning, the main objective of this series of books has been to contribute to reduce the gap between research evidence and clinical practice in the management of the most common mental disorders. This objective appears particularly relevant in the case of phobic disorders. Indeed, phobias are among the most common mental disorders: in the National Comorbidity Survey, covering a national probability sample of adults in the USA, the rates of phobic disorders in the past 12 months were 8.8% for specific phobia, 7.9% for social phobia, 2.8% for agoraphobia without panic, and 2.3% for panic with or without agoraphobia. In the Netherlands Mental Health Survey, the corresponding figures were 7.1%, 4.8%, 1.6% and 2.2%.

The burden placed by phobic disorders on the patients, the families and the society at large is very significant. For instance, social phobia has been consistently associated with a lower educational attainment, a lower employment rate, a decreased work productivity and an increased financial dependency. Due to their frequently early onset, phobic disorders may interfere with the development of personal, sexual, social and intellectual functioning, and there is evidence that early-onset social phobia increases the risk for the subsequent occurrence of alcohol or drug abuse as well as major depression.

Efficacious treatments now exist for all types of phobias. Consistent evidence is available for the efficacy of *in vivo* exposure in treating agoraphobia, social phobia and specific phobia, and of exposure therapy plus cognitive restructuring in treating social phobia. There is good evidence for the efficacy and tolerability of a number of selective serotonin reuptake inhibitors (SSRIs) in the treatment of social phobia, and panic disorder with agoraphobia responds to SSRIs, tricyclic antidepressants and, in a selected group of patients, to benzodiazepines.

In spite of all the above, only a small minority of people with phobic disorders receive adequate treatment (among major mental disorders, only just sexually transmitted ones). The most useful classifications "carve nature at the joints" so that several attributes which we consider important are present in all members of one class but absent in members of other classes. A class is called a diagnosis when its attributes are shared symptoms and signs, etiology, pathophysiology, prognosis or response to a particular treatment (rather than, say, need for hospitalization rather than ambulatory or home care).

Diagnostic classifications may stem from political as well as scientific processes. DSM's demotion of agoraphobia into an aspect of "panic disorder" reflects two political processes in the late 20th century. One was US psychiatry's bid for more mainstream medical status. This strengthened its view of panic and other problems as signs of brain dysfunction needing drug therapy. The second political process was the pharmaceutical industry's successful bid for US Food and Drug Administration (FDA) approval to market "antipanic" drugs for "panic disorder" (the FDA approves drugs for particular diagnoses [12]). The industry sponsored professional meetings to boost that diagnostic entity and funded research worldwide into "antipanic" drugs for "panic disorder". In addition, cognitive therapists jumped onto the panic disorder bandwagon by claiming that panic stemmed from "catastrophic cognitions" which required cognitive restructuring.

Ideally, in a given class all the subsets of common attributes should coincide, but few classifications approach this ideal. At the other extreme are nosologies whose assignment to classes tells us only about one subset of features and no other. There is little point to dividing phobics into those with and without a squint, or those who are left- or right-handed, or phobics who support or oppose their country's government. Such classes predict nothing more about other attributes shared among phobics in those classes. Fortunately we can discern patterns of phobic problems presenting to clinicians that are less arbitrary, because the phobic features tend to co-occur and to cohere over time without treatment (phenomenological and prognostic bases of classification) and may hint at an aspect of etiology.

The patterns may look different when fuller data are collected about *all* phobics in the community, including the majority who do not seek treatment and those who see only primary care professionals.

Whatever classification is adopted is, of course, provisional like every scientific theory and requires revision as knowledge advances and the taxonomy's purpose changes.

CONUNDRUMS IN CLASSIFYING PHOBIAS

Several snags are encountered in evolving different bases for a taxonomy of phobic symptoms.

Phobias May be Cued (Triggered, Evoked) by Almost Anything

A classification based entirely on the triggers of terror leads to an endless terminology telling us little beyond the label. Such a classification was prominent in the past. Numerous Greek and Latin prefixes were attached to -phobia according to the object or situation that was feared (for a long table of such phobias, see [13]). Today's enquirers from the media often ask: "What do you call a phobia of spiders (or heights or blushing or whatever)?" and rest content with the label "arachnophobia" or "acrophobia" or "erythrophobia". Such dry scholasticism has little merit, though below we will see value in the terms "agoraphobia" (fear of public places) and "social phobia", because clinicians commonly see phobias of particular clusters of public or social situations, each cluster having its own correlates (e.g. a fear of crowds often associates with certain other agoraphobic and non-phobic features, and a fear of blushing with other social fears). Particular clusters of phobia-inducing situations overlap yet are helpful guides to description, etiology, treatment and prognosis. The type of cue (trigger, stimulus, evoking situation) is thus not entirely irrelevant as a predictor of other features of the phobia. Indeed, DSM's downplaying of which particular cues induce panic is a major snag in its concept of "panic disorder", of which more later.

Phobias Can Occur Alone or as Part of a Wide Range of Mental Health Problems

Examples include children's transient terrors of darkness or animals, fears of cancer that wax and wane with a depressive illness, worry about going out as part of paranoid schizophrenia, apprehension of being fat in anorexia nervosa, preoccupation with other aspects of one's appearance or smell in dysmorphophobia (body dysmorphic disorder) and persistent panic in various public places in a housebound agoraphobic. Some regard phobias as maladaptive "habits" that themselves constitute the problem without any underlying cause, while others think of them as a surface aspect of deeper pathology. The varying significance of different phobic phenomena is hard to grasp if we posit a unitary origin for all of them instead of recognizing that varied factors may play a role in their genesis.

Many Mild Fears are Normal and Protective Rather than a Phobia

Examples are wariness at the top of a cliff or in a dark street at night or in very enclosed or open spaces or when meeting strangers or dangerous creatures. The most common phobias are undue intensifications of fears that promoted survival in our evolutionary past and probably still do. This insight, however, does not help us to classify phobias in a meaningful clinical manner.

Normal fears that do not require treatment and abnormal worries that do are at opposite ends of a continuum and shade into one another at some point. (In the 15th century Erasmus fled from a plague epidemic as people died from it in swarms, and wrote to a fellow fugitive: "Really, I consider total absence of fear, in situations such as mine, to be the mark not of a valiant fellow but of a dolt.") When fears are severe enough to interfere with everyday life, then these are called disabling phobias that are an abnormal disorder. They are less common than normal mild fears. Only a minority of people would not venture into the countryside for fear of snakes or stay away from work for fear of the bus ride to get there or avoid company for fear of blushing.

The tendency for particular phobic patterns to appear and persist in many sufferers justifies calling them "syndromes" (literally "running together"). Several aspects of those patterns could each form the basis for a taxonomy of phobias.

POTENTIAL BASES FOR A TAXONOMY

Presence of Avoidance

This is part of the definition of a phobia and so cannot be a basis for classifying phobias. People whose phobia is mild may not avoid or even tend to avoid the feared stimulus, experiencing only fear in its actual or imagined presence. If avoidance develops, then disability may ensue from reluctance to contemplate or engage in needed activities. Cued discomfort and/or avoidance is the essence of a phobia, yet some syndromes of anxious avoidance are not listed as phobias in the two most widely used diagnostic classification systems (ICD-10 and DSM-IV-TR).

Subjective Experience of the Cue

Few aspects of the phobic experience are known as yet to predict the presence of enough other features to be a basis for classifying phobias. More mapping is needed of which cues evoke which ranges of feelings in phobics.

Contact with whatever brings on the phobia evokes unpleasant feelings called fear, panic, apprehension, worry, dread, discomfort, disgust, nausea, being contaminated, etc. Agoraphobics, social phobics and most specific phobics report fear, and panic if that becomes intense. Certain feelings may be evoked by particular cues: dizziness by public places in agoraphobics, being drawn to a cliff edge in height phobics, a sense of falling in space phobics, disgust in those who fear worms, spiders and snakes. Nausea with *actual* fainting is almost unique to blood phobia, though a feeling of faintness without actually fainting is frequent in agoraphobia. Nausea with disgust is usual in food aversions. Disgust with fear is common in many kinds of phobia. Actual vomiting occurs, rarely, in intense agoraphobia or social phobia. An urge to urinate or defecate occasionally troubles intense phobics of diverse kinds, though actual incontinence is seldom seen. A sense of contamination or of impending doom is common in obsessive–compulsive disorder (OCD). Tingling in the fingers and shivers down the spine ("scroopy" feelings) are typical of touch and sound aversions.

Experience of Panic

Intense fear such as panic is part of the definition of phobia and so cannot guide classification. Panic is sudden terror lasting at least a few minutes with typical manifestations of intense fear, e.g. palpitations, sweating, trembling, dry mouth, sense of choking, difficulty breathing, chest or abdominal discomfort, nausea, urge to micturate or defecate, faintness/dizziness (not vertigo), paraesthesiae, derealization or depersonalization, urge to escape from the site of the panic, sense of going mad, losing control or dying. At least four such somatic or cognitive symptoms are required by both ICD-10 and DSM-IV-TR for the episode to be called "panic", though the empirical basis for this proviso is unclear. The proviso gives a spurious sense of accuracy when in reality there is no clear divide. At different times anyone may feel frightened to various degrees along a continuum from slight twinges of apprehension to paralysing panic, with the number as well as the force of different symptoms growing as fear intensifies.

DSM-III began an emphasis on the tautologous term "panic attacks" that continues in DSM-IV-TR (ICD-10 refers to them at F41.0). Adding "attack" to "panic" is redundant, as dictionaries define "panic" anyway as terror of sudden onset. Typical panic is seen when any severe phobic encounters the evoking cue in reality or in imagination. Panic also occurs in acute and post-traumatic stress disorder, OCD, depression and in many people who have none of the foregoing problems.

DSM-IV-TR differentiates three kinds of panic: cued (situationally bound—i.e. phobic), cued but not on every exposure to the cue (situationally predisposed), and uncued (unexpected, spontaneous, out of the blue—"unpredictable" in ICD-10). It is more realistic to join situationally bound and situationally predisposed panic, as the cue evokes fear rising to panic criteria more consistently as the phobia worsens, and even severe phobics may not experience panic *every* time they encounter their feared cue(s).

DSM-IV-TR requires the presence of uncued panics for the diagnosis of panic disorder (with or without agoraphobia). It claims that cued panics are most characteristic of social and specific phobias. However, cued panics typically also come on when relevant real or imagined cues are encountered in "panic disorder with agoraphobia", "agoraphobia without panic disorder", "post-traumatic stress disorder" and, sometimes, "OCD".

Whether the Cues are Specific or Multiple

At the Same Time

Adults who complain of a disabling phobia of animals or heights or blood or darkness usually have few other phobias—their phobia is fairly specific (focal). Specific phobias are a category (diagnosis) in ICD-10 and in DSM-IV-TR, which recognizes five subtypes: animal, natural environment (e.g. heights, storms, water), blood–injection-injury, situational (e.g. aeroplanes, elevators, closed places) and other.

Although specific phobias are far more focal than agoraphobia, sufferers tend to have further lesser fears in addition to the one for which they sought help, a raised risk of other anxiety disorders and a greater family history of parental depression, substance dependence and antisocial personality disorders [5,14]. Despite this, many specific phobias are remarkably focal. Adults with an animal phobia do not fear all animals, only certain creatures (e.g. large dogs or flapping birds or scurrying spiders). People may fear urinating but not defecating in a public toilet. One woman feared only helmets worn by firemen, not helmets worn by policemen.

In contrast, adults with a disabling phobia of crowds usually also panic in a cluster of other situations such as leaving home alone, travelling by public transport, shopping and enclosed places. This is the agoraphobic cluster of situations. Being phobic of any one situation within that cluster commonly predicts the presence of another phobia of situations within that cluster. A few people fear, say, only enclosed spaces (claustrophobia), but no other situations within that cluster—they have a specific phobia rather than agoraphobia. The more situations that are feared from the agoraphobic cluster, the more the problem can be called agoraphobia, but there is no sharp dividing line.

Two other clusters of multiple phobias at the same time are common. One involves fears of several illnesses (the hypochondriasis cluster): sufferers may at the same time fear that pain in their chest indicates heart disease and coexisting constipation suggests cancer. Some people fear just one illness and no other, in which case it is more a specific nosophobia than hypochondriasis. As with agoraphobia, the more numerous the fears the sufferer has from within the hypochondriasis cluster, the more the problem can be called hypochondriasis, and again there is no sharp dividing line. Another frequent cluster of fears is that seen in OCD: sufferers may worry that touching the floor without washing their hands five times afterwards will cause their parents to get a terrible disease and that they themselves will die if they don't check ten times that the radio is off.

Knowing that a sufferer's complaint of panic on leaving home is far more likely to predict the further presence of a phobia of shopping and public transport rather than the presence of a fear of cancer or of AIDS is a good reason for having a diagnostic category of agoraphobia. A similar argument holds for other clusters like social phobia, hypochondriasis and OCD.

Evidence of Clusters of Agoraphobia, Social Phobia and Other Phobic Clusters (Factors). In many multivariate analyses of questionnaire answers, a factor (cluster, component) emerged of agoraphobic fears, e.g. "fear of fainting in public", "nervous on a train" in: (a) clinical phobics ([15–17], reviewed by [18–20]), (b) phobia club members [20,21], (c) neurotic patients [22], (d) psychiatric inpatients [23], (e) psychiatric inpatients with affective illness [24], (f) community samples and hospital patients [25–27] and (g) post-injury chronic pain sufferers [28]. Where this was reported, agoraphobia accounted for much the largest variance among the factors [25]. Also where this was examined, a first-order agoraphobia factor [25] emerged independent of a lifetime history of panic disorder, panics or panic-like symptoms, whereas DSM relegates agoraphobia to being a complication of panic disorder, panics or panic-like symptoms. A study of adolescents and young adults also reported that agoraphobia often existed independently of panic disorder, panics or specific phobia [29].

Loadings on an agoraphobia or a social phobia factor separated agoraphobics from social phobics (e.g. "fear of expressing myself in case I make a foolish mistake", "feel awkward with strangers") [25,30–33]. A second-order social phobia factor split into two first-order factors ("speaking in public" and "being observed") in the analysis of Cox *et al.* [25]. Social phobia split similarly into "speaking in public" and other social fears in another analysis of the National Comorbidity Survey [34].

In the Cox *et al.* [25] analysis five first-order factors emerged (speaking, being observed, heights or water, threat [including bridges and water/lake/pool] and agoraphobia), with the first two first-order factors melding into one second-order factor of social phobia and the second two into a second-order factor of specific fears, and all the factors melding into a third-order "general fear" factor. Cox *et al.* think this supports Taylor's [35] idea that some influences affect the origin of all phobias while others are unique to particular fears. This shows the uncertainties involved in basing classification solely on factor analyses. It is unclear what the import may be of particular factors emerging as first, second or third order. Moreover, which particular factors emerge depends partly on which items are entered into the analyses and the population being studied.

Hard to Say When Various Fears within a Cluster Are from the Same or Different Syndromes. When people fear several situations from within the agoraphobia, social phobia, hypochondriasis or OCD cluster, it can be hard to judge which feared situations are separate from and which connected to one another, i.e. whether they are part of one or several phobia syndromes or hierarchies. If an agoraphobic fears riding on both a bus and a train, does that imply two separate phobias or one phobia of public transport? If a hypochondriasis sufferer fears he has both heart disease and cancer, does he have two different fears of illness or a general fear of disease? If an OCD patient fears that not checking the door will spell doom for his family and not checking that the radio is off will harm someone else, are those two separate fears or part of one and the same problem? The issue of stimulus generalization bedevils giving a satisfactory answer. Careful experimental work is needed to illuminate this issue.

Persistently over Years

It is more usual for the external cues which frighten a phobic to remain similar over the years than to change at random. This is true whether the phobias are specific or multiple. An adult who is phobic of spiders is unlikely to become phobic of blood or darkness or public places. The same is true for people with several phobias from the agoraphobia, hypochondriasis or OCD cluster [36]. As in OCD, sufferers tend to retain phobias from within the same cluster over the years rather than to switch from one symptom cluster to another. They are more likely to change from one phobia within a cluster to another within that same cluster, e.g. in the case of the agoraphobia cluster, to cease fearing public transport, say, but start to panic in shops; in the case of the hypochondriasis cluster, to stop having a phobia of cancer but become terrified of AIDS. Similarly, in OCD, symptoms tend to change within rather than between symptom dimensions [36], e.g. contamination concerns may change over time but a washer is less likely to become a hoarder.

The coherence of particular patterns over the years (tendency for the phobias to remain specific or to remain multiple, and for the particular specific phobia or particular cluster of phobias to remain similar), helps the delineation of a meaningful rather than an arbitrary classification of phobias.

Whether the Cues are External or Internal

External cues (triggers, stimuli, evoking situations) for phobias may be animals, public places, strangers, sight of blood, etc. There are often internal (interoceptive) cues too. Specific phobics may say the animal they fear is disgusting or threatening in a way most people do not recognize. Agoraphobics often say that when they panic in public places they fear they may look stupid or go mad or lose control or die, and that their accompanying palpitations or dizziness or overbreathing or other obvious sensations of fear make them worse. They fear fear itself. Cognitive therapists assume that such internal fears (catastrophic cognitions) are the heart of the problem.

Cognitions (thoughts) need not be primary. They might just be the cognitive part of the whole phobic response, which also includes components that are subjective (sense of dread, etc. without reason), motor (avoidance, freezing, trembling) and physiological (palpitations, sweating, dizziness, urge to urinate etc.). Once cognitions occur, however, they might secondarily augment the phobic response, so dealing with them could be therapeutic even if they are not the primary part of the response.

It remains to be seen whether classifying phobias according to whether they are mainly of internal or mainly external cues predicts much else in sufferers. We saw above that knowing the external cues for a phobia allows one to make important other predictions about its likely phenomenology. Studies are needed to see if particular internal cues for a phobia are as or more predictive of important other features than are particular external cues.

Whether Non-Phobic (Uncued) As Well as Phobic (Cued) Symptoms are Present

The absence of non-phobic (uncued, unexpected, unpredictable) anxiety or depression is *per se* insufficient to classify a phobia, but its presence strengthens the chance that one is seeing agoraphobia or social phobia. Whereas specific phobics rarely have other mental health problems, many agoraphobics also have non-phobic panics and anxiety without any particular trigger, often during depressive episodes [4,5,16,21]. The more diffuse forms of social phobia too are liable to low mood. Calling such associated non-phobic symptoms comorbidities seems premature, as that would imply their being separate from the phobia. Until this issue has been better explored, we prefer to call them associations rather than comorbidities.

The association of phobias with non-phobic anxiety and depression was noted yet again in recent multivariate analyses. A higher order "internalizing" factor comprising several phobic and other anxiety disorders and mood disorders emerged in analyses of a US national "comorbidity" survey [37], including its clinical subsample [38], and in an unselected New Zealand birth cohort that stayed stable from age 18 to 21 [39]. Very high internalizing scores related to more hospital stays and recently impaired days [38], resembling past findings that more initial non-phobic pathology predicted poorer outcome [19].

In Krueger's 1999 analysis the internalizing factor broke down into two subfactors—"anxious-misery" (major depressive episode, dysthymia, generalized anxiety disorder) and "fear" (social phobia, simple phobia, agoraphobia, panic disorder)—similar to factors found previously elsewhere [16,17,20,21] and to the association noted without a multivariate analysis [18]. Krueger's internalizing factor resembles Carl Jung's idea of introversion a century ago and Hans Eysenck's notion of neuroticism 50 years ago, which was a higher-order factor comprising lower-order factors of depression, general anxiety and phobias.

Krueger saw internalizing as a "core psychopathological process" underlying its component phobic and other syndromes, but did not report the detailed comparisons of specific phobia with agoraphobia, social phobia and other phobias that are needed to detect their differential long-term associations with non-phobic anxiety, depression and other variables [4,5,18,19]. Working out what may be "core" to phobias requires more detailed ongoing surveys of large cohorts over many years and careful testing of rival putative mechanisms to test how well particular first-, second- or third-order factors predict other important features.

Onset Age and Gender

Early onset age predicts certain other phenomenological features likely to be present, but is not enough to be a main basis for classifying phobias. In adults with specific phobias of animals or insects or of blood, the specific phobia usually began in childhood before age 8 and often even earlier [19,40]. The same is true for the diffuse shyness which is called avoidant personality disorder in DSM-IV-TR. In contrast, specific social phobias and agoraphobia tend to begin in young adult life (social phobias slightly earlier on average), and space phobia in middle age or later. Adults who have a coexisting animal phobia and agoraphobia almost always say their animal phobia began in childhood while their agoraphobia started after puberty. This points to separate origins for those two phobias and is another reason for regarding them as separate diagnostic categories (along with the far smaller association of multiple phobias and of non-phobic symptoms with animal phobia than agoraphobia).

Gender predicts too little else to be a basis for classification. Most adults seeking help for phobias are female. Exceptions are that those who consult therapists for social phobias are as often men as women, except for those who have diffuse social phobia starting in childhood (avoidant personality disorder), who are far more often men than women.

High Familiality and Bradycardic Fainting

Two features that are unique to blood–injury phobia in addition to the evoking cue are a reason for classifying it as a special type of specific phobia. First, blood–injury phobics usually remember far more relatives with the same problem than do other phobics—blood–injury phobia is the most familial of all phobias, and indeed of all anxiety disorders. Being so strongly familial may relate to its second unique feature: the tendency of blood–injury phobics to actually faint on seeing blood or even just hearing it spoken about. This follows marked slowing of the heart rate on seeing blood, perhaps after an initial brief tachycardia (a diphasic cardiovascular response). It is unclear if this vasovagal phenomenon indicates a homology with the tonic immobility (death feigning) that is seen in many vertebrate and invertebrate species [19]. Actual fainting as opposed to just feeling faint (which is common in agoraphobia) is rare in phobias other than blood–injury phobia.

Fear of Falling (Space Phobia)

Space phobics have a fear of falling with rescue reactions which are triggered by the absence of visuospatial support, and have six associations apart from the trigger that are not shared with other phobic syndromes. These associations are more than enough to regard space phobia as a special kind of specific phobia and to classify it as different from agoraphobia:

(a) Space phobia is rarely associated with other specific phobias.
(b) Space phobia typically begins in the elderly, unlike most specific and other phobias, which usually start several decades earlier. Even when someone has agoraphobic fears (e.g. public transport, crowds) together with space phobia, the agoraphobic fears usually began long before the space phobia did and were much milder than the space phobia.

(c) Intense fears of falling and/or open space without visual support are a central feature of space phobia but are usually mild or absent in agoraphobia. Unlike agoraphobics, space phobics often actually fall if they do not see potential support nearby and even crawl on the floor to cross a room. In some cases, space phobia is a transient phase in a developing disorder of balance that progresses to the point where the person cannot stand unaided even in the presence of visuospatial cues. A few space phobias are triggered by space and depth cues while driving rather than walking.
(d) Unlike agoraphobics, space phobics seldom have accompanying non-phobic panic or depression.
(e) Unlike agoraphobics, space phobics frequently have diverse neurological and/or cardiovascular disorders that suggest disturbed integration of vestibular–ocular reflexes from diverse lesions in or above the neck.
(f) Unlike agoraphobics, space phobics improve relatively little with exposure therapy.

Response to Treatment

With a few exceptions, the response of phobias to particular treatments is an uncertain guide to classification: the fact that amitriptyline is both an analgesic and an antidepressant is not a good reason to classify pain with depression. Various phobia syndromes that differ in other important ways improve similarly with a given treatment approach. Agoraphobia, social and specific phobias, and OCD with phobic features all respond well to exposure therapy and (except for specific phobias) improve too with certain drug therapies. The improvement in all these syndromes tends to continue long after the end of exposure therapy but to dwindle after medication is stopped.

The tendency for blood–injury phobics to faint at the sight of blood affects how certain treatment should be done: sufferers should lie down when they first expose themselves to the sight of blood until their tendency to faint habituates and disappears. Knowing the usual features of each phobia syndrome helps therapists to guide patients to tailor exposure therapy to their own needs, and the same might apply to cognitive therapy. This issue, however, is not an example of response to treatment guiding classification.

The search for syndromes with particular treatment responses has some merit. It was especially energized by political influences over the last generation. The search so far, however, has generated fewer scientific advances in the mental health field than financial advances for pharmaceutical companies. Although the FDA approves specific drugs for particular syndromes, selective serotonin reuptake inhibitors (SSRIs) and other "antidepressants" have broad-spectrum effects across several syndromes of anxious avoidance as well as mood disorders, with cross-syndrome similarities of effect exceeding between-syndrome differences in effect. The broad-spectrum cross-syndrome effect of medication resembles that of psychotherapies. This is not to say that an effective treatment works equally well in all disorders, but rather that it often works well in more than one disorder and perhaps even more than one group of disorders. Achievement of the dream of classifying phobias by treatment response lies in the future.

CURRENT CLASSIFICATIONS OF PHOBIC DISORDERS AND THEIR SIMILARITIES AND DIFFERENCES

The two most widely used classifications today are ICD-10 and DSM-IV-TR (Tables 1.1–1.4).

ICD-10 lists, under the heading "Neurotic, stress-related and somatoform disorders", F40 Phobic anxiety disorders, the diagnoses F40.0 Agoraphobia, 40.1 Social phobias and 40.2 Specific (isolated) phobias, which closely resemble those that DSM-IV-TR lists under the heading "Anxiety disorders" (300.21, 300.22, 300.23 and 300.29).

ICD-10 and DSM-IV-TR are similar in excluding from their list of phobia diagnoses other syndromes with phobia-like features of anxious avoidance, such as dysmorphophobia (non-delusional) and hypochondriasis, OCD and touch/sound aversions.

ICD-10 lists, under F40 Phobic anxiety disorders, two diagnoses (F40.8 Other phobic anxiety disorders and F40.9 Phobic anxiety disorder unspecified) that have no counterpart in DSM-IV-TR.

ICD-10 lists a diagnosis F41.0 Panic disorder (episodic paroxysmal anxiety) under F41 Anxiety disorders rather than F40 Phobic anxiety disorders (and excludes from it F40.0 Panic disorder with agoraphobia). DSM-IV-TR lists its counterpart 300.01 Panic disorder without agoraphobia under "Anxiety disorders".

THE MAIN PHOBIC SYNDROMES

The rest of this chapter outlines each syndrome of anxious avoidance that has a phobia diagnosis in ICD-10 (F40) and DSM-IV-TR (300.2). Thereafter it notes more briefly other syndromes of anxious avoidance. Almost all the syndromes are detailed in Marks [19,41]. They are described in the order in which they appear in the left-hand column of Table 1.1.

TABLE 1.1 Phobias coded under anxiety disorders in ICD-10 [11] and DSM-IV-TR [8]

ICD-10	DSM-IV-TR
F40–48 NEUROTIC, STRESS-RELATED AND SOMATOFORM DISORDERS F40 Phobic anxiety disorders	ANXIETY DISORDERS No 'Phobic anxiety disorders' or 'Phobias' 'Agoraphobia' is not codable as a diagnosis; instead:
F40.0 Agoraphobia	300.21 Panic disorder with agoraphobia 300.22 Agoraphobia without history of panic disorder
F40.1 Social phobias	300.23 Social phobia (social anxiety disorder)
F40.2 Specific (isolated) phobias Subtypes: animal type, nature forces, blood–injection–injury, enclosed spaces, [sphincteric], other	300.29 Specific (*formerly simple*) phobia Subtypes: animal, natural environment (e.g. storms, heights, water), blood–injection–injury, situational (e.g. public transport, tunnels, bridges, elevators, flying, driving, enclosed places)
F40.8 Other phobic anxiety disorders F40.9 Phobic anxiety disorder, unspecified Phobia NOS, Phobic state NOS	

TABLE 1.2 Phobia-like syndromes not called phobias in ICD-10 [11] or DSM-IV-TR [8]

ICD-10	DSM-IV-TR
F42 Obsessive–compulsive disorder	300.3 Obsessive–compulsive disorder
F43 Reaction to severe stress, and adjustment disorders	
F43.1 Post-traumatic stress disorder	309.81 Post-traumatic stress disorder
F45 Somatoform disorders	SOMATOFORM DISORDERS
F45.2 Dysmorphophobia (non-delusional)	300.7 Body dysmorphic disorder
F45.2 Hypochondriacal disorder ?nosophobia	300.7 Hypochondriasis
	PERSONALITY DISORDERS 301.82 Avoidant personality disorder
Touch and sound aversions (not in ICD–10 or DSM–IV-TR)	

In all the syndromes the relevant cues evoke fear or other discomfort and perhaps avoidance if the phobia is mild, and evoke panic or other discomfort, marked avoidance and physiological and cognitive manifestations as the phobia grows in severity. Phobics are less likely to seek help if

TABLE 1.3 Non-phobia-like syndromes often associated with phobias

ICD-10	DSM-IV-TR

F41 Other anxiety disorders
  F41.0 Panic disorder (episodic paroxysmal anxiety)
  F41.1 Generalized anxiety disorder
  F41.2 Mixed anxiety and depressive disorder
  F41.3 Other mixed anxiety disorders
F48 Other neurotic disorders
  F48.0 Neurasthenia
  F48.1 Depersonalization–derealization syndrome
F32 Depressive episode
F33 Recurrent depressive disorder
F34 Persistent mood (affective) disorder
  F34.1 Dysthymia
F38 Other mood (affective) disorders
	ANXIETY DISORDERS
	300.01 Panic disorder without agoraphobia
	300.02 Generalized anxiety disorder

TABLE 1.4 Non-phobia-like syndromes with some aspects vaguely like those of phobias

F50.0 Anorexia nervosa
F64 Gender identity disorders
  F64.0 Transsexualism

they can avoid the cue easily in everyday life (e.g. snakes in the UK), than if they cannot avoid the evoking cue without incurring handicap (e.g. leaving home in most societies other than women in purdah).

Agoraphobia (F40.0; Panic Disorder with Agoraphobia 300.21, Agoraphobia without History of Panic Disorder 300.22)

This is a cluster of phobias like leaving home, shops, crowds, public places, travel by train, bus or plane, with accompanying dizziness (not vertigo), faintness and sense of losing control. The fear worsens if it is hard to make a dignified escape from wherever panic strikes. In addition, non-phobic anxiety, panics and depression are common, as are day-to-day fluctuations of intensity of the agoraphobia. Agoraphobia is more common in women than men. It starts mostly in young adult life and can persist for years or decades, though a third had remitted at 11-year follow-up [42].

Onset and Course

The onset of agoraphobia can be sudden within minutes, or gradual over weeks, or slowly over years after initial vague intermittent anxiety. Some people start with an acute sustained panic, followed by phobias confining them to their homes within a few weeks. Others begin with vague fluctuating anxiety that gradually becomes agoraphobic over many years. Many feel uneasy for decades about going about alone but dextrously manage to hide their fears until the fear increases rapidly in new situations, when they seek help because the family cannot cope any longer. All kinds of variations appear between these two extremes.

Agoraphobia may clear up after a few weeks or months without treatment. Other sufferers may progress slowly or rapidly to severe disability with loss of job and becoming housebound for decades. For example, a woman aged 18 suddenly came home one day from work and screamed she was going to die. She spent the next two weeks in bed and thereafter refused to walk beyond the front gate of her home. She did not improve after four months in a psychiatric hospital and after discharge left her home only twice in the next seven years. She spent her time gossiping with neighbours, listening to the radio, and with a boyfriend by whom she had a child at age 27, though she continued to live with her mother. From age 32 until last seen at 36 she improved slowly and became able to go on short bus rides and shopping expeditions. Although she had wet and soiled her bed until age 12, before her phobias started she was a good mixer, had many friends, and often went dancing. She was sexually cold until age 32, after which she had normal orgasm with her boyfriend.

By way of contrast, agoraphobia developed very gradually in a young woman of 17. She slowly developed fears of leaving home at 17, which improved at 20 when she had psychiatric treatment. They became more marked after she gave birth, at 26, to a son, when she became afraid of meeting people and of getting lost in a crowd. For the next two years she was limited to travelling by bike or car to her mother's home a mile away, and thereafter did not go beyond her own home and stopped shopping. She improved when admitted to hospital at age 29, became pregnant after discharge, and improved a bit more after her second child was born. For the next six years, until last seen, she only did local shopping, fetched her child from school, and went out with her husband. She had always been a shy, dependent person dominated by her mother.

Panics in Agoraphobia

Some agoraphobia starts with repeated episodes of panic away from home. The panic can become so intense that the sufferer is glued to the spot for minutes until it diminishes, after which he/she may just want to run to a safe haven—a friend or home. As one woman said:

> At the height of a panic I just wanted to run anywhere. I usually made towards reliable friends...from wherever I happened to be. I felt, however, that I must resist this running away, so I did not allow myself to reach safety unless I was in extremity. One of my devices to keep a hold on myself was to avoid using my last chance, for I did not dare to think what would happen if it failed me. So I would merely go nearer my [escape route] and imagine the friendly welcome I should get. This would often quiet the panic enough for me to start out again, or at least not to be a nuisance or use up any good will. Sometimes I was beaten and had to feel an acute shame and despair of asking for company. I felt the shame even when I hadn't to confess to my need.

The panic may go on for a few minutes to several hours. Once it is over the sufferer may be reluctant to return to the scene of the panic. In other cases the panic can pass, leaving the person feeling as fit as before, and many months may go by before another panic strikes. Panic episodes can be followed by periods of normal activity, and a succession of panics may occur for years. Such episodes may lead to consultation with a doctor, who will find nothing abnormal except for signs of anxiety. Eventually the agoraphobic will begin to avoid certain situations for fear they might precipitate further panic. Because he cannot get off an express train immediately a panic starts, he restricts himself to slow trains; when these too become the setting for panic, he restricts himself to buses, then to walking, then just to walking across the street from home; finally he will not venture beyond the front gate without a companion. Rarely, he may become bedridden for a while, as bed is the only place where the anxiety feels bearable. Typically agoraphobics have periods when they feel better and times when they feel worse.

Differential Diagnosis

Conditions with which agoraphobia might be confused are discussed below roughly in the order of the frequency with which they might present.

- *Social phobia.* Social phobics tend to hate being looked at even by another person, whereas agoraphobics fear crowds rather than scrutiny from individuals *per se*. Social phobics feel fine in deserted public transport,

whereas agoraphobics might be as phobic in a deserted train or bus as in crowded public transport. A minority of sufferers have both agoraphobia and social phobia.
- *Depression.* Episodes of mild to moderate non-suicidal depression commonly accompany more enduring agoraphobia in cases consulting psychiatrists, and may merit a diagnosis of depression as well as agoraphobia. If the agoraphobic symptoms wax and wane with the depression and are absent between the episodes of low mood, then one diagnoses only depression.
- *Panic disorder (panic disorder without agoraphobia).* In this diagnosis the panics are not triggered by any particular cues, so there is no fear or avoidance of agoraphobic situations.
- *Sphincteric phobia.* A phobia of leaving home similar to that of agoraphobia is seen in people who fear urinating or defecating in public toilets or fear the opposite of being "caught short" and becoming incontinent when far from a toilet. These "sphincteric phobics" [19] do not have other agoraphobic fears that are the hallmark of agoraphobia or the generalized anxiety, uncued panic and non-suicidal depression that are common in agoraphobia.
- *Dysmorphophobia (body dysmorphic disorder).* Leaving home may be shunned by people who think inconsolably that they look grotesque or smell bad, contrary to all the evidence. The diagnosis is made from the presence of distorted ideas about their body.
- *Post-traumatic stress disorder.* Leaving home or going to certain places or using certain forms of transport might be avoided after an accident or rape or other trauma people have suffered. The diagnosis of post-traumatic stress disorder depends on the fact that the sufferer fears situations mainly related to the trauma and had no such fears before the trauma occurred.
- *Depersonalization–derealization syndrome.* Here the sense that one is unreal or things around one are unreal is the main focus of the complaint rather than an incidental symptom among other major agoraphobic complaints.
- *Obsessive–compulsive disorder.* If the subject avoids leaving home alone or crowds or shops or public transport because these situations lead to urges to engage in washing, checking or other rituals, this earns a diagnosis of OCD, not of agoraphobia.
- *Space phobia.* See above (p. 12).
- *Paranoid syndromes.* People with paranoid delusions from any cause might stop leaving home for fear of persecution. The diagnosis is made from the fact that the sufferer is housebound due to paranoid feelings rather than because going out triggers inexplicable fear, panic, sense of losing control etc.

Social Phobia (F40.1, 300.23)

When the normal slight anxiety at social occasions becomes so great as to disrupt everyday life, then it is a social phobia. Social phobia may be very focal, or involve several situations (mostly separate from agoraphobic ones), or be diffuse. Social phobia largely concerns a fear of scrutiny, of what other people think. A glance from someone else precipitates panic about being thought stupid.

Sufferers may fear eating and drinking in front of others; their fear may be of their hands trembling as they hold their fork or cup, or feeling nauseous or a lump in their throat and inability to swallow as long as they are watched: "When I go out to eat in strange places I can't eat, my throat feels a quarter of an inch wide, and I sweat". The fear is usually worse in smart crowded restaurants and less at home, but a few cannot even eat with their spouse. They avoid going out to dinner or having friends home for fear that their hands will tremble when drinking coffee or handing a cup to a friend. Social life becomes restricted.

For fear of shaking, blushing, sweating or looking ridiculous, some people will not face another passenger in a bus or train or walk past a queue of people. They are terrified of attracting attention by seeming awkward or fainting. Some may leave their house only under cover of darkness or fog. They will avoid talking to superiors and stage fright prevents them performing to an audience. They stop swimming to avoid strangers looking at their bodies. They shun parties and are too embarrassed to talk to others. "I can't have normal conversation with people. I break out in a sweat, that's my whole problem even with the missus," said a man, who still continued normal sex with her. The fear may appear only in the presence of the opposite sex, or manifest equally in front of men and women.

Social phobics may fear writing in public and so avoid banks or shops as they are terrified their hand will tremble when signing something or handling money in company. For fear of shaking, a secretary may cease typing, a teacher may no longer write on a blackboard or read aloud in front of a class, a seamstress will stop sewing in a factory, an assembly line worker will become unable to work on a production line. Knitting or buttoning a coat can induce agonizing panic when done in front of others.

Generally the fear is that their hands or heads *might* shake: social phobics rarely actually tremble or shake so that they write with a scrawl, rattle their coffee cup against the saucer, spill soup when raising their spoon to their lips, or nod their head visibly when talking. This contrasts strikingly with sufferers from brain diseases which actually cause obvious shaking. People with Parkinson's disease, for example, do not fear doing things in public despite the shaking of their head and hands. Similarly, fear of blushing, which is common in social phobics, is irrespective of their actual facial colouration [43,44].

Some fear they might vomit in public or see others vomiting. Sufferers may avoid anything that might remotely make them or others vomit, such as travelling on a bumpy bus or coach, going on a boat or eating onions. A woman of 34 had feared vomiting for 13 years:

> As a child my mother couldn't help the kids when they vomited and instead would ask my father to clean up the mess. I remember being upset by other children vomiting when I was only about five, but didn't develop the phobia until much later, at age 21. At that time I became afraid that other people or I myself would vomit on the train, so I began avoiding travelling to some places. This fear got worse over the last five years. I wake at 5:15 a.m. daily to travel to my office before the rush hour. With a great effort I might rarely manage to return during rush hour. Over the last two years I've drunk a bottle of brandy a week to calm my fear of travelling, and also take sedatives at times. I worry that I drink ever larger amounts of brandy. In the last five years I've avoided eating in public places, in restaurants, or in strangers' homes. I've also stopped going to theatres with friends if I can help it because it's easier to leave the theatre if I'm alone when I get this awful fear of vomiting. The funny thing, though, is I've never vomited in a public place nor have I seen anyone else vomit for many years.

When alone, she was not anxious and worked well.

A few social phobics fear hearing rather than seeing people. They may not go through a door if voices are heard from the other side, and may avoid answering a knock on the door. They may not use the phone:

> I have a code with my husband and children so that if the phone rings I know it's them. If it's anyone else, I can't answer the phone. I used to be able to when I was working because I knew then it would be about business, but I'm frightened at home.

Sufferers may give up work as a secretary or in a call centre.

Some social phobics may not only fear social situations but be anxious and depressed at other times too. A woman of 20 had had social phobias for three years, which reduced her socializing. She had not been out alone for a year except to travel to work, and since stopping work two months previously she had been out nowhere alone. She came to hospital with her mother. She dreaded people looking at her, that she might shake while drinking or walking out in public, or any other social situation. Even at home she was on edge, shaky and restless, and unexpected panics punctuated her background anxiety. She only relaxed after alcohol or sedative drugs. For two years she had also been depressed and wanting to cry at times.

Lack of Self-Assertion, Shyness

Lack of self-assertion is common even in otherwise well-adjusted people. It may stop them accepting promotion at work and restrict their lives—e.g. a man's shyness since childhood worsened when at 18 he was beaten up by youths after a row in a dance hall. He worked so well in a garage that he was offered the post of manager, but declined this because he could not assert himself with juniors. He was nevertheless quick-tempered at home and had a happy sex life.

Extreme shyness can prevent people from making friends and lead to great loneliness. Many persons are isolated because they fear contacting others, worry they might seem foolish and look silly, and never make the first move towards companionship. They might tread a lonely path between working in a boring office where they keep to themselves and a room in lodgings where they speak to nobody and spend their time reading or watching TV and going for solitary walks. In a few a fear of others or lack of social skills leads them to become hermits, shut up, isolated and unemployed in a dark room, living on a pittance from social security. They might draw down the blinds or dark curtains so nobody can see inside their home.

Extreme shyness in adults can be a continuation of marked childhood shyness that never cleared up, whereas most focal social phobias start in young adult life. Extreme shyness or diffuse social phobia is thus also called anxious (avoidant) personality disorder (F60.6, 301.82).

Onset and Course

Though most other phobias are more frequent in women, social phobias are equally common in men and women, except for extreme shyness, for which help is sought far more often by men than by women.

Social phobias usually start between ages 15 to 25 and develop slowly over months or years with no obvious cause. A few start suddenly after triggering events, as with a young man at a dance who felt sick at the bar and vomited before reaching the toilet, making an embarrassing mess, after which he became afraid of going to dances, bars or parties. As with agoraphobia, once the social phobia has been present for at least a year it tends to continue for many years if untreated.

Differential Diagnosis

Conditions with which social phobia might be confused appear below roughly in the order of the frequency with which they might present.

- *Agoraphobia.* Unlike social phobics, agoraphobics fear crowds *per se* rather than scrutiny/criticism from other people in the crowd and might be as phobic in a deserted train or bus as in crowded public transport. A minority of sufferers have both agoraphobia and social phobia.
- *Depression.* Episodes of mild to moderate non-suicidal depression commonly accompany more enduring social phobia in cases consulting mental health personnel, and may merit a diagnosis of depression as well as social phobia.
- *Sphincteric phobia.* Social situations may be avoided for fear of urinating or defecating in public toilets or the opposite fear of becoming incontinent when far from a toilet. These specific "sphincteric phobics" [19] do not have other social phobias.
- *Dysmorphophobia (body dysmorphic disorder).* Social situations may be shunned by people who think inconsolably that they look grotesque or smell bad, contrary to all the evidence. The diagnosis is made from the presence of distorted ideas about their body.
- *Anxious or avoidant personality disorder (F60.6, 301.82).* See above (p. 22).
- *Post-traumatic stress disorder.* Some people fear and avoid social situations after suffering an accident or rape or other trauma. The diagnosis of post-traumatic stress disorder depends on the fact that the feared situations relate to the trauma and were not feared before the trauma occurred.
- *Obsessive–compulsive disorder.* A subject who avoids social situations because they lead to urges to engage in washing or checking rituals earns a diagnosis of OCD, not of social phobia.
- *Paranoid syndromes.* Paranoid delusions can cause people to become hermits for fear of persecution. Diagnosis depends on the social avoidance being a consequence of the paranoid feelings.

Specific (Isolated) Phobias (F40.2, 300.29)

The presenting complaint is a phobia focusing mainly on well-defined situations with relatively little phobia of anything else. Examples are certain animals or insects; darkness, storms, heights, enclosed spaces, lifts; water, noise; flying or other specific forms of travel; certain foods; blood, injury, injection or other medical or dental procedures; a particular illness; triggers of anger that is hard to manage.

Encountering or thinking about the feared object or situation may evoke striking distress—panic, sweating, trembling in terror. Sufferers may have recurrent nightmares of the feared object or situation, and search for it wherever they go. Blood–injury phobics, unlike other phobics, may faint at the sight of blood.

The slightest evidence of presence of the phobic object is disturbing where most people never notice it. A woman screamed on finding a spider at home, ran to find a neighbour to remove it, shook fearfully, and kept a neighbour at her side for two hours before she could remain alone at home again. Another found herself on top of her refrigerator in the kitchen with no memory of how she had got there; terror at the sight of a spider had made her lose her memory for a moment. Yet another jumped out of a boat (though she could not swim) to avoid a spider she found in it; once she jumped out of a speeding car and on another occasion off a galloping horse to escape spiders she had found near her.

The phobia may severely restrict where phobics live, walk or work. A pigeon phobia may cause avoidance of parks, gardens, waiting at bus stops or shopping. A flying phobic might change his job if the work comes to involve flying. A lift phobic roofing expert who had to complete work on the roof of a 600-foot-high tower walked to the top twice a day rather than go up in the lift. A filmmaker who was phobic of human whistling at a particular frequency could not return to the studio for days after someone whistled there. If the phobia is of medical procedures or blood, it can become life threatening due to avoidance of health care or lead to rotting teeth if dentists are shunned, and women may avoid having children. A phobia of swallowing solid food may force the adoption of a liquid diet. A hypersensitive gag reflex may cause people to avoid wearing ties and dentistry. Sphincteric phobics avoid being far from public toilets for fear that they might wet or soil their pants.

Depression and/or general anxiety is not a common complaint in specific phobics. Away from the feared situation, specific phobics tend to feel normal.

Onset and Course

Adults presenting with a specific phobia of animals or insects or blood–injury or certain other situations usually report that they began in early childhood and continued without much fluctuation thereafter. Most other specific phobias may start at any age. A few specific phobias may start after a bad experience concerning the relevant situation (e.g. driving cars after a traffic accident, a dog phobia after a dog bite). Disability from restrictions to everyday activities caused by changes in living or working arrangements may prompt the seeking of help.

Differential Diagnosis

Conditions with which a specific phobia might be confused will depend on the particular phobia.

- *Agoraphobia.* Unlike people with a specific phobia of travelling in a car or a bus or a train or a plane or being in an enclosed space, agoraphobics have several such phobias, and often also have anxiety or panics in no particular place, and depressive episodes. In certain cases it is arbitrary to distinguish certain specific phobias from a focal form of agoraphobia.
- *Social phobia.* Unlike people with a specific phobia only, say, of eating or writing in front of other people, social phobics tend to have a wider variety of feared situations but, as with agoraphobia, the distinction is sometimes arbitrary.
- *Post-traumatic stress disorder.* Where, say, a specific dog phobia began after a dog bite or specific driving phobia after a traffic accident, post-traumatic stress disorder becomes a more accurate label if there are also other non-phobic features of the disorder, such as anxiety away from the phobic situation.
- *Obsessive–compulsive disorder.* A few OCD sufferers may fear and avoid just one situation, but if that situation evokes washing, checking or other rituals the diagnosis is OCD, not specific phobia.
- *Hypochondriasis.* If a worry concerns only one unchanging illness, like lung cancer or heart disease, then it is an illness phobia or nosophobia, a form of specific phobia, but if it concerns several illnesses or it changes over time then it is best termed hypochondriasis.

Dysmorphophobia (F45.2, Body Dysmorphic Disorder 300.7)

Dysmorphophobic worry about how one looks or smells can cause handicap like that from social phobia. The phobia may be of being too short or too tall, too thin or too fat, being bald or having a big nose or bat ears or a protruding bottom, or being too flat-chested or too bosomy as a woman. Sufferers are endlessly preoccupied with minor or totally imagined body defects that are not evident even to the keenest observer. Severe dysmorphophobia can lead to avoidance of public transport or going on holiday or looking in a mirror, to dropping one's friends, to becoming a recluse, and to a quest for plastic surgery. Anxiety about one's body odour may cause excessive washing, endless use of deodorants and social avoidance.

The fixity of conviction about the abnormality of bodily appearance or smell can be of delusional strength. When the fixed delusion about bodily appearance concerns gender, it may be called transsexualism or anorexia nervosa.

Onset and Course

Onset can be at any age. Once the problem has been present for more than a year, if untreated it can continue unchanged for many years.

Differential Diagnosis

- *Social phobia*. If the social fear and avoidance are not linked to worries about one's appearance or smell, then the condition is social phobia rather than dysmorphophobia.
- *Hypochondriasis or multiple illness phobia*. If the worry concerns not bodily appearance or smell *per se* but rather that the bodily appearance suggests illness, then the problem is hypochondriasis rather than dysmorphophobia.
- *Obsessive–compulsive disorder*. If the concern over bodily appearance or smell is linked to marked checking or other rituals it seems more appropriate to call it OCD.
- *Transsexualism*. If the patient feels that he/she was born as a man trapped in a woman's body, or vice versa, and should have his/her physical gender changed by sex hormones and sex reassignment surgery, then the problem is called transsexualism, not dysmorphophobia.
- *Anorexia nervosa*. If the sufferer starves herself because she is convinced she is too fat despite being very underweight in reality, then the problem is called anorexia nervosa, not dysmorphophobia.

Hypochondriasis (Multiple Illness Phobias) (F45.2, 300.7)

Fears of multiple bodily symptoms and a variety of illnesses are called hypochondriasis. Fear focusing on a single symptom or illness in the absence of another psychiatric problem is an illness phobia, a kind of specific phobia. The distinction is arbitrary at some point.

Sufferers worry endlessly that they have various diseases. They fear that minor pain in the abdomen or chest or a tiny spot on the hand or penis denotes stomach or lung or skin cancer or a sexually transmitted disease. They may constantly search their body for evidence of disease. No skin lesion or body sensation is too trivial. They misinterpret normal tummy rumblings. Their worry itself produces fresh symptoms, such as abdominal pain and discomfort due to gut contractions, which reinforce their gloomy prognostications. Women may examine their breasts for cancer so vigorously and often that they bruise their breasts. Repeatedly normal examinations and investigations that would satisfy the average person allay the worry only briefly, with further reassurance-seeking soon following. Sufferers may make hundreds of phone calls and visits to doctors throughout their district in a vain quest for reassurance.

A physical illness might trigger hypochondriasis or sensitize someone to develop symptoms later, but commonly there is no history of past disease to explain it. Indeed, in a few cases development of the feared disease resolved the fear. One man was so frantic with fear of sexually transmitted disease that he was admitted to a mental hospital. After discharge he got syphilis with a visible ulcer. From that moment his fear disappeared and he attended happily for regular anti-syphilitic treatment.

Illness fears might be triggered by circumstances which sufferers start to avoid, as in a woman with a fear of epilepsy who would not go out alone lest she have a seizure. A man who had had so many X-rays that he thought he might get leukaemia refused to be out of contact with his wife more than a moment in order to get her constant reassurance.

Some illness phobias reflect currently fashionable worries about disease, so we can expect now a surge in phobias of SARS (severe acute respiratory syndrome) just as the last few years of the 20th century saw the advent of AIDS fears and its earlier years saw many fears of tuberculosis. Some illness fears may simply reflect a failure of patient and doctor to communicate well; a taciturn doctor's silence may be misinterpreted as an ominous sign of frightening information being concealed.

Hypochondriasis can cause extreme distress and disability. A woman had gone to 43 hospital casualty departments over three years and had every part of her body X-rayed. At various times she was scared she would die of stomach cancer, a brain tumour, thrombosis. Examinations never revealed any abnormality and she emerged each time from the hospital "rejuvenated—it's like having been condemned to death and given a reprieve". But within a week she would seek out a new hospital "where they won't know I'm a fraud. I'm terrified of the idea of dying, it's the end, the complete end, and the thought of rotting in the ground obsesses me—I can see the worms and maggots." She was petrified of sex with her husband, imagining she could rupture and burst a blood vessel, and afterward would get up at two in the morning and stand for hours outside the hospital so she knew she was in reach of help.

Differential Diagnosis

- *Specific (illness) phobia.* Worry about a single illness can be called a specific illness phobia, and of several illnesses hypochondriasis, but, as noted, the distinction becomes arbitrary at some point.
- *Obsessive–compulsive disorder.* The more the worry generates repeated stereotyped checks and requests for reassurance and investigations, the more the hypochondriasis overlaps with OCD.
- *Depression.* The more the worry about illness began at the time the low mood began, and the more it waxes and wanes as the depression does, the more accurate it is to call the problem depression rather than hypochondriasis.

Post-Traumatic Stress Disorder (F43.1, 309.81)

When the normal reaction to severe trauma lasts longer than a month and is particularly severe, then it is called post-traumatic stress disorder. Sufferers feel tense, irritable, spaced out, startle easily, cannot sleep, and have nightmares and flashbacks about the trauma. Depression and a sense of numbing are frequent, as is grief from any loss associated with the trauma. Patients avoid places, people, thoughts and other reminders of what happened, and this often-prominent aspect of post-traumatic stress disorder is a phobia and merits its inclusion in this chapter.

Onset and Course

Post-traumatic stress disorder is usually a continuation of the usual acute response to stress, and might alter somewhat over time just as grief does. The proportion of survivors continuing to suffer from the disorder diminishes rapidly in the first few months after a trauma and more slowly thereafter. In some the disorder continues for decades and may never clear up if the trauma had been particularly horrible and drawn out. Occasionally there is a delay of up to several years between the time of the trauma and the start of the distress. The more intense and prolonged the trauma, the worse the disorder. People who have had previous anxiety or depressive problems are likely to suffer more.

Differential Diagnosis

- *Specific phobia of traumatic onset.* This is an appropriate label where the non-phobic aspects of post-traumatic stress disorder are absent even though there is a marked phobia of covert and overt reminders of the initiating trauma.
- *Depression* is a sensible diagnosis where the depressive features overshadow all the others.
- *Generalized anxiety* is the most accurate term where the generalized anxiety dominates the clinical picture.

Aversions (not in ICD-10 or DSM-IV-TR)

A common problem that attracts little medical attention and is not in disease classification systems is a strong dislike of touching, tasting or hearing things which most people are indifferent to or may even enjoy. The ensuing discomfort differs from that of fear. Aversions set our teeth on edge and shivers down our spine, make us suck our teeth, go cold and pale, and take a deep breath. Our hair stands on end, and we feel unpleasant and sometimes disgust but not frightened. There may be a desire to wet or wash our fingers or cover them with cream. Some aversions are made worse when our skin is rough or the nails are unevenly clipped so that our fingertips catch as they pass over a surface.

Examples are intense dislike and avoidance of touching fuzzy textures such as those of cotton wool, wire or steel wool, velvet and peach skins, with avoidance of rooms containing new carpets with that texture, and wearing of gloves to handle new tennis balls until the fuzz wears off. Other people avoid handling old pearly buttons or slimy slugs, the latter causing a sense of disgust. Similar discomfort is produced by the squeak of chalk on a blackboard or the scrape of a knife on a plate. Aversions of certain tastes or smells cause avoidance of foods such as onions.

Aversions can disable. A woman disliked the sound of chalk scraping on a blackboard so much that she gave up a cherished ambition to be a teacher. Another found velvet so unbearable that she avoided children's parties. A third said, "All kinds of buttons make me squeamish. I've been like this since I was a young baby and my uncle had the same thing. I can only wear clothes with zip fasteners and hooks, not buttons."

As with phobias, aversions involve discomfort from and avoidance of particular objects or situations, but the discomfort is not fear. Aversions seem to habituate to repeated encounters with the avoided situation, as happens with phobias, but systematic studies are needed.

SUMMARY

Consistent Evidence

The main international and US disease classifications have consistently recognized phobias over the last half century, with subdivisions into agoraphobia, social phobia and specific phobias. Such phobias are common and, if they become chronic, more often stay true to type for many years rather than change into other kinds of problems. Some phobias have, apart from characteristic triggering situations, particular onset ages, gender prevalence, types of discomfort, thoughts and physiological reactions, and associated non-phobic symptoms. Phobias can occur alone or as part of a wide range of problems.

Incomplete Evidence

There is uncertainty about the classification of: (a) panic as opposed to phobia, and agoraphobia in particular; (b) the fluctuating non-suicidal depression that commonly associates with phobias; (c) phobias that are common within other syndromes, such as hypochondriasis, post-traumatic stress disorder, dysmorphophobia and OCD; and (d) touch and sound aversions.

Areas Still Open to Research

In addition to the clarification of the relationship between panic and agoraphobia and between depression and phobias, further research is needed about how far particular subjective feelings, thoughts and physiological features associate with particular phobias.

REFERENCES

1. Stengel E. (1959) Classification of mental disorders. *WHO Bull.*, **21**: 601–663.
2. American Psychiatric Association (1952) *Diagnostic and Statistical Manual of Mental Disorders*. American Psychiatric Association, Washington, DC.
3. American Psychiatric Association (1968) *Diagnostic and Statistical Manual of Mental Disorders*, 2nd edn. American Psychiatric Association, Washington, DC.
4. Marks I.M. (1969) *Fears and Phobias*. Heinemann, London.
5. Marks I.M. (1970) The classification of phobic disorders. *Br. J. Psychiatry*, **116**: 377–386.

DIAGNOSIS AND CLASSIFICATION OF PHOBIAS: A REVIEW

6. American Psychiatric Association (1980) *Diagnostic and Statistical Manual of Mental Disorders*, 3rd edn. American Psychiatric Association, Washington, DC.
7. American Psychiatric Association (1994) *Diagnostic and Statistical Manual of Mental Disorders*, 4th edn. American Psychiatric Association, Washington, DC.
8. American Psychiatric Association (2000) *Diagnostic and Statistical Manual of Mental Disorders*, 4th edn., text revised. American Psychiatric Association, Washington, DC.
9. World Health Organization (1957) *Manual of the International Statistical Classification of Diseases, Injuries and Causes of Death*, 7th revision. World Health Organization, Geneva.
10. World Health Organization (1978) *Mental Disorders: Glossary and Guide to their Classification for Use in Conjunction with the Ninth Revision of the International Classification of Diseases*. World Health Organization, Geneva.
11. World Health Organization (1992) *The ICD-10 Classification of Mental and Behavioural Disorders: Clinical Descriptions and Diagnostic Guidelines*. World Health Organization, Geneva.
12. Maser J.D., Patterson T. (2002) Spectrum and nosology: implications for DSM-V. *Psychiatr. Clin. North Am.*, **25**: 855–885.
13. Tuma A.H., Maser J.D. (1985) *Anxiety and the Anxiety Disorders*. Lawrence Erlbaum, Hillsdale, NJ.
14. Curtis G.C., Magee W.J., Eaton W.W., Wittchen H.-U., Kessler R.C. (1998) Specific fears and phobias: epidemiology and classification. *Br. J. Psychiatry*, **173**: 212–217.
15. Cox B.J., Parker J.D.A., Swinson R.P. (1996) Confirmatory factor analysis of the Fear Questionnaire with social phobia patients. *Br. J. Psychiatry*, **168**: 497–499.
16. Hallam R.S. (1985) *Anxiety: Psychological Perspectives on Panic and Agoraphobia*. Academic Press, New York.
17. Hallam R.S., Hafner R.J. (1978) Fears of phobic patients: factor analyses of self-report data. *Behav. Res. Ther.*, **16**: 1–6.
18. Marks I.M. (1967) Components and correlates in psychiatric questionnaires. *Br. J. Med. Psychol.*, **40**: 261–272.
19. Marks I.M. (1987) *Fears, Phobias and Rituals: Panic, Anxiety, and their Disorders*. Oxford University Press, New York.
20. Marks I.M., Mathews A.M. (1979) Brief standard self-rating for phobic patients. *Behav. Res. Ther.*, **17**: 263–267.
21. Arrindell W.A. (1980) A factorial definition of agoraphobia. *Behav. Res. Ther.*, **18**: 229–242.
22. Dixon J.J., De Monchaux C., Sandler J. (1957) Patterns of anxiety. *Br. J. Med. Psychol.*, **30**: 34–40, 107–112.
23. Fleiss J.L., Gurland B.J., Cooper J.E. (1971) Some contributions to the measurement of psychopathology. *Br. J. Psychiatry*, **119**: 647–656.
24. Schapira K., Roth M., Kerr T.A., Gurney C. (1972) The prognosis of affective disorders: the differentiation of anxiety from depressive illness. *Br. J. Psychiatry*, **121**: 175–181.
25. Cox B.J., McWilliams L.A., Clara I.P., Stein M.B. (2003) The structure of feared situations in a nationally representative sample. *J. Anxiety Disord.*, **17**: 89–101.
26. Derogatis L.R., Cleary P.A. (1977) Factorial invariance across gender in the SCL-90. *Br. J. Soc. Clin. Psychol.*, **16**: 347–356.
27. Lipman R.S., Covi L., Shapiro A.K. (1979) The Hopkins Symptom checklist (HCSL). *J. Affect. Disord.*, **1**: 9–24.

28. Frombach I., Asmundson G.J.G., Cox B. (1999) Confirmatory factor analysis of the Fear Questionnaire in injured workers with chronic pain. *Depress. Anxiety*, **9**: 117–121.
29. Wittchen H.-U., Reed V., Kessler R.C. (1998) Relationship of agoraphobia and panic in a community sample of adolescents and young adults. *Arch. Gen. Psychiatry*, **55**: 1017–1024.
30. Cottraux J., Bouvard M., Messy P. (1987) Validation et analyse d'une échelle de phobias. *Encéphale*, **13**: 23–29.
31. Cox B.J., Swinson R.P., Shaw B.F. (1991) Value of the Fear Questionnaire in differentiating agoraphobia and social phobia. *Br. J. Psychiatry*, **159**: 842–845.
32. Stravynski A., Basoglu M., Marks M., Sengun S., Marks I.M. (1995) The distinctiveness of phobias: a discriminant analysis of fears. *J. Anxiety Disord.*, **9**: 89–101.
33. Van Zuuren F.J. (1988) The Fear Questionnaire: some data on validity, reliability and layout. *Br. J. Psychiatry*, **153**: 659–662.
34. Kessler R.C., Stein M.B., Berglund P. (1998) Social phobia subtypes in NCS. *Am. J. Psychiatry*, **155**: 613–619.
35. Taylor S. (1998) Hierarchic structure of fears. *Behav. Res. Ther.*, **36**: 205–214.
36. Mataix-Cols D., Rauch S.L., Baer L., Shera D., Eisen J., Goodman W.K., Rasmussen S., Jenike M.A. (2002) Symptom stability in adult obsessive–compulsive disorder: data from a two-year naturalistic study. *Am. J. Psychiatry*, **159**: 263–268.
37. Krueger R.F. (1999) The structure of common mental disorders. *Arch. Gen. Psychiatry*, **56**: 921–926.
38. Krueger R.F., Finger M.S. (2001) Using item response theory to understand comorbidity among anxiety and unipolar mood disorders. *Psychol. Assess.*, **13**: 140–151.
39. Krueger R.F., Caspi A., Moffitt T.E., Silva P.A. (1998) The structure and stability of common mental disorders (DSM-III-R): a longitudinal-epidemiological study. *J Abnorm. Psychol.*, **107**: 216–227.
40. Marks I.M., Gelder M.G. (1966) Different ages of onset in varieties of phobia. *Am. J. Psychiatry*, **123**: 218–221.
41. Marks I.M. (2001) *Living With Fear*, 2nd edn. McGraw-Hill UK, Maidenhead.
42. Swoboda H., Amering M., Windhaber J., Katschnig H. (2003) Long-term course of panic disorder—an 11 year follow-up. *J. Anxiety Disord.*, **17**: 223–232.
43. Mulkens S., de Jong P.J., Bögels S.M. (1997) High blushing propensity: fearful preoccupation or facial coloration? *Personal. Indiv. Diff.*, **22**: 817–824.
44. Mulkens S., de Jong P.J., Dobbelaar A., Bögels S.M. (1999) Fear of blushing: fearful preoccupation irrespective of facial coloration. *Behav. Res. Ther.*, **37**: 1119–1128.

Commentaries

1.1
Two Procrustean or One King-Size Bed for Comorbid Agoraphobia and Panic?

Heinz Katschnig[1]

Besides being known as an impassioned behaviour therapist, Isaac Marks is one of the most influential psychopathologists and psychiatric diagnosticians of the outgoing 20th century. His subdivision of the phobias into agoraphobia, social phobia and the specific phobias [1] was directly taken over by the DSM (from its 3rd edition in 1980 onwards) and the ICD (since its 10th revision in 1992).

Isaac Marks may not like the comparison: he reminds one of Sigmund Freud, who besides being a passionate psychoanalyst was also a most influential psychopathologist and psychiatric diagnostician. Sigmund Freud silently (and with a sleeper effect) revolutionized classificatory thinking in psychiatry in the beginning of the 20th century by separating anxiety neurosis from neurasthenia [2] and by defining obsessive–compulsive disorder [3]. The former survived nearly 100 years (until ICD-10 abolished it); the latter concept is still in use today.

Both Marks and Freud are firmly based in clinical practice and are astute observers of psychopathological phenomena. This is documented by their rich and brilliant descriptions of neurotic conditions. In the studies on hysteria, for instance, Freud, together with Breuer [4], portrays vividly what is today called "panic disorder" (in case 4, called "Katharina", where one could in fact apply the operational diagnostic criteria of DSM to make the diagnosis). Similarly, Marks' writings abound with clinical examples and the subdivision of the phobias is based on his intimate clinical knowledge of these conditions.

However, since both Freud and Marks also have their specific theories about the origins and the appropriate treatments of these conditions, it is inconceivable that their theories have not influenced their diagnostic thinking. In the second part of his "Case Katharina" article, Freud goes on to explain the condition with his controversial sexual theories, and one wonders to what extent Freud's diagnostic concepts served his theories.

---

[1] *Department of Psychiatry, University of Vienna, Austria*

And Marks, a virtuoso of exposure therapy, has not by chance focused on exactly those conditions for which exposure therapy is efficacious, i.e. agoraphobia, social phobia and the specific phobias.

One could argue that the diagnosis of panic disorder is beyond the scope of a paper discussing the diagnosis of phobias. But the fact is that the majority of patients in clinical settings suffer from both panic attacks and agoraphobia and that ICD-10 and DSM-IV offer diametrically opposed hierarchical solutions to the problem. It is a pity that this issue is insufficiently and even one-sidedly discussed in Marks and Mataix-Cols' paper.

In DSM-IV the comorbid condition is classified under "panic disorder" (300.21 Panic disorder with agoraphobia), thereby degrading *agoraphobia* to a secondary phenomenon. In ICD-10, instead, it comes under "agoraphobia" (F40.01 Agoraphobia with panic disorder)—here *panic attacks* are demoted to a secondary phenomenon. Each of the two diagnostic systems offers its own Procrustean bed for accommodating the frequent comorbid condition of panic and agoraphobia. And Marks and Mataix-Cols clearly favour the ICD-10 bed, i.e. the "agoraphobia first" approach.

As Marks and Mataix-Cols rightly point out for the DSM approach, the American pharmaceutical industry pressed for a large category of "panic disorder" which included agoraphobia in the 1980s. At that time pharmacological treatments for panic attacks became available, but not for agoraphobia, for which a specific form of psychotherapy—"exposure *in vivo*"—had been shown to be efficacious. The advocates of pharmacotherapy proposed that, if panic attacks are regarded as the core diagnostic feature and agoraphobia as a secondary phenomenon, successful treatment of panic attacks with pharmacotherapy should also wipe out agoraphobia. In fact, clinical trials in DSM-defined patient populations have shown this to be the case (see the review in Chapter 3 of this volume).

In contrast, if agoraphobia is primary and panic attacks are only part of the whole syndrome—a position held by Marks and reflected in ICD-10—the appropriate treatment of the comorbid condition would have to focus on agoraphobia, and successful treatment of agoraphobia by "exposure *in vivo*" would also make panic attacks disappear. There is evidence that this is also true (see the review in Chapter 4 of this volume).

However, what looks like a classical "pharmacotherapy versus psychotherapy" or "biology versus psychology" controversy is more complicated. The issue is not just "pharmacotherapy of panic disorder" versus "psychotherapy of agoraphobia", but also one of "cognitive therapy for panic disorder" versus "exposure *in vivo* for agoraphobia", i.e. an antagonism between different schools of psychotherapy. It is well documented that cognitive therapy works in panic disorder without and with agoraphobia (see the review in Chapter 4 of this volume).

Marks and Mataix-Cols have obviously no commercial interests, but they do have interests: let's call them intellectual, which are more noble than financial ones, but are still interests. They favour one of the two Procrustean diagnostic beds for comorbid panic and agoraphobia. But the differences between ICD-10 and DSM IV are there and practically relevant, whatever one thinks of each of the two approaches. In practice, depending on where one lives, works or intends to publish, one is forced to choose either DSM or ICD. Publication of a scientific paper in US journals, for instance, is nearly impossible if DSM has not been used. In our case this implies that the main diagnosis is panic disorder with an often unknown percentage of patients with agoraphobia.

The reliability of psychiatric diagnosis might be improved by hierarchical and categorical operational diagnostic criteria. But reliability is not identical with validity. At best, the diagnostic definitions of ICD and DSM are hypotheses or "working concepts" which might be *useful* for the clinician, but nothing more and nothing less [5].

The need for hierarchical rules comes from devotees to specific theories, but also from health statisticians and administrators who look for simple diagnostic systems. However, the high comorbidity between all types of presently defined psychiatric disorders, the many common treatments and common psychological mechanisms question the validity of the diagnostic definitions and the hierarchical rules applied, not only those concerning panic and agoraphobia. At a WPA Conference in June 2003 in Vienna on "Diagnosis in Psychiatry—Integrating the Sciences", a symposium entitled "Are all anxiety disorders the same?" has precisely pointed the finger at this issue [6]. Psychiatry is shooting itself in the foot, if it continues to use hierarchical rules in diagnostic systems at a stage, when things are not yet clear.

At least for research purposes, the hierarchical diagnostic rules for comorbid panic and agoraphobia should be abandoned and comorbidity explicitly allowed and documented as such (perhaps by adding degrees of severity, which may be important for choosing or combining treatments). This approach might seem difficult for clinicians, but for research it is feasible. Not *two Procrustean* beds, but *one king-size* for comorbid anxiety disorders!

In sum: we should approach psychopathological phenomena with a humbler attitude. The emphasis on multi-axial and dimensional diagnostic systems reflects such a stance—and many speakers at the above mentioned WPA conference stressed this point [7]. As a great American psychiatrist, Adolf Meyer [8], rightly put it nearly one hundred years ago: "An orderly presentation of the facts alone is a real diagnosis."

REFERENCES

1. Marks I.M. (1970) The classification of phobic disorders. *Br. J. Psychiatry*, **116**: 377–386.

2. Freud S. (1953) The justification for detaching from neurasthenia a particular syndrome: the anxiety neurosis. Collected Papers, vol. 1, pp. 76–106. Hogarth Press, London.
3. Freud S. (1895) Obsessions et phobies: leur mecanisme psychique et leur étiologie. Rev. Neurol., 3: 33–38.
4. Breuer J., Freud S. (1895) Studien über Hysterie. Deuticke, Leipzig.
5. Kendell R., Jablensky A. (2003) Distinguishing between validity and utility of psychiatric diagnoses. Am. J. Psychiatry, 160: 4–12.
6. Katschnig H., Faravelli C. (2003) Are all anxiety disorders the same? World Psychiatry, 2 (Suppl. 1): 38–39.
7. Katschnig H., Maj M., Sartorius N. (Eds) (2003) Diagnosis in psychiatry: integrating the sciences. World Psychiatry, 2 (Suppl. 1).
8. Meyer A. (1906) Principles of Grouping Facts in Psychiatry. Reports of the Pathological Institute, State of New York, New York.

1.2
Politics and Pathophysiology in the Classification of Phobias
Franklin R. Schneier[1]

Marks and Mataix-Cols have reviewed the diagnosis and classification of phobias, noting that modern categorizations of phobias emerged following the identification in the 1960s of key demographic and course of illness validators of phobic subtypes. Isaac Marks was himself a key contributor to this work.

In considering political influences on diagnostic classification, Marks and Mataix-Cols argue that the emergence of panic disorder as primary to the development of agoraphobia was influenced by US psychiatry's bid for mainstream medical status and the pharmaceutical industry's desire to market antipanic drugs. Politicization of agoraphobia may also have resulted from scientific conflicts, i.e. the concurrent emergence of effective medication and behavioural therapies and their respective divergent scientific models. The relationship of panic attacks to agoraphobia remains controversial, but most patients with agoraphobia report that initial panic attacks preceded or coincided with phobic onset (see [1] for review), unlike most patients with other phobias.

A leading scientific proponent of the primacy of panic disorder in most patients with agoraphobia has been Donald Klein. Klein has recounted his early observations from the late 1950s that imipramine seemed to directly block panic attacks but not phobic anxiety in severe agoraphobia patients [2].

---

[1] Anxiety Disorders Clinic, New York State Psychiatric Institute, 1051 Riverside Drive, Unit 69, New York, NY 10032, USA

Subsequent findings that lactate infusions provoked panic attacks in agoraphobic patients but not in healthy subjects led to the discovery of a variety of panicogenic agents and hopes that the pathophysiology of panic attacks might be uncovered. While a comprehensive understanding of panic attacks remains elusive, the approaches of pharmacological dissection and symptom provocation have increased understanding of the physiology of panic and have been a model for the field with respect to the search for biological markers that might enhance the classification of psychiatric disorders.

Although panic attacks can occur in all phobic disorders, the quality of panic attacks may help differentiate subtypes of phobias, with symptoms of dizziness and fear of dying occurring more commonly in agoraphobia, symptoms of blushing and twitching more common in social phobia [3], and fainting more common in blood–injury phobia. Marks and Mataix-Cols note that many medications and psychotherapies have non-specific effects across disorders, but differential responsivity of panic disorder (but not social phobia or specific phobias) to tricyclic antidepressants, and performance anxiety (but not generalized social phobia or panic disorder) to beta-adrenergic blockers has also helped to validate diagnostic categories [4].

Twin studies have supported the validity of five phobia subtypes (social, agoraphobia, animal, situational and blood–injury), with aggregation due largely to genetic factors [5,6]. It has been argued, however, that the future development of a "genetic nosology" that can classify individuals in terms of the heritable aspects of psychopathology should incorporate both categorical diagnoses and biological trait markers [7]. Such markers, or endophenotypes, may be closer to underlying pathophysiological processes, and may be amenable to further exploration through animal models as well. One promising approach involves measurement of individual variation in fear conditioning, a model for the acquisition of phobias. Fear conditioning has recently been shown to have significant genetic heritability [8], but its relationship to categories of phobias needs further study.

In regard to social fears, Marks and Mataix-Cols refer to early onset diffuse shyness as avoidant personality disorder. DSM-III-R and DSM-IV, however, have incorporated these individuals into the generalized subtype of social phobia, defined by fear of most social situations, and frequently overlapping with avoidant personality disorder. Although reasonably well validated [9], generalized social phobia straddles the border between discrete social phobia (with which it shares the core feature of fear of scrutiny and embarrassment) and broader trait social anxiety and shyness. Most patients seeking treatment for social phobia have this pervasive and impairing generalized subtype, leading some to advocate use of the alternative term "social anxiety disorder" [10]. Our classification of phobias continues to evolve with the social needs, politics and science of our times.

REFERENCES

1. Pollack M.H., Smoller J.W., Otto M.W., Scott E.L., Rosenbaum J.F. (2002) Phenomenology of panic disorder. In *Textbook of Anxiety Disorders* (Eds D.J. Stein, E. Hollander), pp. 237–246. American Psychiatric Publishing, Washington, DC.
2. Klein D.F. (1987) Anxiety reconceptualized. *Mod. Probl. Pharmacopsychiat.*, **22**: 1–35.
3. Hazen A.L., Stein M.B. (1995) Clinical phenomenology and comorbidity. In *Social Phobia: Clinical and Research Perspectives* (Ed. M.B. Stein), pp. 3–42. American Psychiatric Press, Washington, DC.
4. Schneier F.R., Marshall R.D., Erwin B.A., Heimberg R.G., Mellman L. (2001) Social phobia and specific phobias. In *Treatments of Psychiatric Disorders* (Ed. G.O. Gabbard), pp. 1485–1514. American Psychiatric Publishing, Washington, DC.
5. Kendler K.S., Karkowski L.M., Prescott C.A. (1999) Fears and phobias: reliability and heritability. *Psychol. Med.*, **29**: 539–553.
6. Kendler K.S., Myers J., Prescott C.A., Neale M.C. (2001) The genetic epidemiology of irrational fears and phobias in men. *Arch. Gen. Psychiatry*, **58**: 257–265.
7. Smoller J.W., Tsuang M.T. (1998) Panic and phobic anxiety: defining phenotypes for genetic studies. *Am. J. Psychiatry*, **155**: 1152–1162.
8. Hettema J.M., Annas P., Neale M.C., Kendler K.S., Fredrikson M. (2003) A twin study of the genetics of fear conditioning. *Arch. Gen. Psychiatry*, **60**: 702–708.
9. Mannuzza S., Schneier F.R., Chapman T.F., Liebowitz M.R., Klein D.F., Fyer A.J. (1995) Generalized social phobia: reliability and validity. *Arch. Gen. Psychiatry*, **52**: 230–237.
10. Liebowitz M.R., Heimberg R.G., Fresco D.M., Travers J., Stein M.D. (2000) Social phobia or social anxiety disorder: what's in a name? *Arch. Gen. Psychiatry*, **57**: 191–192.

1.3
A Critical Evaluation of the Classification of Phobias
David V. Sheehan[1]

The paper by Marks and Mataix-Cols is a useful updated summary of the seminal contributions of Isaac Marks from the 1960s to the present on the classification of phobias. It outlines the evidence, both old and new, in

---

[1] *University of South Florida Psychiatry Center, 3515 East Fletcher Ave., Tampa, FL 33613, USA*

support of the classification he first proposed in his 1969 book on fears and phobias [1] and which he further elucidated in many contributions since, notably in his 1987 book on fears, phobias and rituals [2]. In spite of many official national and international classifications of anxiety and phobic disorders since that time, his views on this topic have remained consistent over time. Many of his ideas were incorporated into both the ICD and DSM systems, although he outlines points of difference with both, particularly with the DSM classification since 1980 (DSM-III).

Marks and Mataix-Cols' review selectively supports one position without also critically evaluating its limitations. This is puzzling, since at the outset the authors state that "classifications are fictions imposed on a complex world to understand and manage it". The rest of the chapter leaves the impression that the authors take their own classification more seriously than a fiction but regard competing classifications as fictions.

They invoke conspiracy theories to dismiss the DSM classification: in particular, they argue that the "demotion of agoraphobia into an aspect of 'panic disorder'" was a bid by the pharmaceutical industry to get the Food and Drug Administration (FDA) approval for antipanic medications. This is a view widely repeated at European meetings. However, it is not correct. The DSM-III was already in print before the first study on an antipanic medication in pursuit of an FDA indication for panic disorder was ever started in the US.

The section on response to treatment ignores a large body of evidence that has contributed substantially to our understanding of several anxiety and phobic disorders. This is given short shrift, with sweeping statements like "SSRIs and other 'antidepressants' have broad-spectrum effects across several syndromes of anxious avoidance as well as mood disorders". However, some approved antidepressants (e.g. bupropion) have no anxiolytic, antipanic or broad-spectrum effects. The comment "The broad-spectrum cross-syndrome effect of medication resembles that of psychotherapies" is also not correct. Psychotherapy has no known clinically meaningful effect in obsessive–compulsive disorder (OCD), and the effect sizes for SSRIs across the spectrum of anxiety disorders are higher than the effect sizes for psychotherapies in the same disorders. This reader does not share the authors' enthusiasm that "OCD with phobic features... respond[s] *well* to exposure therapy" (my italics). At best, exposure therapy and medications are quite mediocre in their effects in the majority of OCD patients, providing about a 30% symptom relief overall in such patient populations. On the other hand, the time to meaningful therapeutic benefit with SSRIs is different across the disorders, the dose needed to separate the SSRI from placebo is different across the disorders, and the magnitude of benefit at all time points is different across the disorders even with the same SSRI.

Although there are clearly many parts of this review which are at variance with views held by most psychiatrists in the US, the authors do draw our attention to many neglected points of interest. For example, they criticize the decision by both ICD-10 and DSM-IV to require four symptoms in the definition of a panic attack. They are correct in stating that the demarcation between a panic attack (four or more symptoms) and a limited symptom attack (three or fewer symptoms) was an arbitrary, even whimsical, decision made in the absence of any empirical justification, "when in reality there is no clear divide". This demarcation line should be eliminated. However, such a move would pose major problems in the current classification of some anxiety and phobic disorders and would result in a major realignment of our current thinking that would present problems not only for ICD-10 and DSM-IV but also for Marks' own classification. Eventually this writer believes that point will be pivotal. However, it is unlikely that this classification debate will be resolved with scientific confidence until we better understand the genetics and proteomics of anxiety and phobic disorders. In the meantime Isaac Marks continues to play a valuable role as polemicist and gadfly by provoking debate and stimulating us to find more compelling evidence to reject or support the differing classification systems.

REFERENCES

1. Marks I.M. (1969) *Fears and Phobias*. Heinemann, London.
2. Marks I.M. (1987) *Fears, Phobias and Rituals*. Oxford University Press, New York.

1.4
The Role of Spontaneous, Unexpected Panic Attacks in the Diagnosis and Classification of Phobic Disorders

Giulio Perugi[1,2] and Cristina Toni[2]

The review by Marks and Mataix-Cols raises once again the theoretical issue whether or not a spontaneous, unexpected panic attack is essential for the diagnosis of agoraphobia. This question arises primarily because many agoraphobic patients seen in a clinical setting initially display spontaneous panic attacks. Others argue that the requirement for spontaneous panic attacks is stipulated primarily on the grounds of a specific biological theory

---

[1] *Department of Psychiatry, University of Pisa, Via Roma 67, 56100 Pisa, Italy*

[2] *Institute of Behavioural Science G. De Lisio, Carrara-Pisa, Italy*

of panic disorder–agoraphobia, which is unproven. However, arguments for retention of the requirement for a spontaneous panic attack centre on its usefulness in defining boundaries with other phobic disorders in a pharmacotherapeutic perspective.

The current US official position, since DSM-III, is that spontaneous panic attack represents the hallmark of panic disorder with agoraphobia (PDA) and plays a major role in the development of the polyphobic syndrome which these patients display during the course of their disorder. On the other hand, according to European tradition [1,2], neurotic personality and/or prodromal features such as mild depression or excessive worries precede agoraphobia. According to this point of view, agoraphobia is a complex syndrome which should not be considered as a subset of panic disorder.

Most clinical studies [3,4] support the view that panic attacks represent the first psychopathological manifestation of PDA and that anticipatory anxiety, hypochondriacal fears and phobic avoidance develop subsequently. The onset of PDA is often abrupt, giving the impression that a qualitative shift in emotional life has taken place. However, there are several lines of evidence suggesting that this impression may obscure sporadic subthreshold manifestations of anxiety in the development of these anxiety states. Research on prodromal symptoms [5] in patients with PDA has provided some empirical support for this viewpoint. Some of the prodromal features reported may be viewed as a result of comorbidity phenomena, but other aspects would seem to indicate a putative phobic–anxious life-lasting temperamental style [6].

The main problem in the study of the prodromes of PDA is the definition of the first panic attack. Many patients may suffer from sporadic and isolated minor attacks, which Sheehan and Sheehan [7] call "sub-panic attacks", which precede by many years the onset of the full-blown PDA clinical picture. Convergent data from epidemiological [8] and clinical studies [9] indicate the existence of a significant number of individuals with "infrequent panic". Although infrequent panic can be associated with avoidance, there are insufficient data to assess whether phobias are as common in this population as in disorder-level subjects. Examples in which limited-symptom attacks are associated with avoidance have been provided [10,11]. In these cases, patients report major fears concerning the possibility of their having limited-symptom, mostly somatic, attacks while away from home. Most of them do not recognize the anxious origin of these dysautonomic manifestations, and the identification of the precise onset of the illness is, therefore, not always easy, even for an experienced interviewer. In other cases, spontaneous full-blown panic attacks may be present in the early phases of PDA, but later may become less frequent or disappear and be replaced by situational attacks. These are some of the reasons why high rates of agoraphobia without panic attacks are reported in epidemiological studies, while a diagnosis of agoraphobia without a history of panic is rarely made in clinical practice.

We would agree with Marks and Mataix-Cols that the importance of a classification depends upon its purpose. From a pharmacotherapeutic perspective, the subtypification of panic attacks (unexpected, situationally bound and situationally predisposed) constitutes an essential key to the differentiation of PDA and related illness and social phobic behaviour from other phobic disorders. Unexpected panic attacks are not associated with situational triggers and are prototypical of PDA; situationally-bound panic attacks are exclusively associated with situational triggers and are prototypical of social and specific phobias. Situationally predisposed panic attacks are more likely to occur upon exposure to certain situational triggers; they tend to be associated with PDA but not exclusively. Some controversy may arise with regard to certain situational phobias (driving, flying, heights, bridges, tunnels, enclosed spaces). In these cases, the mode of onset is a key factor in differential diagnosis. Any situational phobia, of which the onset was due to an unexpected panic attack and regarding a situation which had never previously caused the subject any anxiety, should be viewed as a form of PDA even if the official definitions of agoraphobia (DSM-IV and ICD-10) exclude fears of single situations.

In medicine, in the absence of an established etiopathogenetic basis, treatment-oriented classifications have an unquestionable practical value. Pharmacotherapeutic observations have largely supported the essential role of unexpected, spontaneous panic attacks in the delineation of different phobic disorders. In fact, on the basis of the presence of spontaneous panic attacks, different phobic disorders often require different pharmacotherapeutic strategies. Antidepressants such as monoamine oxidase inhibitors (MAOIs) (phenelzine), tricyclics (imipramine, clomipramine) or selective serotonin reuptake inhibitors (SSRIs) (paroxetine, citalopram, sertraline) are mostly effective against spontaneous panic attacks, showing little activity against situational attacks. The principal goal of the pharmacological treatment of PDA is the complete remission of major and minor unexpected panic attacks, while the remission of agoraphobic behaviour is considered to be a secondary consequence of self-exposure. For these reasons, antidepressants have been successfully utilized in PDA, but often with disappointing results in the case of specific phobic disorders. For social phobia, only MAOIs (phenelzine) and SSRIs (fluoxetine, paroxetine, sertraline) have proved to be effective while tricyclics have not, and this effectiveness has been shown in a lower proportion of cases compared with PDA (50% versus 70%), which raises the issue of the existence of different subtypes of social anxiety [12].

REFERENCES

1. Tyrer P. (1986) Classification of anxiety disorders: a critique of DSM-III. *J. Affect. Disord.*, **11**: 99–107.
2. Roth M. (1988) Anxiety and anxiety disorders—general overview. In *Handbook of Anxiety*, vol. 1: *Biological, Clinical and Cultural Perspectives* (Eds M. Roth, G.D. Burrows, R. Noyes Jr), pp. 1–45. Elsevier, Amsterdam.
3. Breier A., Charney D.S., Heninger G.R. (1986) Agoraphobia with panic attacks: development, diagnostic stability, and course of illness. *Arch. Gen. Psychiatry*, **43**: 1029–1036.
4. Noyes R. (1988) The natural history of anxiety disorders. In *Handbook of Anxiety*, vol 1: *Biological, Clinical and Cultural Perspectives* (Eds M. Roth, G.D. Burrows, R. Noyes Jr), pp. 115–133. Elsevier, Amsterdam.
5. Fava G.A., Grandi S., Canestrari R. (1988) Prodromal symptoms in panic disorder with agoraphobia. *Am. J. Psychiatry*, **145**: 1564–1567.
6. Perugi G., Toni C., Benedetti A., Simonetti B., Simoncini M., Torti C., Musetti L., Akiskal H.S. (1998) Delineating a putative phobic–anxious temperament in 126 panic agoraphobic patients: toward a rapprochement of European and U.S. views. *J. Affect. Disord.*, **37**: 11–23.
7. Sheehan D.V., Sheehan K.H. (1982) The classification of phobic disorders. *Int. J. Psychiatr. Med.*, **12**: 243–266.
8. Vollrath M., Koch R., Angst J. (1990) The Zurich Study. IX. Panic disorder and sporadic panic: symptoms, diagnosis, prevalence, and overlap with depression. *Eur. Arch. Psychiatry Neurol. Sci.*, **239**: 221–230.
9. Katon W., Vitaliano P.P., Russo J., Jones M., Anderson K. (1987) Panic disorder: spectrum of severity and somatization. *J. Nerv. Ment. Dis.*, **175**: 12–19.
10. Klein D.F., Klein H.M. (1989) The nosology, genetics and theory of spontaneous panic and phobia. In *Psychopharmacology of Anxiety* (Ed. P.J. Tyrer), pp. 163–195. Oxford University Press, New York.
11. Weissman M.M., Merikangas K.R. (1986) The epidemiology of anxiety and panic disorders: an update. *J. Clin. Psychiatry*, **47**: 11–17.
12. Perugi G., Nassini S., Maremmani I., Madaro D., Toni C., Simonini E., Akiskal H.S. (2001) Putative clinical subtypes of social phobia: a factor-analytical study. *Acta Psychiatr. Scand.*, **103**: 1–9.

1.5
Anxiety and Phobia: Issues in Classification
George C. Curtis[1]

In their review Marks and Mataix-Cols use the term "phobia" in two ways. One needs to keep straight which usage is intended. For example, "Phobias can be triggered by almost anything" is true of irrational fears in general

---

[1] *Department of Psychiatry, Anxiety Disorders Program, University of Michigan Medical Center, 1500 East Medical Center Drive, Ann Arbor, Michigan 48103, USA*

but not of phobias in DSM/ICD usage. Many of the older lists of "phobias" with Greek prefixes were part of what we would now call obsessive–compulsive disorder.

The Greek prefixes did not predict much. Marks and Gelder [1] and Marks [2] led the way out of this blind alley. They showed that a four-category system comprising animal, social, agora-, and miscellaneous specific phobias predicted a number of things, including age of onset, gender ratio, comorbidity patterns, treatment response and perhaps some psychophysiological properties. This does not necessarily predict etiology, but does appear to tap into something meaningful. DSM/ICD adopted this system, with one change, which, however, may have been a step backward rather than forward.

Miscellaneous specific phobias was the residual category in the Marks system. Residual categories tend to be mixtures, since they contain the leftovers that one is uncertain what to do with. The age of onset data supported this, since only the miscellaneous specific phobia class had a flat distribution of ages of onset, i.e. they began at any and all ages. However, rather than refining the category, DSM enlarged it by combining it with animal phobias, thus making it more of a mixture than it already was. The new category was named simple phobia and, finally, specific phobia.

Some evidence suggests how the specific phobia category might be refined. As Marks points out in his paper, the blood–injury subtype of specific phobias is unique in its high association with vasovagal fainting and its high familiality. In most studies animal phobias have the earliest onset, the highest prevalence, the least comorbidity, the highest proportion of females, the best response to exposure therapy and some evidence of genetic predisposition [3]. Other disorders, such as panic disorder and post-traumatic stress disorder, may land in this category because of arbitrary truncation of their severity dimension. Marks notes that some agoraphobic fears follow uncued panics occurring in the to-be-feared situation. This was an old observation which DSM lost sight of, focusing exclusively on situations where escape would be difficult or embarrassing. A subgroup of so-called specific phobias also begin in this way [4], most being situations from the agoraphobic cluster, and could arguably be considered mild versions of panic disorder with agoraphobia. The distribution of their ages of onset resembles that of panic disorder with agoraphobia more than that of other specific phobias [5]. Also so-called specific phobias which begin with an actual fright or injury, such as height phobias after being injured by a fall or dog phobias after being attacked by a dog, are often accompanied by subdiagnostic features of post-traumatic stress disorder and perhaps should be so classified. In these disorders the age of onset is, of course, determined by the time of the trauma rather than the nature of the phobia.

Marks accepts the notion of uncued panics but maintains that the term "attack" adds nothing more. This should not be true, though arguably it may be, if one adheres to DSM usage. As Marks states, the term "panic" conventionally means sudden, intense fright. "Attack" originally meant sudden and apparently uncued. However, DSM now applies both terms to all intense frights whether cued or not and to all uncued attacks whether intense or not. Mild attacks receive the strange phrase "limited symptom panic attack". In reality not all attacks are panics, and not all panics are attacks. So-called "situationally bound panic attack" only reaches panic proportions if exposure to the feared situation is sudden and close. These considerations plus the fact that real panic attacks can be either frequent or very infrequent may have complicated the debate about whether "agoraphobia without panic disorder" (or panic attacks) is real. DSM describes the condition as fear of situations where one might "develop symptoms", which actually sound like low intensity anxiety attacks. Thus, agoraphobia without panic disorder may usually be triggered by low intensity "panic attacks" with perhaps infrequent real panic attacks.

Marks remains neutral on some key theoretical questions. One is whether cognition is primary to fear and avoidance. Neutrality is wise, because there are serious theories, all backed by evidence [6], for the primacy of cognition, the primacy of behaviour and the primacy of feeling. Another is whether each phobia has a separate etiology or whether there is a general predisposition for all. Some of the best genetic evidence suggests both to be true [3]. This may be distasteful for seekers of theoretical parsimony, but probably conforms better to reality.

REFERENCES

1. Marks I.M., Gelder M.G. (1966) Different ages of onset in varieties of phobia. *Am. J. Psychiatry*, **123**: 218–221.
2. Marks I.M. (1970) The classification of phobic disorders. *Br. J. Psychiatry*, **116**: 377–386.
3. Kendler K.S., Neale M.C., Kessler R.C., Heath A.C., Eaves L.J. (1992) The genetic epidemiology of phobias in women: the interrelationship of agoraphobia, social phobia, situational phobia, and simple phobia. *Arch. Gen. Psychiatry*, **49**: 273–281.
4. Himle J.A., Crystal D., Curtis G.C., Fluent T.E. (1991) Mode of onset of simple phobia subtypes: further evidence of heterogeneity. *Psychiatry Res.*, **36**: 37–43.
5. Himle J.A., McPhee K., Cameron O.G., Curtis G.C. (1989) Simple phobia: evidence for heterogeneity. *Psychiatry Res.*, **28**: 25–30.
6. LeDoux, J. (1996) *The Emotional Brain*. Simon & Schuster, New York.

1.6
Nosology of the Phobias: Clues from the Genome
Raymond R. Crowe[1]

Genetic studies provide a potentially informative tool for guiding classification efforts of psychiatric disorders. Monozygotic (MZ) twins share the same genome, whereas dizygotic (DZ) twins on average share half their genome and are thus genetically equivalent to ordinary siblings. If disorders A and B are each more concordant in MZ than in DZ twins, but neither one increases the occurrence of the other in MZ over DZ co-twins, the evidence supports their nosological separation. On the other hand, if each does increase the occurrence of the other in MZ over DZ co-twins, the two disorders share a common genetic diathesis, and, biologically at least, they are not completely distinct illnesses.

Fortunately, there are large epidemiological samples of twins to provide data on the major phobic syndromes in ICD-10 and DSM-IV: agoraphobia, social phobia, specific phobia of the animal and situational types, as well as blood and injury phobias [1,2]. The genetic variance can be partitioned into common and specific components. *Common* genetic factors are risk factors for developing any phobia, whereas *specific* genetic factors are unique to each type of phobia. Environmental variance can be partitioned in the same way. Thus, regardless of whether the transmission of a phobia is largely genetic or largely nongenetic, one can ask whether the predisposition is a general liability to develop any phobia or specific to individual phobic disorders. Since the variance components sum to 100%, common genetic and environmental components can be combined as common variance, and likewise with specific variance. By examining the proportion of the variance in transmission due to diagnosis-specific factors, we can see to what extent twin data support diagnostic boundaries around each phobia: 100% would indicate no overlap with other phobias and 0% no diagnostic boundary.

- *Agoraphobia.* For agoraphobia, diagnosis-specific factors accounted for 30% of the variance in female and 40% in male twins, providing weak evidence for a diagnostic boundary between agoraphobia and other phobias.
- *Social phobia.* In the case of social phobia, specific factors accounted for a somewhat greater proportion of the variance; 57% in female and 48% in male twins.

---

[1] *Department of Psychiatry, University of Iowa Carver College of Medicine, Iowa City, IA 52242-1000, USA*

- *Animal phobia.* Specific animal phobia had still stronger support for a diagnostic boundary; 59% of the variance in female twins and 64% in males was specific to animal phobia.
- *Situational phobia.* Diagnosis-specific factors accounted for 53% of the variance in female and 76% in male twins.
- *Blood and injury phobia.* Data on blood/injury phobia are only available from male twins and they indicate that 55% of the variance is due to specific factors.

These twin data support the DSM-IV classification of phobias to the extent that the etiology of all five is to some degree diagnosis-specific. The strongest evidence for syndrome specificity was found for the specific phobias, animal and situational; the support for agoraphobia was the weakest; social phobia and blood/injury phobia fell in between. Possibly, if generalized social phobia could have been looked at separately the evidence for specific etiological factors might have been stronger, because family data indicate that the familiality of social phobia is due largely to that subtype [3]. Yet diagnosis-specific factors did not approach 100% of the variance for any of the phobias, the highest being in the 50–75% range for specific phobias. Thus considerable room for syndromal overlap remains.

REFERENCES

1. Kendler K.S., Neale M.C., Kessler R.C., Heath A.C., Eaves L.J. (1992) The genetic epidemiology of phobias in women: the interrelationship of agoraphobia, social phobia, situational phobia, and simple phobia. *Arch. Gen. Psychiatry*, **49**: 273–281.
2. Kendler K.S., Jyers J., Prescott C.A., Neale M.C. (2001) The genetic epidemiology of irrational fears and phobias in men. *Arch. Gen. Psychiatry*, **58**: 257–265.
3. Stein M.B., Chartier M.J., Hazen A.L., Kozak M.V., Tancer M.E., Lander S., Furer P., Chubaty D., Walker, J.R. (1998) A direct-interview family study of generalized social phobia. *Am. J. Psychiatry*, **155**: 90–97.

1.7

Clusters, Comorbidity and Context in Classification of Phobic Disorders

Joshua D. Lipsitz[1]

Current DSM-IV and ICD-10 phobia classifications bear a striking resemblance to the categories proposed by Marks in 1970 [1]. The diagnoses of agoraphobia and social phobia have become generally accepted as valid

---

[1] *Anxiety Clinic, Unit 69, New York State Psychiatric Institute, 1051 Riverside Drive, New York, NY 10032, USA*

and are widely appreciated for their clinical utility. Both diagnostic categories have generated large independent bodies of research and have been the focus of specified treatment approaches. However, it is equally striking that the past three decades have generated relatively little in the way of progress toward further refinements in phobia classification.

Because the third phobia category, specific phobia, was created through subtraction, it was not surprising to find that specific phobias differed from one another along a variety of dimensions. These include some of those dimensions outlined by Marks and Mataix-Cols as a potential basis for taxonomy. Clinical features such as focus of fear, presence of unexpected panic attacks and distinct physiological response have been taken as evidence of phobia heterogeneity in some studies [2]. However, other studies have failed to replicate findings of clinical difference [3].

Several limitations may be responsible for a lack of progress in refining the residual category of specific phobia. One problem is that research has focused on phobia heterogeneity but not on the extent to which phobias within each proposed subcategory cluster. To show that new diagnostic categories are valid, it is not sufficient to show that phobias in one category differ from those in another category. It must also be the case that different phobias within the same category are more similar to each other along the same dimensions. This type of analysis would require very large samples with a range of representative phobias from each proposed category. Instead, most studies have attempted to draw conclusions from a single representative group (e.g. spider phobia for animal category) as contrasted with another representative group.

In addition, most studies to date have failed to control for the impact of comorbidity. Clinical samples comprised of patients seeking treatment for a specific type of phobia may also have a variety of other phobias [4] as well as other comorbid anxiety disorders [5] such as panic disorder. These may quietly influence observed clinical features (e.g. presence of panic attacks) attributed to specific phobias in these samples. However, since relatively few patients with pure (non-comorbid) specific phobia seek treatment, it is challenging to obtain pure samples of sufficient size for study.

Finally, studies of specific phobia have taken observations at face value and do not consider the role that external context might play in observed patterns. While all medical and psychological disorders occur within an external context, phobias, like allergies, are entirely defined by their context. A large majority of phobias are direct responses to an external object or situation. However, even for those phobias in which the focus of fear is internal (e.g. fear of vomiting, choking or falling), it is typically through the external context that the fear becomes relevant and clinically meaningful (e.g. eating a certain type of food or walking on an icy pavement). As such, phobias are only partially a function of the individual and his or her symptoms. Equally important to diagnosis, impairment and treatment seeking are incidental characteristics of the external context.

Consider, for example, the interpretation of observed differences in age of onset across phobias [6]. Marks and Mataix-Cols point out, for example, that fear of falling (space phobia) has onset in advanced years. They present this as a feature that distinguishes this phobia from others. However, it is an open question whether this late age of onset is intrinsic and informative about the phobic reaction or whether it is a function of external factors in the individual's context (e.g. increased potential for injury as one gets older, if a fall takes place). Social phobia of dating typically precedes a social phobia of speaking up at parent–teacher meetings, but we would not see this incidental sequence as evidence that the two fears reflect distinct syndromes. Similarly, Antony et al. [3] question the implications of later age of onset of situational fears in a sample of individuals with driving phobias: since most people do not have an opportunity to drive prior to 16 or 17, this "feature" is incidental to the phobia.

Observed differences in gender distribution across phobias may also be attributable to context. The finding of a roughly even gender distribution for height phobias [7] appears to distinguish this phobia from other specific phobias in which distribution is skewed toward female gender. However, it is possible that height phobias are reported with high frequency in men because cultural norms demand that men experience much higher levels of exposure to heights.

Finally, phobia classification efforts to date may have been overly ambitious. The previous, more deliberate model of identifying a single prominent phobic syndrome (such as social phobia) and keeping the remaining phobias in a residual status for the time being has been abandoned. Comprehensive subtype systems have been advanced and evaluated in an all-or-nothing approach to categorize nearly all of the remaining common phobias. Unfortunately, empirical research is not yet sufficient to inform a comprehensive classification of specific phobias.

REFERENCES

1. Marks I. (1970) The classification of phobic disorders. *Br. J. Psychiatry*, **116**: 377–386.
2. Craske M.G., Zarate R., Burton T., Barlow D.H. (1998) The boundary between simple phobia and agoraphobia: a survey of clinical and nonclinical samples. In *DSM-IV Sourcebook*, vol. 4 (Eds T.A. Widiger, A.J. Frances, H.A. Pincus, R. Ross, M.B. First, W. Davis, M. Kline), pp. 217–244. American Psychiatric Association, Washington, DC.
3. Antony M., Brown T.A., Barlow D.H. (1997) Heterogeneity among specific phobia types in DSM-IV. *Behav. Res. Ther.*, **35**: 1089–1100.

4. Curtis G.C., Magee W.J., Eaton W.W., Wittchen H.U., Kessler R.C. (1998) Specific fears and phobias: epidemiology and classification. *Br. J. Psychiatry*, **173**: 212–217.
5. Magee W.J., Eaton W.W., Wittchen H.U., McGonagle K.A., Kessler R.C. (1996) Agoraphobia, simple phobia, and social phobia in the National Comorbidity Survey. *Arch. Gen. Psychiatry*, **53**: 159–168.
6. Himle J.A., McPhee K., Cameron O.G., Curtis G.C. (1989) Simple phobia: evidence for heterogeneity. *Psychiatry Res.*, **28**: 25–30.
7. Bourdon K.H., Boyd J.H., Rae D.S., Burns B.J., Thompson J.W., Locke B.Z. (1988) Gender differences in phobias: results of the ECA community study. *J. Anxiety Disord.*, **2**: 227–241.

1.8
Comorbidity in Social Phobia: Nosological Implications
Constantin R. Soldatos and Thomas J. Paparrigopoulos[1]

The introduction of operational diagnostic criteria for psychiatric disorders has stimulated interest in comorbidity, which is generally defined as the co-occurrence of two or more disorders over a specified period of time. The study of comorbidity has important implications for both clinical research and practice. It may contribute to the delineation of different disorders and, therefore, validate proposed diagnostic categories. Moreover, given that comorbidity of psychiatric disorders is a very frequent occurrence, confounding symptoms may frequently intrude and blur a prototypal clinical picture. Consequently, reference to comorbidity issues is deemed necessary for an adequate description and improved understanding of the phenomenology of a specific disorder. This applies in particular to anxiety disorders, with as many as 50% of patients having a specific anxiety disorder which may meet diagnostic criteria for another anxiety disorder [1].

Based on clinical studies as well as on general population surveys, social phobia is strongly associated with other anxiety disorders (about 50%), affective disorders (20%) and substance abuse (15%). On average, 80% of patients with social phobia meet diagnostic criteria for another lifetime condition, which is indicative that comorbidity tends to be the rule rather than the exception [2,3]. According to the US National Comorbidity Survey [4], the vast majority of individuals with any phobia in general (83.4%), and primary social phobia specifically (81%), meet the criteria for at least one other lifetime DSM-III-R diagnosed psychiatric disorder. In most cases (76.8%), social phobia precedes the comorbid disorder [3]. In the presence of

---

[1] *University Mental Health Research Institute, Eginition Hospital, 72 Vasilissis Sophias Avenue, Athens GR-11528, Greece*

the diagnosis of social phobia, the odds ratio for other disorders are found to be 7.75 for simple phobia, 7.06 for agoraphobia, 4.83 for panic disorder, 3.77 for generalized anxiety disorder, 3.69 for major depression, 3.15 for dysthymia, 2.69 for post-traumatic stress disorder and 2.01 for substance abuse [4].

Generalized anxiety disorder (GAD) and social phobia frequently co-occur in clinical samples [1] as well as in the general population [4]. It has been reported that GAD may be the most common additional diagnosis among patients with social phobia in clinical populations; conversely, social phobia is most frequently diagnosed in patients with GAD (up to 59% of the cases) [1]. Comorbid social phobia and GAD may merely indicate a shortcoming of our taxonomic systems. In this context, it has been suggested that the "mixed" social phobia/GAD group may represent a distinct subgroup of individuals who are characterized by a fear of negative evaluation as well as chronic worry, both resulting in a greater degree of functional impairment [5].

As far as the comorbidity of social phobia and panic disorder is concerned, it has been reported to be as high as 50% [3]. These two purportedly distinct conditions present with quite similar and overlapping symptoms and at times they are difficult to distinguish on clinical grounds, e.g. when a person experiences a panic attack while giving a speech and afterwards develops social phobia. The differentiation commonly offered by clinicians is that, in contrast to what a patient with social phobia presents, a patient with panic disorder does not fear scrutiny itself but the physical sensations associated with a feeling of being in danger and trapped, yet this distinction is not always easy to make.

Finally, attention should be given to the demarcation of the boundaries of social phobia with avoidant personality disorder and with temperamental make-ups such as shyness. In studies comparing avoidant personality disorder with non-focused social phobia (generalized social phobia), comorbidity rates vary from approximately 25% up to 89%; thus, the ability to diagnose one disorder in the absence of the other is questioned [6]. Comparison of the characteristics of avoidant personality disorder and generalized social phobia has yielded few qualitative differences, although some investigators have shown that avoidant personality disorder may represent a more severe form of generalized social phobia with respect to intensity of symptoms, fear of negative evaluation, anxiety, avoidance and depression; others have concluded that the co-occurrence of generalized social phobia and avoidant personality disorder pertains to persons with the most severe symptoms of social phobia and poorest functioning [7]. Furthermore, personality dimensions such as shyness have been found to be strongly associated with both avoidant personality disorder and generalized social phobia, and there is evidence that individuals suffering from phobicness in social settings also exhibit fears and avoidance across a variety of non-social domains. Indeed, research supports the position that generalized social phobia and avoidant personality disorder belong to a nosological continuum that is artificially divided between axes II and I of the DSM classification system.

In conclusion, based on the above comorbidity features of social phobia, which are based on clinical and epidemiological studies, future refinement of criteria pertaining to the diagnosis of social phobia should be seriously considered.

REFERENCES

1. Sanderson W.C., Di Nardo P.A., Rapee R.M., Barlow D.H. (1990) Syndrome comorbidity in patients diagnosed with a DSM-III-R anxiety disorder. *J. Abnorm. Psychol.*, **99**: 308–312.
2. Merikangas K.R., Angst J. (1995) Comorbidity and social phobia: evidence from clinical, epidemiologic, and genetic studies. *Eur. Arch. Psychiatry Clin. Neurosci.*, **244**: 297–303.
3. Schneier F.R., Johnson J., Hornig C.D., Liebowitz M.R., Weissman M.M. (1992) Social phobia: comorbidity and morbidity in an epidemiological sample. *Arch. Gen. Psychiatry*, **49**: 282–288.
4. Magee W.J., Eaton W.W., Wittchen H.U., McGonagle K.A., Kessler R.C. (1996) Agoraphobia, simple phobia, and social phobia in the National Comorbidity Survey. *Arch. Gen. Psychiatry*, **53**: 159–168.
5. Mennin D.S., Heimberg R.G., Jack M.S. (2000) Comorbid generalized anxiety disorder in primary social phobia: symptom severity, functional impairment, and treatment response. *J. Anxiety Disord.*, **14**: 325–343.
6. Schneier F.R., Spitzer R.L., Gibbon M., Fyer A.J., Liebowitz M.R. (1991) The relationship of social phobia subtypes and avoidant personality disorder. *Compr. Psychiatry*, **32**: 496–502.
7. Holt C.S., Heimberg R.G., Hope D.A. (1992) Avoidant personality disorder and the generalized subtype of social phobia. *J. Abnorm. Psychol.*, **101**: 318–325.

1.9
Giving Credit to "Neglected" or "Minor" Disorders
Charles Pull[1] and Caroline Pull[2]

The masterly overview by Isaak Marks and David Mataix-Cols provides a comprehensive and useful perspective on the diagnosis and classification of

---

[1] *Department of Neurosciences, Centre Hospitalier de Luxembourg, 1210 Luxembourg*

[2] *Association Luxembourg Alzheimer, 45, rue Nicolas Hein, B.P. 5021, Luxembourg*

phobias and on their history. It is impressive to look back on the multitude of descriptions, concepts and classifications of the different phobias that were in use up to a recent past and to see that the two main current classifications of mental disorders, ICD-10 and DSM-IV-TR, adopt positions that are very similar in this field. The current conceptualization of the diagnosis and classification of the phobias is based upon an atheoretical approach. The diagnostic process uses explicit descriptive criteria and algorithms for defining each disorder and relies on structured interview procedures for making diagnoses. The approach has led to a tremendous advance in the diagnostic reliability of the phobias and has had a major impact on the quality as well as on the amount of research that has been done on phobic disorders in the last decades.

In the past, the phobias were either "neglected" or considered as "minor" disorders. The results of recent research in the field have highlighted the prevalence of phobias and the severity of the distress that is frequently associated with these disorders, as well as the impact on quality of life, interference with the person's normal routine, occupational functioning, social activities and relationships. This has led to a new and more adequate appreciation of the phobias in general and of social phobia in particular. In a recent study [1] we compared patients with social phobia to normal controls on measures of avoidance, using the Liebowitz Social Anxiety Scale [2], assertiveness, using the Schedule for Assessing Assertive Behavior developed by Rathus [3], quality of life, using the Quality of Life Rating Scale or WHO-QoL [4], and disability, using the Disability Assessment Schedule, version II or WHO-DAS-II [5]. As was to be expected—Marks and Mataix-Cols emphasize the fact that avoidance is part of the definition of a phobia—patients with a diagnosis of social phobia scored significantly higher on avoidance (37.8 versus 8.7) than normal controls. Patients had significantly lower global scores on assertive behaviour (-25.9 versus $+21.3$), a result that is in line with the statement by Marks and Mataix-Cols that lack of self-assertion is common even in otherwise well-adjusted people. Quality of life was significantly worse in patients according to global assessment as well as for each of the specific domains that are assessed in the WHO-QoL, and patients with social phobia scored significantly higher in each one of the domains of disablement that are assessed in the WHO-DAS-II. These results fully support the statements by Marks and Mataix-Cols on the consequences of social phobia on the sufferers' lives.

The current classification of phobias should not be considered as final. There are some differences between ICD-10 and DSM-IV that need to be clarified through additional research. As an example, social phobia may be very focal, or may involve several situations. When the sufferer's fears are related to most social situations, DSM-IV-TR recommends using the specifier "generalized". According to DSM-IV-TR, individuals with social phobia, generalized, usually fear both public performance situations and social interactional situations, and may be more likely to manifest deficits in social skills and to have severe social and work impairment. This distinction is not made in ICD-10. A related issue concerns the relation between the generalized type of social phobia (coded on axis I) and avoidant (DSM-IV-TR) (coded on axis II) or anxious personality disorder (ICD-10). As stated by Marks and Mataix-Cols, "extreme shyness in adults can be a continuation of marked childhood shyness that never cleared up, whereas most focal social phobias start in young adult life and extreme shyness or diffuse social phobia is thus also called avoidant (DSM-IV-TR) or anxious personality disorder (ICD-10)". According to DSM-IV-TR, the additional diagnosis of avoidant personality disorder should be considered when the fears include most social situations. In our own work [1], we assessed patients with a primary diagnosis of social phobia using a semi-structured interview, the International Personality Disorders Examination [6] and found that a majority of our probands had an anxious (73%) or avoidant (76%) personality disorder in addition to social phobia. Patients with a diagnosis of social phobia and avoidant personality disorder (DSM-IV-TR) had significantly higher global scores on anxiety (43.2 versus 33.7) and avoidance (40.8 versus 28.7) on the Liebowitz Social Anxiety Scale [2] than patients without this diagnosis. Significantly higher scores on anxious (43.3 versus 34.4) and avoidance (39.9 versus 32.0) items were also found in patients with a diagnosis of anxious personality disorder (ICD-10). The results support the position adopted in DSM-IV-TR for differentiating between social phobia and "generalized" social phobia and for differentiating between social phobia with and without an additional diagnosis of avoidant or anxious personality disorder.

REFERENCES

1. Pull C. (2002) Lebensqualität, Behinderung und Selbstsicherheit bei Patienten mit sozialer Angststörung. Diplomarbeit an der naturwissenschaftlichen Fakultät der Leopold-Franzens-Universität Innsbruck.
2. Liebowitz M., Gorman J., Fyer A., Klein D. (1985) Social phobia: review of a neglected anxiety disorder. *Arch. Gen. Psychiatry*, **42**: 729–736.
3. Rathus S. (1973) A 30-item schedule for assessing assertive behavior. *Behav. Ther.*, **4**: 398–406.
4. World Health Organization (1999) *A Rating Scale for Assessing Quality of Life (WHO-QoL)*. World Health Organization, Geneva.
5. World Health Organization (1999) *Disability Assessment Schedule, version II (WHO-DAS-II)*. World Health Organization, Geneva.
6. Loranger A., Sartorius N., Andreoli A., Berger P., Buchheim P., Channabasvanna S., Coid B., Dahl A., Diekstra R., Ferguson B. et al. (1994) The International Personality Disorder Examination. *Arch. Gen. Psychiatry*, **52**: 230–237.

1.10
A Cognitive Approach to Phobias
Jean-Pierre Lépine and Catherine Musa[1]

Marks and Mataix-Cols describe the current problems in classifying phobias as well as the potential bases of their taxonomy. It is important to underline that Isaac Marks' work in this field has been of major historical significance. It permitted the distinction of phobias within the anxiety disorders and the distinction of different phobic syndromes according to their phenomenological components as well as their age of onset. However, this classification has always been based on the behavioural symptoms component and above all on the presence or absence of avoidance. In this paper Marks and Mataix-Cols broaden their perspective and suggest the inclusion in the classification of phobias not only of the so-called classical phobic syndromes but also of other related anxiety syndromes with mostly somatic concerns such as hypochondriasis and, significantly, aversions.

A subject of current debate may remain whether or not such a taxonomy can ignore the cognitive perspective. Indeed, according to this view, biases in information processing are a central feature of phobias. These biases seem to be content specific, i.e. related to the particular concerns of each phobic disorder. Furthermore, different patterns of information processing biases are seen according to the specific phobic disorder in question.

Thus, for example, most studies confirm the existence of an attentional bias in terms of hypervigilance to specific panic- and agoraphobia-related words in agoraphobia with panic disorder (e.g. [1]). Moreover, agoraphobic and panic disorder patients seem particularly vigilant to their own bodily sensations. Ehlers and Bruher [2] find that subjects with panic disorder count their heartbeat with far more precision than specific phobia patients or normal controls. According to a recent review by Coles and Heimberg [3], patients with agoraphobia and/or panic disorder also show evidence of an explicit memory bias in terms of better retrieval of specific threatening information. This is particularly interesting given that no such bias is evident in, for example, generalized anxiety disorder. Interpretation biases have also been found in panic disorder and agoraphobia, and probably contribute to the persistence of this disorder. Thus, for example, McNally and Foa [4] find that agoraphobic patients show a tendency to misinterpret relevant internal and external cues. Baptista *et al.* [5] and Harvey *et al.* [6] confirmed these findings.

---

[1] *Department of Psychiatry, Fernand Widal Hospital, Denis Diderot University, Paris, France*

Interpretation biases may also play an important role in social phobia. Social phobics show a tendency to underestimate their own performances and behaviours. Stopa and Clark [7] showed, for example, that social phobic patients underestimate their performance compared to observers' evaluations. This was not true of their "mixed" anxiety disorders control group. In a more recent study [8] these authors found that patients with social phobia also interpret ambiguous social situations in a more negative fashion than anxious control and normal subjects.

The existence of preferential processing of social-threat-related words in social phobia has been confirmed in several studies. Hope et al. [9] and Mattia et al. [10] found that social phobic patients exhibit interference for social-threat but not physical-threat words in the Stroop task. Recently, Spector et al. [11], using the Stroop test, confirmed the existence of an attentional bias in social phobia for specific social-phobia-related words of two types: negative evaluation words (e.g. criticism) and words concerning anxiety symptoms noticeable to others (e.g. blushing). Using the dot probe task, Musa et al. [12] found vigilance to threatening words in social phobia and confirmed that the attentional bias is specific to social-threat-related words. They also found that the presence of an additional diagnosis of depression abolished the attentional bias, suggesting that the latter is characteristic of social phobia but not depression. However, when using pictures of faces, Chen et al. [13] showed that social phobics preferentially process objects as opposed to faces (i.e. they avoid the faces) in the dot probe task. Clark and McManus [14] suggest that these findings could reflect a specific pattern of information processing in social phobia: a reduction of processing of external cues (such as faces) and increased self-focused attention (rumination about negative judgement or visibility of anxiety symptoms).

Concerning specific phobias, in a study of spider phobics, Watts et al. [15] found interference for spider-related words in the Stroop test. Öhman and Soares [16] also found that snake and spider phobics exhibit unconscious, involuntary processing of pictorial cues depicting the feared animal, as indexed by physiological and self-report measures of fear. Presented with masked and unmasked briefly presented slides of spiders, snakes, mushrooms and flowers, subjects exhibit fear only to slides of their phobic object whether it is masked (subliminal) or unmasked (unmasked). However, Thorpe and Salkovskis [17], using the Stroop test in a masked and unmasked condition, showed an interference effect for spider-related words, but only in the unmasked condition, suggesting strategic but not automatic attentional biases in this disorder. In a later experiment, Thorpe and Salkovskis [18] failed to find evidence of a recall or recognition bias in subjects with spider phobia. Similarly, Sawchuk et al. [19] failed to find a recognition memory bias for relevant phobic pictures in a sample of spider phobics, blood–injection–injury phobics and normal controls. Furthermore, no discrimination bias was found for relevant phobic pictures in a discrimination task. Thus, although there seems to be evidence of an attentional bias for relevant phobic information, no such bias is evident in research on explicit memory in specific phobias. In the same way, no interpretation bias has been found to date in specific phobias.

Taking into account that Marks and Mataix-Cols include hypochondriasis, dysmorphophobia, post-traumatic stress disorder (PTSD) and aversions in their classification of phobias, noting that these disorders also present the symptom of anxious avoidance, it would be interesting to explore information processing in these disorders in order to observe possible similarities or differences with other phobic disorders.

Indeed, for example, several studies of information processing in PTSD patients have been carried out. They show existence of a specific attentional bias for trauma-related words. Bryant and Harvey [20], for example, in a study of car accident survivors, found an attentional bias specific to accident-related words. Also, Vrana *et al.* [21] found evidence of an explicit memory bias for trauma-related words in Vietnam veterans with PTSD. Amir *et al.* [22] found an implicit memory bias in Vietnam veterans with PTSD for specific Vietnam-war-related words.

It should also be noted that Marks and Mataix-Cols do not include obsessive–compulsive disorder (OCD) in their classification of phobias, even though this disorder shares many behavioural (avoidance, for example) and cognitive symptoms with phobias. In a cognitive perspective, it can be mentioned that studies of attention find hypervigilance to specific threat words in OCD subjects (e.g. [23]) and a memory bias in terms of better retrieval of threat material (e.g. [24]).

To conclude, a behavioural perspective remains of essential importance in the definition of a taxonomy of phobic disorders, as well as in the comprehension and treatment of these subtypes of anxiety disorders. Nonetheless, the cognitive approach to phobias, which stresses the importance of information processing biases in these disorders, is currently extending the knowledge of the underlying mechanisms associated with these syndromes. We think, therefore, that a combined perspective should be taken into account when defining a future taxonomy of anxiety disorders. However, although research studies have confirmed the existence of information processing biases as well as a relative specificity in their modalities in the different anxiety and phobic disorders, further research is still needed to investigate the different patterns of these mechanisms as well as their impact on the genesis and persistence of phobias.

REFERENCES

1. McNally R.J., Reiman B.C., Kim E. (1990) Selective processing of threat cues in panic disorder. *Behav. Res. Ther.*, **28**: 407–412.
2. Ehlers A., Bruer P. (1992) Increased cardiac awareness in panic disorder. *J. Abnorm. Psychol.*, **101**: 371–382.
3. Coles M.E., Heimberg R.G. (2002) Memory biases in the anxiety disorders: current status. *Clin. Psychol. Rev.*, **22**: 587–627.
4. McNally R.J., Foa E.B. (1987) Cognition and agoraphobia: bias in the interpretation of threat. *Cogn. Ther. Res.*, **11**: 567–581.
5. Baptista A., Figuiera M.L., Lima M.L., Matos F. (1990) Bias in judgement in panic disorder patients. *Acta Psiqiatr. Portug.*, **36**: 25–35.
6. Harvey J.M., Richards J.C., Dziadosz T., Swindell A. (1993) Misinterpretation of ambiguous stimuli in panic disorder. *Cogn. Ther. Res.*, **17**: 235–248.
7. Stopa L., Clark D.M. (1993) Cognitive processes in social phobia. *Behav. Res. Ther.*, **31**: 255–267.
8. Stopa L., Clark D.M. (2000) Social phobia and interpretation of social events. *Behav. Res. Ther.*, **38**: 273–283.
9. Hope D.A., Rappee R.M., Heimberg R.G., Dombeck M.J. (1990) Representations of the self in social phobia: vulnerability to social threat. *Cogn. Ther. Res.*, **14**: 177–189.
10. Mattia J.I., Heimberg R.G., Hope D.A. (1993) The revised Stroop color-naming task in social phobics. *Behav. Res. Ther.*, **31**: 305–313.
11. Spector I.P., Pecknold J.C., Libman E. (2002) Selective attentional bias related to the noticeability aspect of anxiety symptoms in generalized social phobia. *J. Anxiety Disord.*, **17**: 517–531.
12. Musa Z.C., Lépine J.-P., Clark D.M., Mansell W., Ehlers A. (2003) Selective attention in social phobia and the moderating effect of a concurrent depressive disorder. *Behav. Res. Ther.*, **41**: 1043–1054.
13. Chen Y.P., Ehlers A., Clark D.M., Mansell W. (2002) Patients with generalized social phobia direct their attention away from faces. *Behav. Res. Ther.*, **40**: 677–687.
14. Clark D.M., McManus F. (2002) Information processing in social phobia. *Biol. Psychiatry*, **51**: 92–100.
15. Watts F.N., McKenna F.P., Sharrock R., Trezise L. (1986) Colour naming of phobia related words. *Br. J. Psychol.*, **77**: 97–108.
16. Öhman A., Soares J.J.F. (1994) Unconscious anxiety: phobic responses to masked stimuli. *J. Abnorm. Psychol.*, **103**: 231–240.
17. Thorpe S.J., Salkovskis P.M. (1997) Information processing in spider phobics: the Stroop colour naming task may indicate strategic but not automatic attentional bias. *Behav. Res. Ther.*, **35**: 131–144.
18. Thorpe S.J., Salkovskis P.M. (2000) Recall and recognition memory for spider information. *J. Anxiety Disord.*, **14**: 359–375.
19. Sawchuk C.N., Meunier S.A., Lohr J.M., Westendorf D.H. (2002) Fear, disgust, and information processing in specific phobia application of signal detection theory. *J. Anxiety Disord.*, **16**: 495–510.
20. Bryant R.A., Harvey A.G. (1995) Processing threatening information in posttraumatic stress disorder. *J. Abnorm. Psychol.*, **104**: 537–541.
21. Vrana S.R., Roodman A., Beckham J.C. (1995) Selective processing of trauma relevant words in post-traumatic stress disorder. *J. Anxiety Disord.*, **9**: 515–530.

22. Amir N., McNally R.J., Weigartz P.D. (1996) Implicit memory bias for threat in post-traumatic stress disorder. *Cogn. Ther. Res.*, **20**: 625–636.
23. Tata P.R., Leibowitz J.A., Prunty M.J., Cameron M., Pickering A.D. (1996) Attentional bias in obsessional compulsive disorder. *Behav. Res. Ther.*, **34**: 53–60.
24. Randomsky A.S., Rachman S. (1999) Memory bias in obsessive–compulsive disorder (OCD). *Behav. Res. Ther.*, **37**: 605–618.

1.11
Diagnosis and Classification of Phobias and Other Anxiety Disorders: Quite Different Categories or Just One Dimension?

Miguel R. Jorge[1]

Phobias achieved a separate diagnostic status in psychiatric classifications soon after the Second World War, probably because of their frequent occurrence in soldiers at the battlefront. One of the main questions regarding their classification is related to a major issue among nosologists nowadays, at least for some classes of mental disorders such as anxiety disorders: are they better represented by diagnostic categories or dimensions?

Costello [1] pointed out that research on symptoms may be more fruitful than research on categories or syndromes because of: (a) the questionable validity of psychiatric diagnostic systems; (b) the requirement to assess large number of different types of symptoms rather than adequately measure individual items; (c) the uncertainty about whether there is a true cut off between a psychiatric syndrome and normality; and (d) symptomatological overlap between diagnostic groups. In contrast, Mojtabai and Rieder [2] found little evidence in support of the thesis that: (a) symptoms have higher reliability and validity compared to diagnostic categories; (b) underlying pathological mechanisms are symptom specific; and (c) elucidation of the process of symptom development will lead to the discovery of the causes of syndromes.

Ten years before the publication of the DSM-III and the boom of neuroscience research, Robins and Guze [3] proposed five phases for establishing diagnostic validity in psychiatric diagnosis: clinical description, laboratory studies, delimitation from other disorders, follow-up study, and family study. Until the causes of mental illnesses are identified, measuring psychopathology probably will require a combination of a categorical and a dimensional approach [4]. As Marks and Mataix-Cols

---

[1] *Department of Psychiatry, Federal University of São Paulo, Rua Antonio Felício 85, 04530-060 São Paulo, Brazil*

point out, "certain quantitative changes along dimensions can also mean qualitative categorical changes. Dimensional and categorical classes need not be mutually exclusive."

Evidence has been accumulated in the last 20 years showing that prototypical mental disorders such as major depressive disorders, anxiety disorders, schizophrenia and bipolar disorders seem to merge imperceptibly into one another and into normality [5]. However, it is somewhat unlikely that the next revision of psychiatric classification systems such as the DSM-V will turn from a categorical to a dimensional approach, since "it is probably significant that most of the advocates of dimensional representation are not practicing clinicians but are primarily theoreticians" [6].

Even considering the categorical classification adopted by both ICD-10 and DSM-IV-TR, Marks and Mataix-Cols offer a classification of phobias that roughly supports the idea of a unique dimension for anxiety disorders and also include some other disorders (such as panic, depression and anorexia nervosa) which are often associated with phobias. In a merge to normality states, Marks and Mataix-Cols propose a new category of phobia-like syndromes not called phobias (jointly with obsessive–compulsive disorder, post-traumatic stress disorder, somatoform disorders and avoidant personality disorder) that they call touch and sound aversions.

In conclusion, the classification of anxiety disorders and the relation phobias have to other mental disorders are issues that will benefit much from etiologic and other diagnostic validity studies under way.

REFERENCES

1. Costello C.G. (1992) Research on symptoms versus research on syndromes: argument in favour of allocating more time to the study of symptoms. *Br. J. Psychiatry*, **160**: 304–309.
2. Mojtabai R., Rieder R.O. (1998) Limitations to the symptom-oriented approach to psychiatric research. *Br. J. Psychiatry*, **173**: 198–202.
3. Robins E., Guze S.B. (1970) Establishment of diagnostic validity in psychiatric illness: its application to schizophrenia. *Am. J. Psychiatry*, **126**: 983–987.
4. Maser J.D., Patterson T. (2002) Spectrum and nosology: implications for DSM-V. *Psychiatr. Clin. North Am.*, **25**: 855–885.
5. Kendler K.S., Gardner C.O. (1998) Boundaries of major depression: an evaluation of DSM-IV criteria. *Am. J. Psychiatry*, **155**: 172–177.
6. Rousanville B.J., Alarcón R.D., Andrews G., Jackson J.S., Kendell R.E., Kendler K. (2002) Basic nomenclature issues for DSM-V. In *A Research Agenda for DSM-V* (Eds D.J. Kupfer, M.B. First, D.A. Regier), p. 13. American Psychiatric Association, Washington, DC.

CHAPTER

2

Epidemiology of Phobias: A Review

Gavin Andrews

*Clinical Research Unit for Anxiety and Depression,
School of Psychiatry,
University of New South Wales at St. Vincent's Hospital, 299 Forbes St.,
Darlinghurst, NSW 2010, Australia*

INTRODUCTION

An ambitious corporate lawyer consults you. He says that he has always had a fear of confined spaces and avoids travelling in lifts or elevators because they make him too anxious. "I know it is silly, but I fear that if it stops between floors there will be no air and I will suffocate before I'm rescued." His firm has offices on the 12th floor of a high rise building and he uses the stairs. "It must be good for my health," he says. The firm is relocating to the 37th floor of a new security building in which the stairwell is locked and access to their floor is only by elevator. He asks for help but when he learns that treatment will involve confronting his fears in a planned and graded fashion he never returns. You later learn that he has taken a position in a suburban practice and you wonder how a fear of something not intrinsically dangerous could be so intense that it caused a man to halve his income and give up his ambition. Then you realize that the fear is of suffocating in the lift, not of travelling in the lift.

A woman is brought by her daughter because she is afraid to leave home on her own. She explains that many years ago she had a number of severe panic attacks during which she thought she would collapse and die. She developed a fear of panic and resolved this fear by staying at home where she could get help, and only travelled with a trusted adult who could summon help should a panic occur. It is some years since a severe panic occurred but she is reluctant to test her ability to cope away from help. We explain that she could learn to control her panics and master her fears. She says that she now knows that people do not die from panic attacks and can

---

Phobias. Edited by Mario Maj, Hagop S. Akiskal, Juan José López-Ibor and Ahmed Okasha.
©2004 John Wiley & Sons Ltd: ISBN 0-470-85833-8

recover from agoraphobia but declines treatment, despite her unhappiness with her dependent lifestyle. The risk of challenging her fear is too great; she worries that she might be the exception who died from panic.

A young man in his first year at college consults because of his fear of embarrassing himself in situations where others could notice. He avoids any social situation and now is avoiding lectures and seminars. He thinks he will have to stop his studies. Asked what he might do, he replies that he has a night job stacking supermarket shelves where he works alone and that he could do this full time: "I can get to and from work in the dark, and I'd work alone so no one would see that I was anxious and think I was weird." He explains that he has taken medication and, while that helps, he still worries that people will notice how nervous he is. You explain that he could learn to confront the fears of negative evaluation and master the feared situations, learning that few noticed him, let alone bothered to judge him. He agrees to treatment but does not keep the next appointment. A year later you discover that he stopped his studies and is working in menial night jobs. Apart from his family he is socially isolated. You marvel that the prospect that others might think negatively about you can be so threatening that all life's opportunities are forgone.

Mental disorders are identified by recognizable sets of symptoms and behaviours associated with distress, and interference with personal functioning. As such, they place a limit on the ability of the individual to function adaptively. The lawyer, the mother and the student all gave up significant life goals because of their fears, despite recognizing that the fears were excessive and despite knowing that they could be treated. They overestimated both probability and cost of the fears, the probability of a negative outcome should they enter the feared situation and the cost of their reaction in that situation. This review is about the epidemiology of phobias, defined as irrational fears of situations that are not intrinsically dangerous, accompanied by anticipatory anxiety about the prospect of encountering the situation, fear of specific consequences should they be in the situation and, most of all, avoidance of the situations. In the classifications panic disorder is often classified with agoraphobia and the two are ascertained as a single combination disorder. We shall include data on panic disorder alone where relevant. We shall explore the following questions:

(a) How many people have panic disorder, agoraphobia or both, social phobia or specific phobias (animals or insects; storms, heights or still water; enclosed spaces; blood–injury phobia) not better explained by agoraphobia or social phobia?
(b) Do people with phobias differ from people without a mental disorder?
(c) Do people with phobias differ from people with other mental disorders?

(d) How disabling are these phobias?
(e) What treatment do they seek and use?
(f) What is the comorbidity with other mental disorders?

Finally, we will note some specific issues in respect to social phobia.

PREVALENCE OF PHOBIAS

Psychiatric epidemiology was facilitated when the American Psychiatric Association's DSM-III [1] provided explicit criteria for the diagnosis of each mental disorder, criteria that were revised in DSM-III-R and DSM-IV [2]. Explicit criteria also appeared in the World Health Organization's ICD-10 [3]. The DSM-III criteria were operationalized by the Diagnostic Interview Schedule (DIS) [4] and respondents were systematically asked whether they had experienced the symptoms required to fulfil the diagnostic criteria. This structured interview enabled well-trained interviewers without clinical expertise to explore symptoms and generate data that could be matched to the scoring algorithms. The DIS and the later development, the Composite International Diagnostic Interview (CIDI) [5], were reliable (inter-rater reliability was near perfect) although test–retest reliability, because of respondent variability, was less so. Most versions of these interviews ask about the occurrence of a symptom at any point in the person's lifetime, which raises severe doubts about the accuracy of recall. Lifetime rates are therefore likely to be underestimates [6]. When rates over a shorter period are derived from a "lifetime" DIS or CIDI, the bias is likely to be the opposite, because a respondent who had the required number of symptoms at some point is asked "when was the last time that you had problems like (the symptoms they had mentioned)?". People could be recorded as being current or 12 month cases when they might only have sub-threshold sets of the symptoms that, at an earlier time, had satisfied the diagnostic criteria. Thus these one-year or one-month prevalence rates will be overestimates of the true state of affairs. Despite these concerns, and given that the under- and overestimate biases might cancel each other, the advent of the explicit criteria and diagnostic instruments that allow people with these symptoms to be identified in community surveys has enabled psychiatric epidemiology to progress.

This review is restricted to data gathered since the advent of the DIS/CIDI-type interviews. Most surveys present data in terms of panic disorder with or without agoraphobia, agoraphobia without panic disorder, social phobia and the specific or simple phobias. The classifications have not always been this straightforward: DSM-III and ICD-10 both identified agoraphobia with and without panic attacks and panic disorder unassociated with agoraphobia, and the latter should not therefore be included in any discussion of the phobias. DSM-IV reversed the emphasis, to panic disorder with and without agoraphobia, and agoraphobia without a history of panic disorder, in which case panic disorder with agoraphobia should be included. Data are seldom presented on agoraphobia alone and so this review will pay attention to panic disorder either alone or in combination with agoraphobia. DSM-III used the term simple phobia but ICD-10 and DSM-IV use the term specific phobia for the same entities. The term specific phobia will be used in this chapter.

Each diagnostic set contains exclusion criteria ("the disorder is not better explained by...") and these hierarchy rules differ considerably between DSM and ICD classifications and have significant effects on prevalence of individual anxiety disorders [7]. Epidemiological studies vary in their application of these rules and the cautious reader is therefore referred to the original papers to ascertain whether such rules were used or not. Variance in the classification used, in the application of the exclusion criteria, variation in diagnostic instrument, the age span sampled, and in the time frame encompassed can all affect prevalence rates. In this review we will focus on the prevalence of a disorder in the 12 months preceding the survey and, because of the method factors that can affect results, refrain from making comparisons between countries, being more interested in overall values as "best estimates".

The exemplar community survey was the Epidemiologic Catchment Area (ECA) programme [8]. This was a five-site multistage probability sampling in which some 20 000 adults were interviewed with the DIS to generate DSM-III diagnoses. The rate of panic disorder was relatively constant across the sites (mean 0.9%, low: 0.8% in Durham, high: 1.1% in St. Louis). The rate of phobias in the 12 months prior to interview in the five sites varied considerably from 6.3% in St. Louis to a high of 16.3% in Baltimore (mean 11.8%). Rates for the individual phobias were not published.

The ECA studies stimulated a number of smaller-scale replications in other countries. In New Zealand, for example, Oakley-Browne et al. [9] used the DIS to interview an urban sample of some 1500 respondents aged between 18 and 64. The rate of any phobia in the previous 12 months was 8.0%; 2.9% met criteria for agoraphobia, 2.8% for social phobia and 4.8% for DSM-III specific phobia. An additional 1.4% met criteria for panic disorder. Except for social phobia, the disorders were more frequent in women. Weissman et al. [10] reported on rates of DSM-III panic disorder in ten countries. The rates in New Zealand were median, and, as such, representative. The median age of onset of first symptoms of panic disorder in these ten countries was 25 years.

The National Comorbidity Survey (NCS) [11] covered a national probability sample of adults aged 15 to 54 years in the USA ($n = 8098$). It used a specific version of the CIDI to identify people who met criteria for a DSM-III-R mental disorder. The rates of respondents meeting criteria for a phobic disorder in the previous 12 months were 2.3% for panic with or without agoraphobia, 2.8% for agoraphobia without panic, 7.9% for social phobia and 8.8% for specific phobia. The rate for "any of the above disorders" was not given. As comorbidity within the anxiety disorders is common, the overall rate of any of the above disorders will be less than the total of 21.8%. The rate for any anxiety disorder was 17.2%, but this included 3.1% of people with generalized anxiety disorder. A proportional reduction based on a transfer factor of 0.67 was used to control for comorbidity, which means that the proportion of people who met criteria for any panic or phobia would be in the region of 15%. This is higher than in the ECA studies. Women were twice as likely as men to meet criteria, and again the sex preponderance was least in social phobia. Magee et al. [12] found that while the age of onset of first symptoms was 15 years for specific phobia and 16 years for social phobia, agoraphobia had a median age of onset of 29 years. They then presented data to show that the first symptoms of specific and social phobia occurred before any other disorder in 40% and 34% of people, respectively, while agoraphobia was temporally primary in only 20% of cases. Curtis et al. [13] explored the occurrence of specific phobias in the NCS data. Most people who met criteria for a phobia had more than one fear. The number of fears and not the type of specific phobia predicted impairment. The eight fears enquired about by the interviewer did not cluster as suggested by the classification, but contributed equally to comorbidity with other anxiety disorders, especially social phobia and agoraphobia. The authors argued that the number of fears might be a marker for subsequent psychopathology.

The National Comorbidity Survey was replicated in Ontario, Canada, with the same version of the CIDI, the same age group and similar sample size [14]. The rates of disorder were lower than in the NCS: 6.7% for social phobia, 6.4% for specific phobia, 1.6% for agoraphobia and 1.1% for panic disorder, with 10.6% for any panic or phobia. Female preponderance was pronounced, but least of all in social phobia. As a consequence of the number of surveys that followed the NCS, Kessler and Ustun established a World Health Organization International Consortium in Psychiatric Epidemiology (ICPE) to pool data from various local surveys. Judging from the rates for any anxiety disorder, the median frequency of panic and phobias was 9.3% [15]. Some of the individual surveys will be reviewed. This consortium led to the establishment of World Mental Health 2000 sets of surveys that use a standard method and are, during 2002–2004, using the same method to conduct epidemiological surveys of mental disorders in some 30 countries. These data are not yet available.

The National Psychiatric Morbidity Surveys of Great Britain [16] included a household survey in which some 10 000 adults aged between 16 and 65 were interviewed with a Clinical Interview Schedule of neurotic symptoms. These symptoms were mapped onto ICD-10 categories using hierarchical rules to determine the allocated diagnosis when a symptom threshold was exceeded and two or more anxiety or depressive disorders were likely. Social, specific or agoraphobia in the previous week was reported by 1.1% of respondents, panic by 0.8%, 1.9% of respondents in total. These one-week prevalences can be extrapolated to 12-month prevalences (transfer factor 2.0) but, even so, at 3.8%, the results are less than the surveys previously mentioned. Phobias, but not panic disorder, were more frequent among women. It is difficult to compare the results of this study with those with DIS/CIDI-derived diagnoses. This survey noted the occurrence of symptoms in the past week and relied on 14 symptom clusters, whereas the DIS/CIDI interviews used some 80 questions to determine whether diagnostic criteria were met. The use of ICD-10 is not the issue; the somewhat arbitrary mapping of the 14 clusters onto the 9 diagnostic categories is a matter for concern.

The Early Developmental Stages of Psychopathology (EDSP) programme [17] surveyed 3021 respondents aged 14 to 24 in Munich. A specific version of the CIDI was used to identify mental disorders. In the previous 12 months, 1.2% of respondents met criteria for panic disorder with or without agoraphobia, 1.6% for agoraphobia without panic disorder, 2.6% for social phobia and 1.8% for specific phobia. Diagnoses were more frequent in females. Diagnostic exclusion rules were not used and an arbitrary decision was made to create a "panic not otherwise specified" category. Comorbidity within the anxiety disorders was less than in the NCS and the sum of the diagnostic prevalences for any anxiety disorder was 77% of the observed total for "any anxiety disorder". On that basis, the prevalence of panic and phobias listed above would be in the region of 5.5%. Reed and Wittchen [18] argued that late onset panic attacks (over the age of 18) are associated not just with the development of panic disorder and agoraphobia but with a range of other mental disorders. Wittchen *et al.* [19] further questioned the necessary relationship between panic attacks and agoraphobia in these young people and reported that the majority of their sample with carefully documented agoraphobia did not have a prior history of panic.

The Netherlands Mental Health Survey [20] used the CIDI to determine DSM-III-R diagnoses in a random sample of residents aged 18 to 64. Some 7000 were interviewed. In the previous 12 months, 2.2% of respondents met criteria for panic disorder with or without agoraphobia, 1.6% for agoraphobia without panic disorder, 7.1% for specific phobia and 4.8% for social phobia, and from their data we estimate that the rate of any panic or phobia would be about 11%. Female preponderance was least in social phobia.

The Australian National Mental Health Survey [21] used the CIDI to determine DSM-IV and ICD-10 diagnoses in a random sample of household residents aged 18 and over. Some 10 600 persons were interviewed with a 12-month version and not the lifetime version of the CIDI. The rates of anxiety disorders were low. This may be a reflection that all people were required to have all the necessary symptoms in the 12 months and not merely, as occurs in the lifetime surveys, to report that some symptoms had occurred in the last 12 months. The operation of the exclusion criteria materially altered the DSM-IV prevalences. Rates with exclusion criteria operationalized are in parentheses. In the previous 12 months 2.2% (1.1%) of respondents met criteria for DSM-IV panic disorder with or without agoraphobia, 1.6% (0.5%) met criteria for agoraphobia without panic disorder and 2.3% (1.3%) met criteria for social phobia. The prevalence of specific phobias was not ascertained. Corresponding rates for ICD-10 exclusion criteria operationalized were 1.1%, 1.1% and 2.7%, respectively, and the reasons behind these differences between DSM and ICD have been discussed [22,23]. Female preponderance was least in social phobia. Andrews and Slade [24] reviewed the data from the survey on the characteristics of panic disorder, panic disorder with agoraphobia and agoraphobia without panic disorder. They argued that panic disorder and agoraphobia are equally common, comorbid and disabling, but panic disorder is more likely to lead to treatment seeking. Panic disorder with agoraphobia, it was argued, should be regarded as a "double" or comorbid disorder, because it is more disabling and distressing than either panic disorder alone or agoraphobia alone, exactly like most pairs of comorbid disorders. They therefore concur with the position taken by Wittchen *et al.* [19].

In Brazil, Andrade *et al.* [25] administered the CIDI to some 1500 residents of São Paulo aged 18 years and older. In ICD-10 terms, the rate in the previous 12 months for panic disorder was 1.0%, for agoraphobia 1.2%, for specific phobia 3.5%, and for social phobia 2.2%, rates quite similar to the Australian ICD-10 rates. Yet again, female preponderance was evident in all disorders but least so in social phobia.

The changes in the emphasis of the classification between DSM-III and DSM-IV and between DSM-IV and ICD-10 make rates for the members of the panic/agoraphobia group of disorders difficult to compare. Nevertheless the median rates in these eight surveys for any panic/agoraphobic disorder was 2.8%, for social phobia 2.8% and for specific phobia 5.6%. The comorbidity-adjusted median for any of the above disorders would be in the region of 8%; that is, in any 12-month period, one in 12 adults could be expected to meet criteria for one of these disorders.

PEOPLE WITH PANIC AND PHOBIAS

Sociodemographic Characteristics

What type of people suffer from panic and phobias? Sociodemographic data restricted to panic and phobias are uncommon, but data on the demographic correlates of anxiety disorders do exist. People with panic and phobias comprise 80% of the people with anxiety disorders in most surveys, so data for anxiety disorders will be presented as a proxy for people with panic and phobias. The NCS found significantly increased odds ratios (an odds ratio of 2 means that the characteristic is twice as common in the nominated group) between a DSM-III-R diagnosis of an anxiety disorder and female gender, youth, poor education and low income but not with race or urbanicity [11]. The Australian survey [21] found significant adjusted odds ratios between ICD-10 diagnosis of an anxiety disorder and female gender, youth, separated/divorced/widowed, poor education and employment status, but not with race or urbanicity. Thus the results of the NCS and the Australian survey concur: anxiety disorders, like affective disorders, are more frequent in women, and in those with lesser education and poorer incomes or work roles, and are less frequent in the elderly and those who are married. Actually these are the demographic correlates of any mental disorder. The substance use disorders are different, and are more frequent in young males, less frequent in blacks in the US or in people of non-English-speaking background in Australia, otherwise the associations with marital status, education and income are the same. Remember that these are correlates, and no issue of causation can be argued on the basis of such cross-sectional data. Nevertheless, some suggestion that a train of adversity could follow the onset of the disorder comes from the age of onset in the seven countries in the ICPE surveys [15]. The median age of onset of symptoms of anxiety disorders was 15 years (range 12–18), occurring before education is finished or occupational or marital choices are made.

Chronicity

We were unable to locate chronicity data on the individual panic and phobias. One can estimate the chronicity of a disorder from the proportion of people who have ever met criteria for an anxiety disorder and who report symptoms in the past 12 months. In the seven countries in the ICPE surveys [15], 68% of people who had ever met criteria had symptoms in the past 12 months, while of people with symptoms in the past 12 months, 60% reported symptoms in the past month. The results from the Australian survey [21] were similar: 58% of people who had met criteria for an anxiety disorder in the past year were still troubled by their disorder. This level of chronicity is average for the mental disorders as a whole. Neurasthenia and personality disorders are more chronic, affective and substance use disorders less so. Anxiety disorders thus occupy some middle ground on this indicator of chronicity. This level of chronicity, following onset in adolescence, means that the anxiety disorders have the potential to seriously disrupt life trajectories.

Comorbidity

When patients with a mental disorder consult a doctor, they describe their principal complaint, and while there may be other disorders present that complicate or are more important, the wise clinician will pay attention to the disorder that troubles the patient the most. Structured diagnostic interviews are impervious to the person's principal complaint and ask about each disorder in turn. Regier et al. [26] examined the two waves of the ECA data and concluded that anxiety disorders, especially social and specific phobias, have an early onset in adolescence and predispose individuals to later major depression and addictive disorders. Andrews et al. [27] looked at the comorbidity between six anxiety and depressive disorders and concluded there must be some common etiological factor that accounted for comorbidity being four times as frequent as one would expect if disorders co-occurred by chance, that is co-occurrence being determined only by the frequency of each disorder. They postulated that this tendency to co-occur must be part of a general neurotic syndrome driven by some underlying risk factor. Kessler [28] examined the lifetime odds ratios of pairs of disorders occurring in the NCS and concluded that "virtually all of the odds ratios were greater than 1.0. This means that there is a positive association between the lifetime occurrences of almost every pair of disorders." They found the strongest comorbidities between the anxiety and affective disorders.

Lifetime comorbidity is interesting but many things might contribute to this. Of more interest is the probability of disorders co-occurring. Kessler [28] also examined the probability of disorders (exclusion criteria deleted) co-occurring in the six months prior to the NCS survey. The odds ratios were larger than the lifetime odds ratios, with panic having odds ratios greater than 10 with the affective disorders, and with the phobias having a similar but less extreme pattern. The association with substance use disorder was significant but more modest. Andrews et al. [29] used data from the Australian survey to carry the argument one step further. Controlling for the general tendency for comorbidity to occur (i.e. the general neurotic syndrome), they examined the multivariate odds ratios between pairs of disorders occurring in the past year. In panic/agoraphobia there were highly significant odds ratios for the co-occurrence of social phobia, generalized anxiety disorder and cluster A personality disorder, and significant odds ratios with post-traumatic stress disorder (PTSD) and alcohol abuse and dependence. In social phobia there were highly significant odds ratios with panic/agoraphobia and generalized anxiety disorder, and significant associations between PTSD and cluster A personality disorder. In neither disorder did the association with the affective disorders remain significant once the probability of any comorbidity was controlled.

Nevertheless, the combination of affective disorders and anxiety disorders was frequent and more predictive of disability and service utilization than any other combination of diagnostic groups. To elucidate which combination was most important, Andrews et al. [29] had respondents nominate, when they had met criteria for more than one disorder, which disorder "troubled them the most" exactly as DSM-IV suggests. In that survey the affective and anxiety disorders taken together, whether they were a person's only or main disorder, accounted for 72% of the disability days and 78% of consultations for a mental problem reported by all people identified with a mental disorder in the Australian survey. Forty per cent of people who identified an anxiety disorder as their only or main complaint during the previous 12 months were comorbid for another disorder in that time, 17% for an affective disorder, 28% for a personality disorder and 9% for a substance use disorder. Thus, many of those who were comorbid met criteria for more than one group of comorbid disorders. Data on comorbidity among the individual phobias were not provided.

Disability Attributed to Panic and Phobias

Comorbidity, especially concurrent comorbidity, makes it difficult to attribute current disability and service utilization. Mendlowicz and Stein [30] reviewed the use of quality of life instruments in people with anxiety disorders and noted that they markedly compromise quality of life and psychosocial functioning. Importantly, they noted that treatment can reduce this disability. Goering et al. [31], reporting from the Ontario survey, noted that people with single affective disorders typically have more disability than people with single anxiety or substance use disorders and that people with multiple disorders have disability rates comparable with those with affective disorders. Stein and Kean [32] from the same survey reported that people with social phobia were impaired on a broad spectrum of measures, including low functioning on a "quality of well-being scale". Bijl and Ravelli [33] obtained a similar result from the

Netherlands survey. Eating disorders and schizophrenia were associated with most days ill in bed, disability days, and Short Form-36 (SF-36) role limitations due to emotional problems. On each of these measures the affective disorders ranked third, with the anxiety and substance use disorders fourth and fifth, respectively. The substantial minority of people with comorbid disorders were comparable in disability level to people with schizophrenia or eating disorders.

The Australian survey used the Short Form-12 (SF-12) [34] and the disability days measure [35] to assess disability. Sanderson and Andrews [36] used a regression technique to control for comorbidity, sociodemographic factors and physical illness, and found that depression, panic disorder, agoraphobia, social phobia, generalized anxiety disorder, and alcohol and drug dependence were all independently associated with disability. Schizophrenia was not included in this analysis. On the mental health summary scale of the SF-12, 57% of respondents who met criteria for social phobia scored below 40, that is were moderately or severely disabled, as did 69% of people with panic, and 46% of people with agoraphobia. In comparison, 72% of people with generalized anxiety disorder and 75% of people with an affective disorder scored as moderately or severely disabled. Obsessive–compulsive disorder (OCD) and PTSD were not independent predictors of disability.

Regression strategies are cumbersome. As mentioned above, Andrews et al. [29] used the principal complaint technique to circumvent the problem posed by comorbidity. They studied the four largest diagnostic groups in their survey: affective, anxiety, personality and substance use disorders. Anxiety disorders ranked second, after the affective disorders, as determinants of disability as measured by the mental health summary scale of the SF-12 (mean score 40; affective 33, personality disorder 46 and substance use disorder 49). Anxiety disorders also ranked second as determinants of disability days (affective 11 days per 30, anxiety 9, personality 5 and substance use disorders 3 days out of 30). Anxiety disorders were the most frequent of all four and accounted for 38% of all the disability days, with panic and the phobias important contributors to this total. Affective disorders accounted for 34% of disability days, so that the anxiety and affective disorders together account for more than 70% of the disability recorded in this sample. Schizophrenia and eating disorders, while more disabling, are rare and account for only a small fraction of the disability attributed to mental disorders.

Service Utilization

In the ECA surveys, Regier et al. [37] found that 59% of people with panic consulted a medical practitioner in the preceding year, a rate comparable to that of people with bipolar disorder or schizophrenia. On the other hand, only 31% of people with a phobia consulted, a rate virtually identical to that for all people with mental disorders. People with panic disorder alone made high use of hospital emergency departments, but people with agoraphobia with panic attacks were also high service users [38].

Kessler et al. [39] reported the use of outpatient services from cases identified in the NCS. A quarter of people who met criteria for any 12 month disorder reported using services. The rates for any anxiety disorder were similar. The rates of service use varied considerably within the anxiety disorders, with panic disorder being associated with the highest utilization rates (46%) and social phobia (23%) with the lowest. Specific phobias and agoraphobia occupied intermediate positions. When the total number of visits to the health care sectors was calculated, there were no significant differences between diagnoses. Kessler et al. [40] reported on the delay between onset of first symptoms and treatment contact in the NCS. More than half of people with panic disorder made contact with health services within the year of onset. In contrast, half the people with phobias never made contact with treatment services, ever. The delay in getting treatment in the phobias was related to age of onset: onset in childhood was related to very low treatment seeking ever, while onset in adult life was still associated with delays of 5–15 years. These results were replicated in the Ontario Survey [41].

In the Munich EDSP survey, 25% of their young people used services for their anxiety disorder, a rate comparable to the NCS [42]. Again, panic disorder had the highest rate but now people with specific phobias were the least likely to access help. In the UK survey [43] rates of treatment were very low: 22% of people with panic and 14% with phobias reported contact with health services. In the Netherlands survey [44], 40% of people with a 12 month anxiety disorder reported some form of health care; three-quarters received help from their family practitioner. As in the previous surveys, people with panic or agoraphobia were more likely to receive care, people with social or specific phobias less likely to receive care, and people with specific phobias were no more likely to receive health care than the general population without a mental disorder.

Issakidis and Andrews [45] analysed the service utilization of people in the Australian survey who identified anxiety as their principal complaint. Tracing people through the system, they showed that while 41% of people with an anxiety disorder reported a consultation for a mental health problem, only in cases of panic disorder was this followed by putatively effective treatment with medication or cognitive-behaviour therapy (CBT). People with agoraphobia or with social phobia rarely consulted and only 39% and 20%, respectively, reported receiving either medication or CBT, the treatments of benefit. The shortfall in service delivery among people with panic and phobias is considerable.

THE EPIDEMIOLOGY OF SOCIAL PHOBIA

It has been convenient to discuss panic, agoraphobia and the specific phobias in the setting of their parent surveys, but there are issues in social phobia that warrant a special section. Kessler *et al.* [46] found that the social fears in the NCS could be disaggregated into a class characterized by speaking fears and a class characterized by a broader range of social fears. Social phobia characterized by speaking fears was less persistent, less impairing and less comorbid than the more generalized social phobia. Heimberg *et al.* [47] subsequently argued that the prevalence of generalized social phobia appeared to be increasing among the white, the educated and the married. Pelissolo *et al.* [48] noted an increase in prevalence in a French sample and attributed this to varying thresholds in the diagnostic criteria. Wittchen *et al.* [49] reported from the EDSP survey that used the DSM-IV classification. This provided some support to the Kessler position: people with generalized social phobia feared a range of situations not necessarily focused on public speaking and their disorder was more persistent, impairing and comorbid. People with a social phobia focused around performance rather than interacting with people seemed to have a milder variant of the disorder.

Furmark *et al.* [50] administered a social phobia questionnaire to some 1200 adults in Sweden. While, based on DSM-IV criteria, the questionnaire essentially set a cut point on a continuum, equal numbers of people identified as suffering from social phobia or not endorsed being distressed by fears of speaking in front of people or maintaining a conversation with someone unfamiliar. Four times as many people without any phobia compared to people with social phobia identified using public lavatories as likely to cause distress. Clearly, while these items are endorsed by people with social phobia at a high frequency, they are also part of the normal range of responses.

A similar community survey in Canada ($n = 1956$) [51] showed that while 7.2% met criteria for social phobia, analysis of the fears failed to yield subtypes: impairment increased linearly as the number of social fears was increased. In the Australian survey [52], rates of social phobia were less than in many other surveys (12 month 1.3% exclusion criteria applied, 2.3% not applied). Considerable comorbidity was identified, the comorbidity with depression and alcohol use being mostly secondary, i.e. occurring after the onset of the social phobia. Comorbidity with avoidant personality disorder was associated with a greater burden of affective disorder. This was the first survey to measure rates for the personality disorders. The authors concluded that avoidant personality disorder was most likely to be a severe variant of social phobia and not an independent disorder.

CONCLUSIONS

It is usual for reviewers to conclude by saying that the disorders they have been reviewing are frequent, disabling, difficult to treat and, because they constitute a major public health problem, more money is required. This invites commentators to take a contrary stand, saying that the disorders in question are "not expensive, and cheap to treat" [53]. Aware of this risk, we will hold that the panic/phobia group of disorders is frequent, disabling, difficult to treat and does constitute a major public health problem. Whether more money is required is doubtful; we should probably plan on doing better with the money we have.

Frequency

The panic/phobia group of disorders is frequent. On the basis of evidence from eight surveys we concluded that 1 in 12 adults would meet criteria for one of these disorders in 12 months. This prevalence rate (8%) is comparable to the prevalence of the affective disorders and 20 times the prevalence of schizophrenia. Panic and phobias are more chronic than depression though less chronic than schizophrenia. The average person with panic or phobia can expect to be troubled for 7 months in 12, and continue to be troubled year after year.

Disability

The panic/agoraphobia group of disorders is disabling. Most reports present data for the anxiety disorders as a single group. In the Dutch study [33] the affective disorders were 1.8 times more disabling (in terms of disability days per person) than the anxiety disorders, schizophrenia on the same measure 5 times more disabling than the anxiety disorders. In the Australian survey [29] with comorbidity controlled, the affective disorders were 1.3 times as disabling as the anxiety disorders, again measured in disability days reported by the average sufferer. There are no data on the disability due to specific phobias but there are data on other phobias and panic. Sanderson and Andrews [36] found that after comorbidity, sociodemographic factors and physical illness were controlled, depression, panic disorder, agoraphobia, social phobia, generalized anxiety disorder, and alcohol and drug dependence were independently associated with disability on the mental health summary scale of the SF-12. Seventy-five per cent of people with an affective disorder scored as moderately or severely disabled (score <40), whereas 58% of people with an anxiety disorder did likewise, an increase in disability (1.3:1) in affective disorders comparable to that found in the disability days data [29]. The proportions of people with the diagnoses of interest who had scores in this moderate or severe disability range were panic disorder 69%, agoraphobia 46% and social phobia 57%, data that suggest that people with panic and phobias are as disabled as those with any anxiety disorder.

The cumulative disability attributed to a disorder is a product of the frequency of the disorder and the average level of disability. If panic and phobias have prevalences that are comparable to those of the affective disorders but are less disabling (1:1.5 to combine the results of the Dutch and Australian studies), then the disability attributed to the panic and phobias will be two-thirds that due to the affective disorders. If schizophrenia is 20 times less common than the panic and phobias yet 5 times more disabling, then the total disability attributed to schizophrenia will be a quarter that due to panic and phobias.

Difficult to Treat

There are effective treatments for panic disorder and the phobias [54]. The problem is that, apart from panic, few people with these disorders attend for treatment and, when they do, few are treated appropriately. In the Australian survey [55], only 39% of people with panic disorder, agoraphobia or panic disorder with agoraphobia as a principal complaint sought a mental health consultation and 61% of them received medication or CBT, the treatments known to be beneficial. Thus only 24% of people with these panic and agoraphobic disorders were being helped. In social phobia the picture was more dismal: 21% received a mental health consultation, and only 32% received medication or CBT, the treatments known to be beneficial. Thus, only 7% of people with social phobia could have been helped by treatment.

In the Munich study [42], the probability of consulting for a mental health problem ranged from a high of 50% for panic disorder through 36% for agoraphobia and 32% for social phobia to a low of 21% for specific phobia. Only 8% of all cases were rated as receiving some form of adequate treatment. "Assuming that scientifically proven treatment recommendations are correct," wrote Wittchen, "this points to a serious mismatch problem and possibly a waste of personnel and financial resources." In the introduction we presented vignettes of three individuals with potentially treatable conditions who declined to come for treatment despite their considerable handicap. At some level they might have been wise, if the probability of getting adequate treatment was as low as was shown in the Australian and German studies. Before we can ask for better coverage, we need to ensure that when people do come for treatment, they get treatments that are known to work, not just treatments that the doctor, through ignorance or bias, likes to give.

A Major Public Health Problem

Panic and the phobias make a significant contribution to the burden of disease. The original Burden of Disease study only included panic disorder, while the estimation of the burden of disease in Australia in 1999 [56] included panic, agoraphobia and social phobia but not the specific phobias. These three disorders accounted for 28 000 Disability Adjusted Life Years lost, 1.1% of the total burden of disease in Australia, and 8% of the burden of all mental disorders. Put in context, the burden of panic and phobias was half the burden of asthma and four times the burden of insulin-dependent diabetes and comparable to the burden of prostate cancer.

There is another reason why phobias constitute a major public health problem. A number of authors reviewed refer to the early age of onset of the phobias, on the propensity of fears to be the forerunners of other mental disorders, and on the possibility that fears in adolescence will lead to a limitation on educational, vocational and marital success. There is adequate evidence that simple school-based programmes can prevent the emergence of anxiety disorders among children at risk [57]. If we had knowledge that could prevent prostate cancer, it would be mandated. We know how to prevent panic and phobias in young people, yet there are no national programmes of prevention. Why do we continue to believe that the phobias are disorders of little importance? Perhaps the remaining chapters in this volume will clarify the problem and illuminate the way forward.

SUMMARY

Consistent Evidence

There is consistent evidence showing that phobias are common, disabling and difficult to treat, and constitute a major public health problem. Their prevalence rate (8%) is comparable to the prevalence of affective disorders and 20 times the prevalence of schizophrenia. Combining the results of the

Dutch and Australian studies, the disability attributed to panic and phobias is shown to be two-thirds that due to affective disorders. Phobias are difficult to treat because sufferers are slow to come for treatment and often afraid of confronting their fears when they get to treatment. The burden of panic and phobias is four times the burden of insulin-dependent diabetes and comparable to the burden of prostate cancer.

Incomplete Evidence

There is incomplete evidence about the patterns of comorbidity and time delay between onset of phobia and the beginning of treatment. When data from the currently ongoing World Mental Health Survey become available, there will be a better understanding of many things about phobias, if only because a common instrument will have been used in all countries.

Areas Still Open to Research

We need to know why only some people develop such intractable phobias in the apparent absence of aversive or traumatic experiences. Mostly we need to know how to intervene in young people so that the tide of disability and subsequent morbidity does not occur.

REFERENCES

1. American Psychiatric Association (1980) *Diagnostic and Statistical Manual of Mental Disorders*, 3rd edn. American Psychiatric Association, Washington, DC.
2. American Psychiatric Association (1994) *Diagnostic and Statistical Manual of Mental Disorders*, 4th edn. American Psychiatric Association, Washington, DC.
3. World Health Organization (1992) *The ICD-10 Classification of Mental Disorders. Clinical Descriptions and Diagnostic Guidelines*. World Health Organization, Geneva.
4. Robins, L.N., Helzer J.E., Croughan J., Ratcliff K. (1981) National Institute of Mental Health Diagnostic Interview Schedule. *Arch. Gen. Psychiatry*, **38**: 381–389.
5. World Health Organization (1997) *Composite International Diagnostic Interview— Version 2.1*. World Health Organization, Geneva.
6. Andrews G., Anstey K., Brodaty H., Issakidis C., Luscombe G. (1999) Recall of depressive episodes 25 years previously. *Psychol. Med.* **29**: 787–791.
7. Andrews G. (2000) The anxiety disorder inclusion and exclusion criteria in DSM-IV and ICD-10. *Curr. Opin. Psychiatry*, **13**: 139–141.
8. Robins L.N., Regier D.A. (1991) *Psychiatric Disorders in America*. Free Press, New York.

9. Oakley-Browne M.A., Joyce P.R., Wells E., Bushnell J.A., Hornblow A.R. (1989) Christchurch Psychiatric Epidemiology Study, Part II. *Aust. N. Zeal. J. Psychiatry*, **23**: 327–340.
10. Weissman M.M., Bland R.C., Canino G.J., Faravelli C., Greenwald S., Hwu H.G., Joyce P.R., Karam E.G., Lee C.K., Lellouch J. et al. (1997) The crossnational study of panic disorder. *Arch. Gen. Psychiatry*, **54**: 305–309.
11. Kessler R.C., McGonagle K.A., Zhao S., Nelson C.B., Hughes M., Eshleman S., Wittchen H.U., Kendler K.S. (1994) Lifetime and 12-month prevalence of DSM-III-R psychiatric disorders in the United States. *Arch. Gen. Psychiatry*, **51**: 8–19.
12. Magee W.J., Eaton W.W., Wittchen H.-U., McGonagle K.A., Kessler R.C. (1996) Agoraphobia, simple phobia, and social phobia in the National Comorbidity Survey. *Arch. Gen. Psychiatry*, **53**: 159–168.
13. Curtis G.C., Magee W.J., Eaton W.W., Wittchen H.U., Kessler R.C. (1998) Specific fears and phobias. *Br. J. Psychiatry*, **173**: 212–217.
14. Offord D.R., Boyle M.H., Campbell D., Goering P., Lin E., Wong M., Racine Y.A. (1996) One-year prevalence of psychiatric disorder in Ontarians 15 to 64 years of age. *Can. J. Psychiatry*, **41**: 559–563.
15. WHO International Consortium in Psychiatric Epidemiology (2000) Crossnational comparisons of the prevalences and correlates of mental disorders. *WHO Bull.*, **78**: 413–424.
16. Jenkins R., Lewis G., Bebbington P., Brugha T., Farrell M., Gill B., Meltzer H. (1997) The National Psychiatric Morbidity Surveys of Great Britain—initial findings from the household survey. *Psychol. Med.*, **27**: 775–789.
17. Wittchen H.-U., Nelson C.B., Lachner G. (1998) Prevalence of mental disorders and psychosocial impairments in adolescents and young adults. *Psychol. Med.*, **28**: 109–126.
18. Reed V., Wittchen H.-U. (1998) DSM-IV panic attacks and panic disorder in a community sample of adolescents and young adults. *J. Psychiatr. Res.*, **32**: 335–345.
19. Wittchen H.-U., Reed V., Kessler R.C. (1998) The relationship of agoraphobia and panic in a community sample of adolescents and young adults. *Arch. Gen. Psychiatry*, **55**: 1017–1024.
20. Bijl R.V., Ravelli A., van Zessen G. (1998) Prevalence of psychiatric disorder in the general population: results of the Netherlands Mental Health Survey and Incidence Study. *Soc. Psychiatry Psychiatr. Epidemiol.*, **33**: 587–595.
21. Andrews G., Henderson S., Hall W. (2001) Prevalence, comorbidity, disability and service utilisation: overview of the Australian National Mental Health Survey. *Br. J. Psychiatry*, **178**: 145–153.
22. Andrews G., Slade T., Peters L., Beard J. (1998) General anxiety disorder, obsessive compulsive disorder and social phobia: correspondence between ICD-10 and DSM-IV. *Int. J. Methods Psychiatr. Res.*, **7**: 110–115.
23. Andrews G., Slade T. (1998) Panic and agoraphobia: sources of dissonance between ICD-10 and DSM-IV. *Int. J. Methods Psychiatr. Res.*, **7**: 156–161.
24. Andrews G., Slade T. (2002) Agoraphobia without a history of panic disorder may be part of the panic disorder syndrome. *J. Nerv. Ment. Dis.*, **190**: 624–630.
25. Andrade L., Walters E.E., Gentil V., Laurenti R. (2002) Prevalence of ICD-10 mental disorders in a catchment area in the city of São Paulo, Brazil. *Soc. Psychiatry Psychiatr. Epidemiol.*, **37**: 316–325.
26. Regier D.A., Rae D.S., Narrow W.E., Kaelber C.T., Schatzberg A.F. (1998) Prevalence of anxiety disorders and their comorbidity with mood and addictive disorders. *Br. J. Psychiatry*, **173** (Suppl. 34): 24–28.

27. Andrews G., Stewart G.W., Morris-Yates A., Holt P.E., Henderson A.S. (1990) Evidence for a general neurotic syndrome. *Br. J. Psychiatry*, **157**: 6–12.
28. Kessler R.C. (1995) Epidemiology of psychiatric comorbidity. In *Textbook in Psychiatric Epidemiology* (Eds M.T. Tsuang, M. Tohen, G.E.P. Zahner), pp. 179–197. Wiley-Liss, New York.
29. Andrews G., Slade T., Issakidis C. (2002) Deconstructing current comorbidity. *Br. J. Psychiatry*, **181**: 306–314.
30. Mendlowicz M.V., Stein M.B. (2000) Quality of life in individuals with anxiety disorders. *Am. J. Psychiatry*, **157**: 669–682.
31. Goering P., Lin E., Campbell D., Boyle M.H., Offord D.R. (1996) Psychiatric disability in Ontario. *Can. J. Psychiatry*, **41**: 564–571.
32. Stein M.B., Kean Y.M. (2000) Disability and quality of life in social phobia. *Am. J. Psychiatry*, **157**: 1606–1613.
33. Bijl R.V., Ravelli A. (2000) Current and residual functional disability associated with psychopathology. *Psychol. Med.*, **30**: 657–668.
34. Ware J.E., Kosinski M., Keller S.D. (1996) A 12 item short form health survey. *Med. Care* **34**: 220–233.
35. Kessler R.C., Frank R.G. (1997) The impact of psychiatric disorders on work loss days. *Psychol. Med.*, **27**: 861–873.
36. Sanderson K., Andrews G. (2002) Prevalence and severity of mental health-related disability and relationship to diagnosis. *Psychiatr. Serv.*, **53**: 80–86.
37. Regier D.A., Narrow W.E., Rae D.S., Manderscheid R.W., Locke B.Z., Goodwin F.K. (1993) The de facto US mental and addictive disorders service system. *Arch. Gen. Psychiatry*, **50**: 85–94.
38. Thompson J.W., Burns B.J., Bartko J., Boyd J.H., Taube C.A., Bourdon K.H. (1988) The use of ambulatory services by people with and without phobia. *Med. Care*, **26**: 183–198.
39. Kessler R.C., Zhao S., Katz S.J., Kouzis A., Frank R.G., Edlund M., Leaf P. (1999) Past-year use of outpatient services for psychiatric problems in the National Comorbidity Survey. *Am. J. Psychiatry*, **156**: 115–123.
40. Kessler R.C., Olfson M., Berglund P.A. (1998) Patterns and predictors of treatment contact after first onset of psychiatric disorders. *Am. J. Psychiatry*, **155**: 62–69.
41. Olfson M., Kessler R.C., Berglund P.A., Lin E. (1998) Psychiatric disorder onset and first treatment contact in the United States and Ontario. *Am. J. Psychiatry*, **155**: 1415–1422.
42. Wittchen H.-U. (2000) Met and unmet need in anxiety disorders. In *Unmet Need in Psychiatry* (Eds G. Andrews, S. Henderson), pp. 256–276. Cambridge University Press, Cambridge.
43. Bebbington P.E., Brugha T.S., Meltzer H., Jenkins R., Ceresa C., Farrell M., Lewis G. (2000) Neurotic disorders and the receipt of psychiatric treatment. *Psychol. Med.*, **30**: 1369–1376.
44. Bijl R.V., Ravelli A. (2000) Psychiatric mobidity, service use and need for care in the general population. *Am. J. Publ. Health*, **90**: 602–607.
45. Issakidis C., Andrews G. (2002) Service utilisation for anxiety in an Australian community sample. *Soc. Psychiatry Psychiatr. Epidemiol.*, **37**: 153–163.
46. Kessler R.C., Stein M.B., Berglund P. (1998) Social phobia subtypes in the National Comorbidity Survey. *Am. J. Psychiatry*, **155**: 613–619.
47. Heimberg R.G., Stein M.B., Hiripi E., Kessler R.C. (2000) Trends in the prevalence of social phobia in the United States. *Eur. Psychiatry*, **15**: 29–37.

48. Pelissolo A., Andre C., Moutard-Martin F., Wittchen H.U., Lépine J.P. (2000) Social phobia in the community. *Eur. Psychiatry*, **15**: 25–28.
49. Wittchen H.-U., Stein M.B., Kessler R.C. (1999) Social fears and social phobia in a community sample of adolescents and young adults. *Psychol. Med.*, **29**: 309–323.
50. Furmark T., Tillifors M., Everz P.-O., Marteinsdottir I., Gefvert O., Fredrikson M. (1999) Social phobia in the general population. *Soc. Psychiatry Psychiatr. Epidemiol.*, **34**: 416–424.
51. Stein M.B., Torgrud L.J., Walker J.R. (2000) Social phobia symptoms, subtypes and severity. *Arch. Gen. Psychiatry*, **57**: 1046–1052.
52. Lampe L., Slade T., Issakidis C., Andrews G. (2003) Social phobia in the Australian National Survey of Mental Health and Well-Being (NSMHWB). *Psychol. Med.*, **33**: 637–646.
53. Andrews G. (2000) Not expensive and cheap to treat: new evidence leads to different conclusions. In *Obsessive–Compulsive Disorder* (Eds M. Maj, N. Sartorius, A. Okasha, J. Zohar), pp. 290–292. Wiley, Chichester.
54. Nathan P.E., Gorman J.M. (2002) *A Guide to Treatments that Work*. Oxford University Press, New York.
55. Issakidis C., Sanderson K., Corry J., Andrews G., Lapsley H. (in press) Modelling the population cost-effectiveness of current and evidence based optimal treatment for anxiety disorders. *Psychol. Med.*
56. Mathers C., Vos T., Stephenson C. (1999) *The Burden of Disease and Injury in Australia*. Australian Institute of Health and Welfare, Canberra.
57. Andrews G., Wilkinson D. (2002) The prevention of mental disorders in young people. *Med. J. Australia*, **177**: S97–S100.

Commentaries

2.1
Risk-Factor and Genetic Epidemiology of Phobic Disorders: A Promising Approach

Assen Jablensky[1]

In his authoritative review, Andrews restricts himself (for good reasons) to a crop of relatively recent population surveys, all using the Composite International Diagnostic Interview (CIDI) [1] or its predecessor, the Diagnostic Interview Schedule (DIS) [2], to assess the prevalence of phobic disorders, the associated burden of disability and the level of service utilization. His conclusion that "phobias are common, disabling and difficult to treat, and constitute a major public health problem" is substantiated by the epidemiological evidence, but the expectation that the currently ongoing World Mental Health Survey will result in a "better understanding of many things about phobias, if only because a common instrument will have been used in all countries" is unwarranted. CIDI-based survey epidemiology is certainly contributing to the population mapping of prevalences and disability rates, but its capacity to unravel the complex issues of etiology is limited.

Epidemiology is not restricted to its descriptive branch (sometimes referred to as "head counting"). The tools of analytical, risk-factor and genetic epidemiology have a better chance of allowing us to understand causation and, ultimately, prevention. To illustrate this point, I choose four examples of incisive and challenging research demonstrating that the etiology of phobias is complex and likely multifactorial, but not intractable.

An example of epidemiological "dissection" of anxiety and depressive disorders is provided by a prospective study by Brown and colleagues [3,4] of a sample of 404 British women considered to be at high risk for depression (being inner-city residents, working class, many of them single mothers, with a child living at home). Following in-depth initial interviews, the women were re-interviewed for psychiatric symptoms at one-year, two-year and (a quarter of the sample) at eight-year follow-up. Indices of childhood adversity (physical or sexual abuse, parental indifference) and adult life adversity (death of a child, death of a partner, multiple abortions,

[1] *Centre for Clinical Research in Neuropsychiatry, University of Western Australia, Perth, Australia*

sexual abuse, domestic violence) were constructed and used in log-linear analyses modelling the relationship between such risk factors and psychiatric disorder. The one-year prevalence of DSM-III-R anxiety disorders (panic disorder, agoraphobia, social phobia, simple phobias, generalized anxiety) was 23.8%. Close to half of the sample had experienced clinically significant depression at some point during the anxiety episode, while only 7.2% had depression without anxiety. Panic disorder was most likely (67%), and simple phobias least likely (11%), to be associated with depression. The time spent in anxiety (8.1% of the one-year period preceding the interview) was double the time spent in depression, and anxiety disorders were more often chronic than depression. Onsets of anxiety disorders within an ongoing depressive episode were rare; however, onsets of depression among those with ongoing anxiety disorder were common.

The analysis of risk factors highlighted different mechanisms of operation for psychosocial factors in depression and anxiety. While adult life adversity and low levels of social support were related to depression, vulnerability to anxiety was less influenced by current adversity or levels of support and more by early adversity, constitutional factors, or both. About half of the women with anxiety disorder (particularly panic disorder and agoraphobia) had experienced early adversity, which remained significantly associated with anxiety after controlling for adult adversity.

The study design allowed teasing out the separate contributions of anxiety and depression to the commonly observed comorbidity of the two conditions. The main contribution to comorbidity (44% of the total rate) resulted from the joint high prevalences of the two conditions, i.e. represented chance comorbidity. However, over 50% of the observed comorbidity was non-chance, suggesting that factors other than childhood and adult life adversity may play an important role. Although involvement of further psychosocial stressors could not be ruled out, the study suggests an underlying common genetic liability, or a single neurodevelopmental process, at the root of the comorbidity problem.

My second example highlights the potential benefits from epidemiological studies of rare isolate populations that are relatively homogeneous, in both genetic and lifestyle respects.

The Hutterites, a Protestant anabaptist sect founded in the 16th century by Jacob Hutter in Switzerland, are a genetic isolate with a high index of consanguinity resulting from a closed-in lifestyle, imposed by religious persecution and group migration that led them first to Russia and later on to the US and Canada, where they settled as small farming communities. The majority of the Hutterites (present number estimated at about 40 000) are the descendants of 89 individuals who formed a "family" at the end of the 18th century. They represent an almost ideal founder population that had experienced a relatively recent bottleneck, ensuring a high degree of genetic homogeneity. The medical and psychiatric profile of the Hutterites was first described in the 1950s by Eaton and Weil in a classic monograph entitled *Culture and Mental Disorders* [5]. The main finding of the study was the extremely low incidence of schizophrenia, which was hypothetically explained as the result of sociogenetic selection: individuals with schizoid traits or other schizophrenia-prone attributes were unlikely to adjust to the highly collectivist ethos of the community and, hence, had low chances of procreation within the sect. A follow-up epidemiological study some 40 years later [6] replicated the original finding of a low incidence of psychoses in the Hutterite communities, but it also revealed something that had escaped the initial survey: an unusually high prevalence of neurotic disorders, including anxiety and phobias. The prevalence rate of neurotic disorders, at 86.7 per 1000, was more than twice the expected rate, based on the general population of the area.

Both cultural and genetic factors may be at work to produce this phenomenon. While providing an extraordinary level of familial and community support, the strict religious indoctrination, lifestyle regimentation and conformity to tradition within the closely knit community may be conducive to excessive anxiety in many individual members—with or without a specific genetic vulnerability. Such an interpretation would be in agreement with the findings of another population survey—that in the Outer Hebrides [7]—which revealed that the rates of chronic anxiety were highest among the most socially integrated members of the community (e.g. churchgoers and owners of small farms) while rates of depression were highest among the least integrated.

The third example concerns the genetic epidemiology of anxiety disorders. A number of studies point to a significant familial aggregation for panic disorder, generalized anxiety and phobias. Genes seem to account for the greater part of this aggregation, although non-shared environmental factors are also likely to play a role [8]. In a major twin study, Kendler *et al.* [9] attempted an evaluation of a stress–diathesis model of anxiety disorders which predicts that the severity of fear-inducing stress is inversely proportional to the level of genetic diathesis.

A total of 7566 twin pairs from the Virginia Twin Registry were included. The majority had face-to-face interviews (DIS-based), and also responded to 12 neuroticism items from the Eysenck Personality Questionnaire. The prevalence of phobias in the twin sample was 26.1%. Five "modes of acquisition" (MOAs) of anxiety disorders were investigated: trauma to self, observed trauma to others, observed fear or avoidance in others, taught to be afraid, no memory of how the fear developed. Those with no memory of a stressful event were assumed to have highest "endogenous" liability, while those reporting trauma to self were considered to have low liability. Two hypotheses were tested: (a) the risk of phobias in co-twins will be highest in twins with the lowest level of environmental trauma; (b) neuroticism (index of phobia-proneness) will be highest in twins whose onset was associated with the lowest level of trauma.

More than 50% of the subjects with agoraphobia, social and situational fears reported "no memory" (but none of the twins with animal or blood/injury phobias). Neither of the hypotheses was confirmed. Lack of memory of trauma did not predict an increased risk of phobia in the co-twin, and there was no significant effect of the reported severity of trauma on the risk of phobias. In fact, the genetic liability to phobia was highest, rather than lowest, in those who had experienced trauma to self (which could indicate that individuals with high liability tend to select themselves into traumatic events). Neuroticism predicted significantly all phobia types but was not associated with severity of trauma. The investigators concluded that the stress–diathesis model might not be applicable to phobias. The results were consistent with a growing body of data suggesting that phobias arise in a non-associative manner (i.e. without learning).

My last example illustrates the unsuspected insights into phenotype–genotype relationships in panic disorder and phobias that can result from a fresh look at the clinical phenotype. Several genome scans of families with multiple cases of panic and phobic disorders had produced, at best, inconclusive findings, until a research group in Barcelona [10] investigated a previously reported but ignored, curious epidemiological finding: a strong association between panic/agoraphobia disorders and the seemingly unrelated comorbid condition of joint laxity and hypermobility [11]. People with panic/agoraphobia/social phobia disorders had been found to have a 16-fold increased risk of joint laxity, yet this highly significant comorbidity had been largely unattended to. When the phenotype was extended to include the joint abnormality, the genome scan revealed a highly significant linkage to a previously unsuspected region on chromosome 15 which turned out to contain an interstitial duplication of a stretch of DNA (termed DUP 25) that includes a number of candidate genes, yet to be investigated. The remarkable implication of this genomic discovery is that panic disorder, agoraphobia, social phobia and joint laxity may be pleiotropic expressions of a single underlying genomic anomaly, estimated to be present in up to 90% of the cases and in less that 7% of the general population [12]. This finding (which calls for replication) may provide an unexpected perspective on the hypothesis, persuasively argued by Andrews *et al.* [13], that "there must be some common aetiological factor" underlying the comorbid anxiety and depressive disorders and manifesting as a "general neurotic syndrome".

REFERENCES

1. Robins L.N., Wing J.K., Wittchen H.U., Helzer J.E., Babor T.F., Burke J., Farmer A., Jablensky A., Pickens R., Regier D.A. et al. (1988) The Composite International Diagnostic Interview: an epidemiologic instrument suitable for use in conjunction with different diagnostic systems and in different cultures. *Arch. Gen. Psychiatry*, **45**: 1069–1077.
2. Robins L.N., Helzer J.E., Croughan J., Ratcliff K. (1981) National Institute of Mental Health Diagnostic Interview Schedule. *Arch. Gen. Psychiatry*, **38**: 381–389.
3. Brown G.W, Harris T.O. (1993) Aetiology of anxiety and depressive disorders in an inner-city population. 1. Early adversity. *Psychol. Med.*, **23**: 143–154.
4. Brown G.W., Harris T.O., Eales M.J. (1993) Aetiology of anxiety and depressive disorders in an inner-city population. 2. Comorbidity and adversity. *Psychol. Med.*, **23**: 155–165.
5. Eaton J.W., Weil R.J. (1955) *Culture and Mental Disorders*. Free Press, Glencoe, IL.
6. Nimgaonkar V.L., Fujiwara T.M., Dutta M., Wood J., Gentry K., Maendel S., Morgan K., Eaton J. (2000) Low prevalence of psychoses among the Hutterites, an isolated religious community. *Am. J. Psychiatry*, **157**: 1065–1070.
7. Prudo R., Brown G.W., Harris T.O. (1984) Psychiatric disorder in a rural and an urban population. 3. Social integration and the morphology of affective disorder. *Psychol. Med.*, **14**: 327–345.
8. Hettema J.M., Neale M.C., Kendler K.S. (2001) A review and meta-analysis of the genetic epidemiology of anxiety disorders. *Am. J. Psychiatry*, **158**: 1568–1578.
9. Kendler K.S., Myers J., Prescott C.A. (2002) The etiology of phobias. *Arch. Gen. Psychiatry*, **59**: 242–248.
10. Gratacos M., Nadal M., Martin-Santos R., Pujana M.A., Gago J., Peral B., Armengol L., Ponsa I., Miro R., Bulbena A. et al. (2001) A polymorphic genomic duplication on human chromosome 15 is a susceptibility factor for panic and phobic disorders. *Cell*, **106**: 367–379.
11. Bulbena A., Duro J.C., Mateo A., Porta M., Vallejo J. (1988) Joint hypermobility syndrome and anxiety disorders. *Lancet*, **2**: 694.
12. Collier D.A. (2002) FISH, flexible joints and panic: are anxiety disorders really expressions of instability in the human genome? *Br. J. Psychiatry*, **181**: 457–459.
13. Andrews G., Stewart G.W., Morris-Yates A., Holt P.E., Henderson A.S. (1998) Evidence for a general neurotic syndrome. *Br. J. Psychiatry*, **157**: 6–12.

2.2
Defining a Case for Psychiatric Epidemiology: Threshold, Non-Criterion Symptoms, and Category versus Spectrum

Jack D. Maser and Jonathan M. Meyer[1]

Gavin Andrews' comprehensive review of the epidemiology of phobias and panic disorder raises a number of issues, many of which are embedded in

---

[1] *Department of Psychiatry, University of California at San Diego and Veterans Affairs San Diego Healthcare System, 3350 La Jolla Village Drive, San Diego, CA 92161-0002, USA*

how accurately ICD-10 and DSM-IV represent the true nature of psychopathology. Nearly all of the prevalence figures cited are based on an assumption that these two nomenclatures accurately represent the breadth of panic and phobia; however, both DSM and ICD are works in progress, periodically revised in light of new data. These manuals bring to epidemiology operational criteria by which to define a case of mental illness, and thereby count it reliably. Yet, the inherent shortcomings of the current nosology introduce an unknown degree of error into epidemiologic findings, mostly in the direction of underestimating the true impact of panic and phobia symptoms among persons who do not meet strict DSM or ICD definitions of disorder. These sources of error have implications for case finding and estimates of the true societal burden of mental illness. We here focus on three issues related to nosology and the definition of "caseness": threshold for a disorder, use of criterion versus non-criterion symptoms, and format of classification.

First, each syndrome defined in DSM or ICD has a threshold of symptom number (and often duration), above which a mental illness is present and below which a mental illness is not recognized. The threshold was achieved by expert clinical consensus, despite evidence of impairment present in individuals with subthreshold symptoms. It may be that a single chronic symptom constitutes a demand for treatment and is worthy of inclusion in a count of the mentally ill. This impact of subthreshold symptoms is seen in data from 1488 subjects assessed in the Duke University Epidemiological Catchment Area Study. This study revealed that counting subthreshold social phobia increased prevalence, and that those with the subthreshold condition reported considerable impairment in work, school, social interactions and other aspects of living [1]. Similarly, Mendlowicz and Stein found that persons meeting criteria for social phobia and those with non-comorbid, subthreshold social phobia had lower psychosocial functioning and reduced quality of life when compared with non-phobic normal subjects [2].

A long-term study of depression also illustrates the impact of subthreshold symptoms on outcomes. Judd *et al.* followed depression symptom expression for over 12 years in a cohort of 431 patients who met Research Diagnostic Criteria for major depressive disorder (MDD). While symptoms varied in this time frame from asymptomatic to the diagnostic threshold of MDD, 87% of the time was *not* spent at the MDD level [3]. Thus, an epidemiological study might have counted only a small percentage of depressives at any one point in time. Importantly, a gradient of psychosocial dysfunction accompanied even one or two symptoms over the 12 years of follow-up [4], and the presence of subthreshold symptoms was also associated with more rapid relapse to MDD [5].

In primary care settings subthreshold symptoms of anxiety appear more often than symptoms of the full-blown disorder, yet associated functional impairment is still present in the subthreshold patients. Olfson et al. [6] found that 6.6% of primary care patients had symptoms of anxiety, but only 3.7% met criteria for a specific disorder. Nevertheless, patients with subthreshold symptoms had significantly higher Sheehan Disability Scale scores (greater impairment) than did patients without psychiatric symptoms.

Second, the symptom lists in ICD/DSM represent "criterion symptoms" required to define the presence of a disorder, but important ancillary or "non-criterion symptoms" that contribute to the clinical picture and possibly the course of the disorder are not mentioned. Criterion symptoms are of central focus in most patients, but atypical cases that present with few or none of the DSM/ICD diagnostic criteria are often observed, especially in primary care settings. These presentations are classified in DSM-IV as "not otherwise specified" (NOS), one of the most used categories in the manual (ICD-10 has a similar designation), and in the clinical arena, psychopathology is often unmistakable in the patient with non-criterion symptoms.

Third, a dimensional approach recognizes the full complement of features associated with a clinical entity, including the importance of and possible impairment in subthreshold patients, as well as the non-criterion symptoms which, at times, are nearly pathognomonic for a disorder (e.g. panic patients who avoid tight-fitting neck wear). Cassano and his colleagues in the International Spectrum Project [7,8] have generated clinical instruments that incorporate criterion and non-criterion symptoms, see subthreshold conditions as clinically relevant, and hold behavioural traits and temperament as important determinants of clinical presentation and outcome [9]. Although epidemiological studies have not assessed non-criterion symptoms, several have recorded subthreshold symptoms and the count, of course, is much higher than that of full-blown disorders [1,10]. Most medical disciplines use categories for identifying cases and severity as a characterizing dimension. Given the clinical material that psychiatrists study and treat, a broader dimensional approach, beyond the severity, may be warranted. A nosology based on a spectrum and dimensional perspective could more accurately represent psychopathology than does the present format.

In conclusion, aggressive case finding should use both subthreshold criteria and non-criterion symptoms, but researchers and health care policy planners may want different thresholds for their different purposes. In the future, phenotypic clinical signs and symptoms may be complemented or replaced by biological markers, ensuring that the concept of caseness revolves around a discrete psychopathological entity. For now, there is recognition, both in clinical practice and research reports, that a continuum exists between asymptomatic, subthreshold symptomatic and symptoms that cross the diagnostic threshold. The accompanying gradient of impairment supports the idea that psychopathology begins before the DSM/ICD thresholds are met and that the definition of a case should be changed. If a spectrum format were to be adopted in DSM-V, the prevalence of disorders might change radically. The epidemiological data on panic and phobic disorders described by Andrews may therefore represent the tip of the psychopathological iceberg.

REFERENCES

1. Davidson J.R., Hughes D.C., George L.K., Blazer D.G. (1994) The boundary of social phobia: exploring the threshold. *Arch. Gen. Psychiatry*, **51**: 975–983.
2. Mendlowicz M.V., Stein M.B. (2000) Quality of life in individuals with anxiety disorders. *Am. J. Psychiatry*, **157**: 669–682.
3. Judd L.L., Akiskal H.S., Maser J.D., Zeller P., Endicott J., Coryell W., Paulus M.P., Kunovac J.L., Leon A.C., Mueller T.I. et al. (1998) A prospective 12-year study of depressive symptoms in major depressive disorders. *Arch. Gen. Psychiatry*, **55**: 694–700.
4. Judd L.L., Akiskal H.S., Zeller P., Paulus M., Leon A.C., Maser J.D., Endicott J., Coryell W., Kunovac J.L., Mueller T.I. et al. (2000) Psychosocial disability during the long-term course of unipolar major depressive disorder. *Arch. Gen. Psychiatry*, **57**, 375–380.
5. Judd L.L., Akiskal H.S., Maser J.D., Zeller P., Endicott J., Keller M.B., Coryell W., Paulus M.P., Kunovac J.L., Leon A.C. et al. (1998) Major depressive disorder: a prospective study of residual subthreshold depressive symptoms as predictor of rapid relapse. *J. Affect. Disord.*, **5**, 97–108.
6. Olfson M., Broadhead W.E., Weissman M.M., Leon A.C., Farber L., Hoven C., Kathol R. (1996) Subthreshold psychiatric symptoms in a primary care group practice. *Arch. Gen. Psychiatry*, **53**: 880–886.
7. Cassano G.B., Banti S., Mauri M., Dell'Osso L., Miniati M., Maser J.D., Shear K., Frank E., Grochocinski V., Rucci P. (1999) Internal consistency and discriminant validity of the Structured Clinical Interview for Panic Agoraphobic Spectrum. *Int. J. Meth. Psychiatr. Res.*, **8**: 138–144.
8. Maser J.D., Patterson T. (2002) Spectrum and nosology: implications for DSM-V. *Psychiatr. Clin. North Am.*, **25**: 855–885.
9. Cassano G.B., Michelini S., Shear M.K., Coli E., Maser J.D., Frank E. (1997) The panic–agoraphobic spectrum: a descriptive approach to the assessment and treatment of subtle symptoms. *Am. J. Psychiatry*, **154**: 27–38.
10. Broadhead W.E., Blazer D.G., George L.K., Tse C.K. (1990) Depression, disability days, and days lost from work in a prospective epidemiologic survey. *JAMA*, **264**: 2524–2528.

2.3
Phobias: A Difficult Challenge for Epidemiology
Carlo Faravelli[1]

An ambitious corporate lawyer has his office at the 12th floor of a high-rise building and he uses the stairs. When he is interviewed for an epidemiological survey, he admits being uneasy when in close spaces, but this does not limit him in any regards. It is true that he uses the stairs, but this is because "it is good for my health". As no other sign of psychopathology appears, and given that the criterion of occupational impairment is not met, he counts as a non-case in the epidemiological analysis. A couple of years later, this same lawyer is interviewed again for the second wave of the same research. At this point he had to leave his previous employment: his firm had relocated to the 37th floor of a new building and he cannot stand travelling in elevators. When asked by the interviewer for how long he has been troubled with this problem, he answers "since when I was a boy" and the interviewer notes the age of onset at, say, 16.

The same case brought by Gavin Andrews at the very beginning of his excellent review may be a good example of the difficulties that the epidemiologist encounters when dealing with phobic states.

Phobias are in fact some of the most difficult challenges for epidemiology. Epidemiology requires clearly defined diagnostic criteria (and this is the reason for the "epidemiological renaissance" after DSM-III), but it also needs precise and reliable definition of the boundary between cases and non-cases. When the existence of a psychiatric pathology is an "all or nothing" phenomenon, then the epidemiologists may give fairly accurate estimates, with low variation (and this is the case with panic disorder). Phobias are instead continuous phenomena, ranging from normality to extreme severity, and the choice of a cut-off point to differentiate normality from pathology is somehow arbitrary. The often discussed issue of social anxiety, ranging from slight shyness to the complete avoidance of social situations, is perhaps the best example. The main criterion suggested by present classifications (namely DSM-III and later nosologies) for differentiating pathological from non-pathological forms is functional impairment. This, however, though it may appear soundly rooted in common sense at first sight, is a severe limitation for the epidemiological studies. The variance due to external, culturally bound factors is in fact so heavy as to prevent reliable indications. The case of the lawyer cited above is a clear example: it would seem that the diagnosis of the disorder is based

---

[1] *Department of Psychiatry, University of Florence, Via Morgagni 85, 50100 Florence, Italy*

on the oscillations of the real estate market (availability of offices) rather than on psychopathological grounds. This is particularly true for agoraphobia and social phobia. The presence of a severe social phobia, for instance, is no obstacle for the life of a nun, while it is a serious limitation for a salesman. When we cross-tabulated the level of social avoidance with the social/occupational impairment, we found that the relationship was much weaker than expected [1]. Moreover, as Andrews points out, even minor changes in the choice of the diagnostic system and interviewing method adopted lead to dramatic changes in the prevalence figures. It is as if phobias represent a pyramid or an iceberg in which the slightest lowering of the point of recognition (or the level of the water in the case of the iceberg) is followed by terrific increases of the emerged part.

Quite often phobics are also phobic about being phobic. In other words the fear of having a psychiatric disorder is such that these subjects deny even to themselves the presence of psychological weaknesses ("I could travel in an elevator, but I prefer to climb the stairs in order to take some physical exercise"). This brings us to another consideration: when some evident and undeniable symptom occurs ("I cannot maintain my job if my office is situated at the 37th floor"), the defences are disrupted and the entire castle of self-deception falls. The probability of eliciting other symptoms previously "protected/defended" then arises, and this could be one of the reasons why the presence of one symptom increases the risk of almost all the other symptoms in psychiatry.

The identification of the age of onset of a phobia is probably influenced by the same fact. When a given pathology is detected, the usual structured interviews ask for the duration (or the age at onset) of the symptoms. It is common for the respondent to go back to the earliest manifestations ("since I remember" is the typical answer of the social phobic subject). It appears clear that recording this as the true age of onset is not appropriate when one adopts precise diagnostic criteria. The age at onset should be, if one wants to be rigorous, the first time that the subject met all the diagnostic criteria. This is either almost impossible to detect for phobic states or is determined by external circumstances, as in the case of the lawyer.

Phobias, especially simple phobias, are common in children, and are considered non-pathological before puberty. A child who is afraid of the dark is no concern: if such a fear persists at the military draft, then it can be a problem! Yet, most epidemiological surveys report lifetime estimates of phobias, without being particularly concerned about this issue.

The main problem with present epidemiological surveys, however, is the one related to the method adopted. Basically the epidemiology of phobias explores the avoidance of the feared objects/situations. Avoidance may also be due to other factors: diminution of drive and loss of interest for the social situations, delusional fears, peculiar beliefs that may be normal in a given cultural context, and others. In particular, the DSM-III, DSM-III-R and DSM-IV almost invariably require the diagnoser to check the criteria "not better accounted for by another disorder" and/or "not due to a medical condition, to a drug etc.". The lay interviewer cannot adhere to this requirement.

A more general issue is whether a psychiatric symptom may be assimilated to the answer to a standardized question. In other words, the main limitation of epidemiological studies in the field of anxiety and mood disorders is the implicit assumption that a standardized screening questionnaire read and recorded by non-clinicians may be equivalent to the clinical interview. So far, the studies of agreement between lay interviewers and clinical psychiatrists clearly demonstrate that the gap is still ample. Though not entering into the disputed issue of validity versus reliability, it seems that the general statement, emerging from all epidemiological surveys, that phobias are under-treated (or not treated adequately) is at least premature. A more cautious conclusion would be that most of the cases diagnosed as phobia are/were not receiving treatment. The push to regard all those falling into the category of phobic disorders as needing treatment is sponsored by those who can make a profit out of it. This is certainly true for some cases (the lawyer, for instance, but not the nun), but cannot be a rule on the basis of the present knowledge.

REFERENCE

1. Faravelli C., Zucchi T., Viviani B., Salmoria R., Perone A., Paionni A., Scarpato M.A., Vigliaturo D., Rosi S., D'Adamo D. et al. (2000) Epidemiology of social phobia: a clinical approach. *Eur. Psychiatry*, 15: 17–24.

2.4
Phobias: Handy or Handicapping Conditions
Peter Tyrer[1]

Gavin Andrews' review confirms what the reader probably suspects already: phobias are common and many are disabling. More disturbingly, the review suggests that many of those with phobias do not seek treatment or, if they do consult, do not receive those treatments that are recommended and evidence-based. It will also disturb the intelligent reader that there is such overlap, graced by the unfortunate term comorbidity, between the phobias and other mood and anxiety disorders. This commentary addresses

[1] *Department of Psychological Medicine, Imperial College, London W6 8RP, UK*

an issue that is very important in clinical practice: does the epidemiological evidence suggest we are failing in our care for this very important group of disorders?

I will deal with the positive answer to this question first. The case vignettes given by Gavin Andrews indicate a degree of handicap that is quite considerable: an ambitious lawyer who fails to achieve his potential because of a ludicrous fear of lifts, a housebound mother who fears a death-delivering panic, and a student who may give up a worthy profession to become a supermarket worker because of social fears. These are not ludicrous cases; they exist all around us and it is unreasonable to expect an ordinary general practitioner to have a significant therapeutic role in overcoming them. Yes, it is possible, but time and expertise are not commonplace in general practice and the relatively straightforward psychological treatments that are undoubtedly effective, including those written about so comprehensively by Gavin Andrews himself [1], can only be delivered with confidence from secondary care.

In practice, at least in the UK, with its relative shortage of psychiatrists, the treatment of phobias is far from satisfactory, as there is a bias towards the treatment of severe mental illness, and only the most severe phobias fall into this category, even though, as Andrews and others have argued [2], the burden created by phobias is great. General practitioners do not particularly want to deal with severe mental illness and have accepted the notion of a "primary care-led National Health Service" in which they are the prime providers for those with non-psychotic disorders and only provide medication and the care of physical illness for the psychotic patients [3]. The notion that phobic patients could be carefully guided back to health with judicious psychological and targeted drug treatment with proper acknowledgement of their work potential [4] is far from a reality.

On the negative side, we do not have as much evidence as we should like that our interventions are effective over the course of a phobic disorder. Despite all our apparent advances in the past 50 years, the prevalence of each of the anxiety disorders has changed very little, if at all. Approximately two out of five of those with common neurotic disorders, and phobias do not differ significantly from anxiety and depressive ones, have a poor long-term outcome [5,6], and even the good results of treatments such as cognitive-behaviour therapy [7] cannot disguise the fact that a minority still do very badly. This minority shows repeated diagnostic shift in their main diagnosis over time [8] and this is more common in those with personality disorder. The notion of the general neurotic syndrome [9,10] combines comorbidity of neurotic diagnoses and personality abnormality and for this group we have less evidence for effective treatments [6]. For this group it may indeed be handy to be able to retreat into phobic avoidance to prevent further distress at times of difficulty and in such instances the failure to seek help is more understandable.

In social anxiety disorder (phobia) there is also a great overlap with avoidant personality disorder [11] and it is therefore not surprising that more of those with social phobia than other anxiety disorders have personality abnormalities or disorder [12,13]; they may be the same condition. A majority of those with personality disorder are treatment resisting (type R) rather than treatment seeking (type S) [14] so do not seek help. In view of this, the alleged mismatch between personnel and resources may not be as great as the epidemiological data suggest, since the assumption that scientifically proven treatment recommendations are correct is unwarranted for a large group that we fail to identify in our fragmented classificatory system.

REFERENCES

1. Andrews G., Creamer M., Crino R., Hunt C., Lampe L., Page A. (2002) *The Treatment of Anxiety Disorders: Clinician Guides and Patient Manuals*, 2nd edn. Cambridge University Press, Cambridge.
2. Lépine J.P., Pelissolo A. (2000) Why take social anxiety disorder seriously? *Depress. Anxiety*, **11**: 87–92.
3. Bindman J., Johnson S., Wright S., Szmukler G., Bebbington P., Kuipers E., Thornicroft G. (1997) Integration between primary and secondary services in the care of the severely mentally ill: patients' and general practitioners' views. *Br. J. Psychiatry*, **171**: 169–174.
4. Boardman J., Grove B., Perkins R., Shepherd G. (2003) Work and employment for people with psychiatric disabilities. *Br. J. Psychiatry*, **182**: 467–468.
5. Tyrer P., Remington M., Alexander J. (1987) The outcome of neurotic disorders after out-patient and day hospital care. *Br. J. Psychiatry*, **151**: 57–62.
6. Tyrer P., Seivewright H., Johnson T. (2003). The core elements of neurosis: mixed anxiety–depression (cothymia) and personality disorder. *J. Personal. Disord.*, **17**: 109–118.
7. Juster H.R., Heimberg R.G. (1995) Social phobia: longitudinal course and long-term outcome of cognitive-behavioral treatment. *Psychiatr. Clin. North Am.*, **18**: 821–842.
8. Seivewright N., Tyrer P., Ferguson B., Murphy S., North B., Johnson T. (2000) Longitudinal study of the influence of life events and personality status on diagnostic change in three neurotic disorders. *Depress. Anxiety*, **11**: 105–113.
9. Tyrer, P. (1985) Neurosis divisible? *Lancet*, **i**: 685–688.
10. Andrews G., Stewart G., Morris-Yates A., Holt P., Henderson S. (1990) Evidence for a general neurotic syndrome. *Br. J. Psychiatry*, **157**: 6–12.
11. Herbert J.D., Hope D.A., Bellack A.S. (1992) Validity of the distinction between generalized social phobia and avoidant personality disorder. *J. Abnorm. Psychol.*, **101**: 332–339.
12. Sanderson W.C., Wetzler S., Beck A.T., Betz F. (1994) Prevalence of personality disorders among patients with anxiety disorders. *Psychiatry Res.*, **51**: 167–174.

13. Bienvenu O.J., Brown C., Samuels J.F., Liang K.Y., Costa P.T., Eaton W.W., Nestadt G. (2001) Normal personality traits and comorbidity among phobic, panic and major depressive disorders. *Psychiatry Res.*, **102**: 73–85.
14. Tyrer P., Mitchard S., Methuen C., Ranger M. (2003) Treatment-rejecting and treatment-seeking personality disorders: type R and type S. *J. Personal. Disord.*, **17**: 265–270.

2.5
Phobic Disorders: Can We Integrate Empirical Findings with Clinical Theories?

Marco Battaglia and Anna Ogliari[1]

From a purely clinical vantage point, a single patient with a phobic disorder (including panic disorder, agoraphobia, social phobia and simple phobias) may be seen as one among the least dramatic and disabling cases to be encountered in clinical practice. We know now how such an oversimplification can be misleading. When one considers the population at large, phobic disorders do constitute a serious problem in public health and can prove challenging to treat. However, when one considers the bulk of information on phobic disorders that comes from basic and applied empirical research and tries to draw connections with clinical wisdom, things become much more complicated. Several of the concepts, models and therapeutic guidelines employed routinely in clinical practice are based on theories, models, common sense, intuitions or assumptions that are sometimes challenged by empirical research. That is why evidence-based medicine is there, but sometimes the contrast is clashing. On the other hand, empirical research is reductive by definition, and needs only limited *a priori* assumptions (some of which can indeed be controlled, or falsified); hypothesis and results do not necessarily need to be related to any given major theory or model, so that each single research paper "must fill a place that before was empty and each contribution must be sturdy enough to bear the weight of contributions to come" [1]. Perhaps that is why empirical research is so hard to order in a comprehensive manner.

This commentary aims at highlighting a couple of apparent idiosyncrasies between clinical concepts and empirical findings in the domain of phobic disorders. It should be noted that the "direction of causation" here is meant to go both ways, i.e. sometimes concepts and expectations rooted in clinical practice are challenged by empirical findings, and other times

---

[1] *Department of Psychology, Vita-Salute San Raffaele University and Department of Neuropsychiatric Sciences, Istituto Scientifico San Raffaele Hospital, Via D'Ancona 20, Milan, Italy*

empirical research appears to proceed largely independently of time-honoured clinical evidence and wisdom. Two brief examples, both confined to a typical phobic disorder, namely panic disorder, will be provided.

First, is the stress–diathesis model relevant for phobias from an empirical vantage point? The stress–diathesis model [2] can be seen as an effort to describe a probabilistic network of causal factors along the pathway to a given illness. One simple prediction based on the stress–diathesis model, i.e. that the magnitude of stress at onset is inversely proportional to the level of underlying diathesis, has been recently controlled in a twin population sample study [3] by assessing the lifetime histories of five phobia subtypes (agoraphobia, social, animal, situational, blood/injury) and the mode of acquisition of the fear in phobic twins, considering five possible categories: trauma to self, observed trauma to others, observed fear in others, taught by others to be afraid, and no memory of how or why fear developed. The underlying diathesis was checked against the co-twin's risk for phobia. Studies of this kind are precious because they allow us to address the question of the ultimate causes of mental disorders based on epidemiological surveys. The results were inconsistent with several traditional etiologic theories for phobias, which assume conditioning or social transmission. Results were more compatible with *non-associative* models, which postulate that the vulnerability to phobias is largely innate and does not arise directly from environmental experiences. These results are consistent with previous findings from the same group [4] that showed how familial aggregation of phobias arise only from genetic determinants, while several traumatic experiences, non-specific in type and unrelated to any individual type of phobia, act as predisposing factors to many different types of phobias. Genetic factors for phobias are partially type-specific, and partially common to all types of phobias [4]. Thus, both genetic and environmentally unique (i.e. not shared within families) determinants are important contributors to influence an individual's liability to develop a phobic disorder. The Kendler *et al.* data [3,4], however, suggest that the influences of environmental variables on the risk of developing phobias take place in a fashion that is largely independent of typical associative mechanisms. Consistently with these results, in an attempt to explain the role of an endophenotype of panic disorder (hypersensitivity to suffocative stimuli and proneness to experience hyperventilation and anxiety after exposure to heightened concentrations of carbon dioxide), we [5,6] have suggested that interactions between aspecific adverse environmental events and a polygenic background can affect the functioning of brain systems that connect some elements of basic respiratory control to the affective states of air hunger and fear that are promoted when respiratory disturbance becomes a salient element of consciousness, via the cholinergic system. Our model is based upon experimental evidence that stressful and potentially harmful stimuli prime relatively long-lasting changes in cholinergic gene expression and cholinergic receptor regulation [7]. The adaptive sequels of these modifications include protection of the brain from overstimulation, and, at the level of the corticolimbic circuitries, promotion of passive avoidance and learning after stress. The extension of the same modifications to the cholinergic receptors involved in chemoception, however, could lower the threshold for reaction to suffocative stimuli, including carbon dioxide. The exaggerated sensitivity to carbon dioxide observed in humans suffering from panic attacks [8] could then be thought of as an evolutionary cost of the involvement of the cholinergic system in shaping otherwise adaptive responses to stress and threatening stimuli [6]. By this chain of events the first panic attacks could then be primed as responses to some *unconditioned* stimuli, while the endophenotype of heightened carbon dioxide responsiveness appears to be relatively specific to people with panic disorder, and occurs independent of a subject trait or state anxiety.

How can this line of reasoning be connected to the clinics of panic disorder? What is the place of learning and conditioning here? Panic attacks at the *onset* of panic disorder typically occur in an out-of-the-blue fashion. The first attacks are so typically characterized by physical symptoms, and so little fear is experienced, that most of these patients seek help for what they perceive as a cardiorespiratory crisis, or a congestion, and few attribute their symptoms to an anxiety disorder from inception. Of course, anxiety, learning, even fear and avoidance are in the picture, but typically occur at a later stage, when a subject gets to know that an attack may occur unpredictably, and learns to associate the occurrence of novel attacks with whatever environmental stimuli they can identify as "triggers". Importantly, however, especially at the onset of panic disorder, the alarm comes from inside the body, not from any external, identifiable source of menace. As consequence, in harmony with research findings, it is suggested that conditioned fear and learning models can only partially help explain panic disorder in the clinical context, and perhaps seeking a specific trauma that allegedly primed panic attacks is a less than optimal strategy in most patients.

Second, are current mouse models of human panic satisfactory from a clinical vantage point? While empirical research on human subjects starts questioning whether, and to what extent, "learning" can have a role in the etiology of phobias, a good deal of animal models (which are priceless tools to study gene–environment interactions in human mental disorders) of phobias seem to capitalize on two key concepts: (a) laboratory tests of anxiety that employ conditioning are better than paradigms based upon non-associative learning, and (b) the animal equivalent of human panic is *fear*.

Consistently with the human data exposed in the first section of this paper, it is suggested here that animal models of human anxiety based on conditioning and fear can be interesting for conditions such as generalized anxiety disorder, but their adoption for a human model of panic disorder can be misleading.

Why are animal researchers so keen on paradigms that imply conditioning? There are at least three important reasons in the mind of the authors of this paper. The first is that a mouse brain is constituted at 45% of its mass by the hippocampus, and "learning" comes easy as an explanation for many response phenotypes. The second is that measures of learning behaviours (e.g. entries in a radial maze) are much more reliable than any measures of emotional behaviour (e.g. heart rate) in the animal. The third is that conditioning-based paradigms are much more laboratory-controllable [9] than unconditioned paradigms.

The inappropriateness of equating human panic disorder to fear, however, has been described from inception, i.e. when panic disorder was differentiated from generalized anxiety disorder on the basis of differential response to benzodiazepines and tricyclics, respectively [7]. Moreover, lack of hypothalamic–pituitary–adrenal axis activation [7] further suggests that equating human panic to fear can be especially misleading for mouse models of human panic. Furthermore, in contrast with the expectation that paradigms that imply conditioning are considered more reliable than paradigms based upon non-associative learning, and somehow ironically, the most successful gene targeting studies of anxiety-related quantitative trait loci in mouse were based on non-associative learning paradigms (e.g. [10,11]).

In conclusion, while many "great models" of psychopathology are now no longer seen as undisputable, at least in part under the challenge of empirical research [12], we can now adopt a broader and critical view, and under the guidance of empirical research constructively criticize several previously uncontrolled assumptions of clinical psychology. Theoretical models and therapeutic paradigms are essential, but are to be controlled and refined by empirical (clinical and preclinical) research, and vice versa. Important contributions to a better integration of knowledge from research and clinical practice can derive from in-depth exploration of valuable endophenotypes, which constitute convenient mid-points between the crucial (but latent) variable of liability and the observed (but tricky) variable of clinical phenotypes. Keeping pace with the progress of empirical research, and integrating its contents with clinical wisdom, is for all of us one of the intellectual endeavours of our time.

ACKNOWLEDGEMENTS

The preparation of this paper was supported in part by a COFIN grant no. 11/2001-113555-004 and a NARSAD Independent Investigator Award.

REFERENCES

1. American Psychiatric Association (1983) *Publication Manual*, 3rd edn. American Psychiatric Association, Washington, DC.
2. Monroe S.M., Simons A.D. (1991) Diathesis–stress theories in the context of life stress research. *Psychol. Bull.*, **110**: 406–425.
3. Kendler K.S., Myers J., Prescott C.A. (2002) The etiology of phobias: an evaluation of the stress–diathesis model. *Arch. Gen. Psychiatry*, **59**: 242–248.
4. Kendler K.S., Neale M.C., Kessler R.C., Heath A.C., Eaves L.J. (1992) The genetic epidemiology of phobias in women: the inter-relationship of agoraphobia, social phobia, situational phobias, and simple phobias. *Arch. Gen. Psychiatry*, **49**: 273–281.
5. Battaglia M., Bertella S., Ogliari A., Bellodi L., Smeraldi E. (2001) Modulation by muscarinic antagonists of the response to carbon dioxide challenge in panic disorder. *Arch. Gen. Psychiatry*, **58**: 114–119.
6. Battaglia M. (2002) Beyond the usual suspects: a cholinergic route for panic attacks. *Mol. Psychiatry*, **7**: 239–246.
7. Kaufer D., Frideman A., Seidman S., Soreq H. (1998) Acute stress facilitates long-lasting changes in cholinergic gene expression. *Nature*, **393**: 373–377.
8. Klein D.F. (1993) False suffocation alarms, spontaneous panic, and related conditions. *Arch. Gen. Psychiatry*, **50**: 306–317.
9. Flint J. (2003) Animal models of anxiety. In *Behavioral Genetics in the Post-Genomic Era* (Eds R. Plomin, J.C. De Fries, I.W. Craig, P. McGuffin), pp. 425–442. American Psychiatric Association, Washington, DC.
10. Gershenfeld H.K., Paul S.M. (1997) Mapping QTLs for fear-like behaviors in mice. *Genomics*, **46**: 1–8.
11. Turri M.G, Datta S.R., DeFries J.C., Henderson N.D., Flint J. (2001) QTL analysis identifies multiple behavioral dimensions in ethological tests of anxiety in laboratory mice. *Curr. Biol.*, **11**: 725–734.
12. Rutter M.L. (1996) Developmental psychopathology: concepts and prospects. In *Frontiers of Developmental Psychopathology* (Eds M. Lenzenweger, I. Haugaard), pp. 209–237. Oxford University Press, New York.

2.6
Social Phobia and Bipolar Disorder:
The Significance of a Counterintuitive and Neglected Comorbidity

Hagop S. Akiskal[1] and Giulio Perugi[2]

Andrews' review of the epidemiology of phobic disorders, based on data gathered by the Diagnostic Interview Schedule (DIS) and the Composite International Diagnostic Interview (CIDI), raises the problem of the low test–retest reliability and validity of the lifetime estimates obtained with

---

[1] *International Mood Center, Department of Psychiatry at the University of California at San Diego, La Jolla, USA*
[2] *Institute of Psychiatry, University of Pisa, Italy*

structured interviews. This problem is particularly relevant in analysing the data on comorbidity between phobic and mood disorders and their interrelationships.

Epidemiological studies have been focused largely on comorbidity between phobias, in particular panic disorder with agoraphobia (PDA), social phobia (SP) and major depression; less attention has been devoted to the comorbidity between phobic and bipolar disorders. The co-occurrence of bipolar disorder in patients with phobias is counterintuitive, but increasing evidence for such a relationship comes from both epidemiological and clinical studies. In the National Comorbidity Survey [1], the reported risk of comorbid PDA and SP is higher in bipolar (odds ratios respectively of 11.0 versus 4.6) compared to major depressive disorder (odds ratios respectively of 7.0 versus 3.6). More recently, in subjects meeting DSM-IV hypomania, recurrent brief hypomania and sporadic brief hypomania, Angst [2] reported elevated rates of comorbidity with PDA and SP over population controls.

The foregoing findings from different epidemiological studies, in both Europe and the US, fly against a common perception that the relationship between anxiety and mood disorders is largely limited to "unipolar" depression and dysthymia. The relative neglect in epidemiological research for the comorbidity between bipolar spectrum disorders and phobic disorders is due to the relative underdiagnosis of bipolar II disorders, often misdiagnosed as unipolar or personality disorders [3]. Dunner and Kai Tay [4] reported that clinicians specifically trained in the recognition of bipolar II disorders outperformed routine interviewers in such structured interviews as the Schedule for Affective Disorders and Schizophrenia (SADS) or the Structured Clinical Interview for DSM-IV (SCID). This methodological point supports earlier recommendations based on research in Memphis [5] that the diagnosis of hypomania among cyclothymic bipolar II subjects should be based on *repeated* expert interviews. Although this point goes against the grain in the literature on structured interviewing, it is consistent in suggesting that the proper identification of bipolar II disorders requires a more sophisticated approach in diagnosis. Therefore, it is likely that bipolar comorbidity, very common in clinical samples [6], is not so easily detected in epidemiological studies utilizing structured interviews based on the diagnostic rules of DSM and ICD systems.

We do agree with Andrews' view that there are clinical issues in SP that warrant special attention. The following case makes that point:

> A 29-year-old single woman was unemployed when she presented for treatment at the clinical centre in Pisa. During her childhood, she was very shy and inhibited. At school, she was very anxious, exhibiting

marked neuro-vegetative symptoms and inability to talk fluently during oral examinations. During adolescence, she reported major problems in speaking in public, coping with the opposite sex, and performing in a lot of social situations, she blushed heavily and made every effort to avoid these situations. She sought psychiatric help for the first time in her life at the age of 26 upon the insistence of her parents. She was treated with paroxetine (40 mg/day) and after a few weeks her social phobia improved. In the following months she appeared less embarrassed in interpersonal contexts, social anxiety completely disappeared and impudence and shamelessness took its place. She felt elated and increasingly self-confident and progressively developed the firm belief that other people could be envious of her because of her qualities and abilities. She started to drink alcohol at night and she became aggressive towards her parents, who prevented her from spending money and having sexual relationships with several boyfriends. After a car accident, while she was drunk and severely agitated, she was hospitalized and treated with lithium and antipsychotics and after 40 days she was discharged. She continued to be treated with mood stabilizers, while antipsychotics were gradually tapered. After a few months, she found a new job and stopped the pharmacological treatment on her own. She was again socially anxious and she had problems with job and interpersonal relationships. Three months ago, she found an article in a newspaper describing SP, and she presented to a centre for treatment of social anxiety and depression. Despite clinical inquiries about past mania and hypomania, during the first psychiatric evaluation she did not report the previous manic episode and she mentioned "depression" as the cause of her hospitalization. According to the SCID-P, completed during the second interview, she was diagnosed as comorbid SP and major depression, with lifetime history of episodic alcohol abuse. The manic nature of her previous episode was evident only after several further interviews, collateral information from her parents, and in-depth review of her psychiatric record from another hospital. This more systematic diagnostic approach also revealed that her maternal grandmother had suffered from documented manic–depressive illness.

This case illustrates the difficulty of bipolar diagnosis with a cross-sectional structured interview. Even greater difficulties are involved in ascertaining the diagnosis of bipolar II disorders where past records on hypomania are usually absent [7,8]. This case also supports Andrews' view that phobias are not disorders of minor clinical importance: they constitute a major public health problem, because they often represent the "fore-runners" of other mental disorders [6]. Actually, in a prospective study [9] of predictors of bipolar II outcome among a large US national cohort of major depressives, phobic anxiety and mood lability were among the most decisive.

The pattern of complex relationships among SP and mood disorders would require better designed prospective epidemiological observations. Nonetheless, the validity of the phenomenon of SP–bipolar comorbidity should no longer be in doubt. In clinical samples, usually SP chronologically precedes (hypo)manic episodes and disappears when the latter episodes supervene [10]. Protracted social anxiety may represent, along with inhibited depression, the dimensional opposite of hypomania [6,11]. The link between bipolarity and SP would seem to be related primarily to a subtype of social anxiety, characterized by fear of multiple social situations, which involve dealing with non-structured or emotionally-laden interpersonal contexts [12]. This, together with a greater avoidance resulting from subtle volitional inhibition, would explain the more severe impairment in bipolar social phobics. Finally, the increased susceptibility to alcohol use in some patients with SP might be related more to the presence of a bipolar diathesis, with marked reactivity to ethanol, than to the social-phobic symptomatology itself [13]. The socializing and disinhibiting effect that many SP patients report with alcohol use might be mediated by increased confidence as part of the hypomania induced by alcohol.

The recognition of bipolar comorbidity in phobic patients has significant theoretical and practical implications. From the theoretical point of view, in hypothesizing a putative common substrate, the fact that not only depression, but also (hypo)mania and mixed states frequently coexist with anxious–phobic disorders should be taken into account in attempts to conceptualize social anxiety. Hypomanic switch on antidepressants or alcohol—and bipolar II disorder—represent prevalent coexisting mood states in the longitudinal history of SP. Such "comorbidity" poses a major problem for Andrews' hypothesis of a "general neurotic syndrome", unless he is prepared to include bipolar II disorders, hypomania and alcohol use among the neurotic conditions! Severity and generalization of the phobic symptoms, multiple comorbidity and alcohol and substance abuse appear to be the most relevant practical consequences of SP–bipolar comorbidity [12], giving rise to complex therapeutic dilemmas.

We submit that the foregoing considerations challenge the view that phobias are isolated syndromes, and enrich the scope of social phobias from psychopathological, clinical, public health and theoretical perspectives.

REFERENCES

1. Kessler R.C., McGonagle K.A., Zhao S., Nelson C.B., Hughes M., Eshleman S. (1994) Lifetime and 12 months prevalence of DSM III-R psychiatric disorders in

the United States: results from the National Comorbidity Survey. *Arch. Gen. Psychiatry*, **51**: 8–19.
2. Angst J. (1998) The emerging epidemiology of hypomania and bipolar II disorder. *J. Affect. Disord.*, **50**: 143–151.
3. Akiskal H.S., Bourgeois M.L., Angst J., Post R., Moller H.J., Hirschfeld R.M.A. (2000) Re-evaluating the prevalence of and diagnostic composition within the broad clinical spectrum of bipolar disorders. *J. Affect. Disord.*, **59** (Suppl. 1): 5s–30s.
4. Dunner D.L., Kai Tay L. (1993) Diagnostic reliability of the history of hypomania in bipolar II patients with major depression. *Compr. Psychiatry*, **34**: 303–307.
5. Akiskal H.S., Djenderedjian A.M., Rosenthal R.H., Khani M.K. (1977) Cyclothymic disorder: validating criteria for inclusion in the bipolar affective group. *Am. J. Psychiatry*, **134**: 1227–1233.
6. Perugi G., Akiskal H.S., Ramacciotti S., Nassini S., Toni C., Milanfranchi A., Musetti L (1999) Depressive comorbidity of panic, social phobic and obsessive–compulsive disorders: is there a bipolar II connection? *J. Psychiatr. Res.*, **33**: 53–61.
7. Hantouche E.G., Akiskal H.S., Lancrenon S., Allilaire J.F., Sechter D., Azorin J.M., Bourgeois M., Fraud J.P., Châtenet-Duchêne L. (1998) Systematic clinical methodology for validating bipolar-II disorder: data in mid-stream from a French national multisite study (EPIDEP). *J. Affect. Disord.*, **50**: 163–173.
8. Benazzi F., Akiskal H.S. (2003) Refining the evaluation of bipolar II: beyond the strict SCID-CV guidelines for hypomania. *J. Affect. Disord.*, **73**: 33–38.
9. Akiskal H.S., Maser J.D., Zeller P., Endicott J., Coryell W., Keller M., Warshaw M., Clayton P., Goodwin F.K. (1995) Switching from "unipolar" to bipolar II: an 11-year prospective study of clinical and temperamental predictors in 559 patients. *Arch. Gen. Psychiatry*, **52**: 114–123.
10. Perugi G., Akiskal H.S., Toni C., Simonini E., Gemignani A. (2001) The temporal relationship between anxiety disorders and (hypo)mania: a retrospective examination of 63 panic, social phobic and obsessive–compulsive patients with comorbid bipolar disorder. *J. Affect. Disord.*, **67**: 199–206.
11. Himmelhoch J.M. (1998) Social anxiety, hypomania and the bipolar spectrum: data, theory and clinical issues. *J. Affect. Disord.*, **50**: 203–213.
12. Perugi G., Frare F., Toni C., Mata B., Akiskal H.S. (2001) Bipolar II and unipolar comorbidity in 153 outpatients with social phobia. *Compr. Psychiatry*, **42**: 375–381.
13. Perugi G., Frare F., Madaro D., Maremmani I., Akiskal H.S. (2002) History of alcohol abuse in social phobic patients is related to bipolar comorbidity. *J. Affect. Disord.*, **68**: 33–39.

2.7
Comorbidity between Phobias and Mood Disorders: Diagnostic and Treatment Implications
Zoltán Rihmer[1]

Andrews' comprehensive review clearly shows that the panic/phobic group of disorders is quite prevalent, disabling and, similarly to many other mental disorders, is under-referred and under-treated. The interaction of these four facts and the universal finding that panic/phobic disorders have an early age of onset can easily explain why these disorders represent a major public health problem everywhere in the world.

The results of a comprehensive epidemiological programme to assess the prevalence of affective and anxiety/phobic disorders showed that panic and phobias are also frequent in Hungary. Investigating the prevalence of anxiety and phobia disorders in a random, representative sample of the Hungarian adult population (aged between 18 and 64 years), it has been found that the past-year prevalences of panic disorder, agoraphobia, social phobia and specific phobia were 3.1%, 10.5%, 4.9% and 4.8%, respectively. The lifetime prevalence rates for the same disorders were 4.4%, 15.3%, 6.4% and 6.3%, respectively [1,2]. These figures are in the same range as reported by Andrews in his review, suggesting that economic and cultural differences have no significant influence on the frequency of panic/phobic disorders. More than half (55%) of the patients with past-year diagnosis of panic disorder also had agoraphobia [2]. Investigating the lifetime comorbidity between panic/phobic disorders and major mood disorders, it has been found that the rate of agoraphobia and specific phobia was the highest in bipolar II patients (20.8% and 37.5%, respectively), social phobia was most prevalent in unipolar major depression (17.6%), while the rate of panic disorder was the same in the unipolar major depressive and bipolar II subgroups (12.4% and 12.5%, respectively). Bipolar I patients, in general, showed a relatively low rate of lifetime comorbidity [3]. In other words, panic disorder, agoraphobia and specific phobia were found to have the greatest tendency to co-occur with unipolar major depression and to show the lowest rate of comorbidity with bipolar I disorder (4.2%). Similarly, Judd et al. [4] found that the lifetime prevalence of phobic disorders was significantly higher in bipolar II than in bipolar I patients (22.5% and 11.8%, respectively).

One possible explanation of the highest degree of comorbidity between panic/phobic disorders and bipolar II illness might be the finding that

---

[1] *National Institute for Psychiatry and Neurology, Budapest 27, POB 1, H-1281 Hungary*

panic disorder and bipolar II disorder are genetically related to each other [5]. The clinical (and theoretical) significance of these different patterns of panic/phobia comorbidity between unipolar major depression, bipolar II and bipolar I disorder is unknown. However, considering the fact that 13–46% of unipolar depressives later convert into bipolar II or bipolar I disorder [6,7], it is possible that panic/phobic disorder in patients with "unipolar" depression is the reflection of bipolar (mainly bipolar II) genotype, and can be an early clinical marker for further bipolar transformation as well. The importance of the early recognition of bipolarity is underlined by the facts that antidepressants are widely used in panic/phobic disorders and, without mood stabilizers, antidepressants can easily induce mixed states, hypomanic/manic switches and rapid cycling in patients with unrecognized bipolarity [8–10].

REFERENCES

1. Szádóczky E., Papp Z., Vitrai J., Rihmer Z., Füredi J. (1998) The prevalence of major depressive and bipolar disorders in Hungary: results from a national epidemiologic survey. *J. Affect. Disord.*, **50**: 153–162.
2. Szádóczky E., Papp Z., Vitrai J., Füredi J. (2000) A hangulat- és szorongásos zavarok elöfordulása a felnött magyar lakosság körében [The prevalence of mood and anxiety disorders in the adult population of Hungary]. *Orvosi Hetilap*, **141**: 17–22.
3. Rihmer Z., Szádóczky E., Füredi J., Kiss K., Papp Z. (2001) Anxiety disorders comorbidity in bipolar I, bipolar II and unipolar major depression: results from a population-based study in Hungary. *J. Affect. Disord.*, **67**: 175–179.
4. Judd L.L., Akiskal H.S., Schettler P.J., Coryell W., Maser J., Rice J.A., Solomon D.A., Keller M.B. (2003) The comparative clinical phenotype and long-term longitudinal episode course of bipolar I and bipolar II: a clinical spectrum of distinct disorders? *J. Affect. Disord.*, **73**: 19–32.
5. MacKinnon D.F., Zandi P.P., Cooper J., Potash J.B., Simpson S.G., Gershon E., Nurnberger J., Reich T., DePaulo J.R. (2002) Comorbid bipolar disorder and panic disorder in families with a high prevalence of bipolar disorder. *Am. J. Psychiatry*, **159**: 30–35.
6. Akiskal H.S., Maser J.D., Zeller P.J., Endicott J., Coryell W., Keller M., Warshaw M., Clayton P., Goodwin F.K. (1995) Switching from "unipolar" to bipolar II: an 11-year prospective study of clinical and temperamental predictors in 559 patients. *Arch. Gen. Psychiatry*, **52**: 114–123.
7. Goldberg J.F., Harrow M., Whiteside J.F. (2001) Risk for bipolar illness in patients initially hospitalized for unipolar depression. *Am. J. Psychiatry*, **158**: 1265–1270.
8. Ghaemi S.N., Boiman E.F., Goodwin F.K. (2000) Diagnosing bipolar disorder and the effect of antidepressants: a naturalistic study. *J. Clin. Psychiatry*, **61**: 804–808.

9. Henry C., Sorbara F., Lacoste J., Gindre C., Leboyer M. (2001) Antidepressant-induced mania in bipolar patients: identification of risk factors. *J. Clin. Psychiatry*, **62**: 249–255.
10. Bottlender R., Rudolf D., Strauss A., Möller H.-J. (2001) Mood-stabilizers reduce the risk of developing antidepressant-induced maniform states in acute treatment of bipolar I depressed patients. *J. Affect. Disord.*, **63**: 79–83.

2.8
Epidemiology of Phobias: Old Terminology, New Relevance
Laszlo A. Papp[1]

In reading a review of recent epidemiological surveys of "phobic" conditions, one should not be surprised by inconsistencies and confusing numbers followed by predictable and somewhat common-sense conclusions. The confusion is partly due to the concept of "phobias". If defined as unreasonable fear and subsequent avoidance of relevant triggers, phobias are part of most anxiety disorders. In fact, one could argue, especially from this side of the Atlantic, that, at least from an epidemiological point of view, a focus on "phobias" has become anachronistic. One of the most important achievements of our evolving diagnostic systems, both DSM and ICD, is that certain historical terms like "neuroses" have been retired and replaced by more meaningful diagnoses. Strictly speaking, the only DSM anxiety disorders remaining in the "phobia" category are specific phobias.

Given that epidemiological surveys are bound by the prevailing diagnostic systems, any current review is thus forced to make arbitrary decisions with regard to which anxiety disorder would qualify as a "phobic condition". Gavin Andrews decided to include panic disorder with or without agoraphobia, social phobia (or social anxiety disorder, as it is now called) and specific phobias. He argues that this choice was dictated by the preponderance of surveys that do not differentiate among phobic conditions, lump panic disorder with and without agoraphobia as one anxiety disorder, and/or follow the diagnostic system of the most current DSM or ICD. While I agree with some of the choices, I disagree with the rationale. For instance, the reason most surveys consider panic disorder with and without agoraphobia as one condition is that research has clearly established basic similarities between them, including no substantive differences in treatment response [1] and neurobiology [2]. One could also question the exclusion of generalized anxiety disorder, obsessive–

---

[1] *New York State Psychiatric Institute, Columbia University, 1051 Riverside Drive, New York, NY 10032, USA*

compulsive disorder and post-traumatic stress disorder, as many patients with these conditions suffer from significant phobic avoidance. To the extent that these concerns are primarily diagnostic, they should be better covered in the appropriate section in this volume. However, it is possible that new developments in neuroscience will again make phobic avoidance an important target for anxiety disorders research. Specifically, recent technology is making it possible to examine the neuroanatomy and neurochemistry of select symptoms of an anxiety disorder such as fear, worry or phobic avoidance. As these symptoms cut across diagnostic categories, future epidemiological studies may focus on avoidance behaviour as a dimension of most anxiety disorders, making the epidemiology of phobias increasingly meaningful once more.

Epidemiological surveys lead to changes in diagnostic thinking, making past surveys obsolete, necessitating new surveys using the new diagnostic categories. Fortunately, progress in epidemiology is not limited to using refined—or simply re-defined—diagnostic categories. As Gavin Andrews' review demonstrates, novel interviewing and data analytic methods, and data from treatment studies, augmented by neuroscience research, will add substantially to the value of these surveys.

In addition to terminology, an important source of potential confusion—and limitation—in epidemiological surveys and reviews is their narrow focus on the general adult population. Rarely do these studies take into consideration the needs of special populations such as the elderly, women and children. This omission is particularly noteworthy in the elderly, which is the fastest growing segment of our population.

According to a recent consensus statement [3], the Epidemiological Catchment Area (ECA) study grossly underdiagnosed psychiatric disorders in the elderly due to the use of age-inappropriate diagnostic criteria [4]. Specifically, because of prominent somatic complaints, concomitant or underlying anxiety disorders are frequently overlooked in older patients [5]. Significant anxiety, as distinct from disorders, may be even more prevalent among the elderly. Up to 52% reported symptoms of anxiety in a survey of 516 elderly patients between the ages of 70 and 103 [6]. Surveys that focus on anxiety symptoms rather than anxiety disorders indicate steadily increasing rates of anxiety as individuals age [7] and confirm that over half of the elderly may suffer from clinically significant anxiety [6,8–10]. Contrary to common belief, a recent large survey also demonstrated that the disability attributable to anxiety in the elderly is comparable to and independent from that of depression [8].

Rather than the nature of the specific anxiety disorder, age-related features of any anxiety disorder in late life, such as possible executive dysfunction, the impact of comorbidity (most importantly depression), and multiple real life-stresses combined with diminishing coping skills and resources, clearly differentiate the needs of the elderly from those of younger adults with comparable pathology. Also due to age-related factors, rates of response and remission are lower in the elderly compared to the general population. Late-life anxiety disorders, frequently complicated with significant phobic avoidance, are some of the most treatment-resistant psychiatric conditions.

My earlier reservations notwithstanding, I do concur with Gavin Andrews'—unstated but implied—conclusion that in spite of the confusion regarding the definition of "phobias", valid and relevant epidemiological statements can be made based on a number of large and diverse surveys. Fortunately for psychiatric epidemiology, these surveys do utilize the increasingly evidence-based categories for specific anxiety disorders rather than ask about "phobias". The best evidence of the validity of these surveys is the relatively consistent figures with respect to prevalence, incidence, age of onset, gender differences, risk factors and comorbidity. The epidemiology of phobic avoidance may become a promising new area based on the dimensional approach of neuroscience to the understanding of anxiety disorders.

There remains a substantial void in addressing the needs of special patient populations with anxiety disorders such as the elderly. Given the enormous economic and social impact of untreated, chronic mental illness in this large and rapidly growing segment of the population, it is imperative that commensurate resources be made available to assess and address their concerns.

REFERENCES

1. Papp L.A. (1999) Somatic treatment of anxiety disorders. In *Comprehensive Textbook of Psychiatry*, 7th edn (Eds H.I. Kaplan, B.J. Sadock), pp. 1490–1498. Williams & Wilkins, Philadelphia, PA.
2. Papp L.A., Martinez J.M., Klein D.F., Coplan J.D., Norman R.G., de Jesus M.J., Ross D., Goetz R., Gorman J.M. (1997) Respiratory psychophysiology of panic disorder: three respiratory challenges in 98 subjects. *Am. J. Psychiatry*, **154**: 1557–1565.
3. Jeste D.V., Alexopoulos G.S., Bartels S.J., Cummings J.L., Gallo J.J., Gottlieb G.L., Halpain M.C., Palmer B.W., Patterson T.L., Reynolds C.F. III *et al.* (1999) Consensus statement on the upcoming crisis in geriatric mental health: research agenda for the next two decades. *Arch. Gen. Psychiatry*, **56**: 848–853.
4. Jeste D.V. (2000) Geriatric psychiatry may be the mainstream psychiatry of the future. *Am. J. Psychiatry*, **157**: 1912–1914.
5. Turnbull J.M. (1989) Anxiety and physical illness in the elderly. *J. Clin. Psychiatry*, **50**: 40–45.
6. Schaub R.T., Linden M. (2000) Anxiety and anxiety disorders in the old and very old—results from the Berlin Aging Study (BASE). *Compr. Psychiatry*, **41** (Suppl. 1): 48–54.

7. Sallis J.F., Lichstein K.L. (1983) Analysis and management of geriatric anxiety. *Int. J. Aging Hum. Develop.*, **15**: 194–211.
8. Kessler R.C., DuPont R.L., Berglund P., Wittchen H. (1999) Impairment in pure and comorbid generalized anxiety disorder and major depression at 12 months in two national surveys. *Am. J. Psychiatry*, **156**: 1915–1923.
9. Beekman A.T., de Beurs E., van Balkom A., Deeg D., van Dyck R., Tillburg W. (2000). Anxiety and depression in later life: co-occurrence and communality of risk factors. *Am. J. Psychiatry*, **157**: 89–95.
10. Szádóczky E., Papp Z., Vitrai J., Füredi J. (2000) The prevalence of mood and anxiety disorders in the adult population of Hungary. *Orvosi Hetilap*, **141**: 17–22.

2.9
Phobias: Reflections on Definitions

Elie G. Karam[1,2] and Nay G. Khatcherian[2]

Although phobias are classified as part of anxiety disorders, what applies to anxiety disorders does not necessarily apply to phobias and what applies to a given phobia does not necessarily apply to another phobia. There are advantages in lumping them together, but they do differ in many aspects. Phobias as a group and anxiety disorders as a family do not have similar "clinical significance", comorbidity, age of onset and treatment outcome.

The issue of "clinical significance" as an essential criterion for diagnosis is still an open question for all mental disorders [1]: there is a true problem in our mind in equating statistical normality with the absence of pathology in the field of phobias and in psychiatry in general. Phobias can be assimilated to allergies: we do not need to be treated for all allergies; we need to be treated for those allergies we most probably will be exposed to or that constitute great danger if we are ever exposed to them. Thus the issue of diagnosis needs to be dissociated in the minds of mental health workers (not only in the field of phobia) from that of necessity for treatment. This does not mean that the proneness to phobia could not by itself be regarded as a marker, even if it has not produced major distress in one's life, the same way most specialists would recognize genetic proneness to allergy even if no anaphylactic reaction has occurred so far in the life of an individual.

While the clinician might not necessarily feel concerned about the above-mentioned dilemma, the issue of clinical significance is of actual importance in large epidemiological studies. We encountered, for example, two problems in this respect in our large ongoing study (World Mental Health

---

[1] *Department of Psychiatry and Psychology, Faculty of Medicine, Balamand University, Beirut, Lebanon*
[2] *Institute for Development, Research and Applied Care (IDRAC), Beirut, Lebanon*

2000/Lebanon). The first is related to the definition of "excessive" as an essential feature of the fear symptoms. The second is related to the assessment of impairment, a criterion to be fulfilled for the person to qualify for phobia: the question "How much did your fear ever interfere with either your work, your social life or your personal relationships?" has led not infrequently in Lebanon to "not at all" answers. How much do we have to probe in a field interview on the clear potential impairment related to the fear of, say, swimming in one's social life? These are not merely theoretical issues. They really lie at the core of the definition and become very important in research for etiology and treatment.

In the same spirit, if phobias are looked at merely as markers, then treatment would depend only on impairment, but if they herald future complications or other disorders then early treatment becomes of paramount importance. One needs to remember that phobias and anxiety disorders in general are among the earliest disorders that appear in one's life. A study by Dadds *et al.* reviewed by Andrews and Wilkinson [2] showed that early intervention with cognitive-behavioural therapy (CBT) among anxious children halves the risk of meeting anxiety disorder criteria (we still have, however, many questions on control groups in psychotherapy studies [3]). But, which phobia, if prevented or treated, would decrease the chance of developing other disorders as adults? While agoraphobia and social phobia are likely candidates, could the same be said about other phobias? We think that early identification of phobias and more specifically the ones that carry more disability (social phobia and agoraphobia) is imperative and this can be achieved through better social awareness, education of teachers (as has been done for attention-deficit/hyperactivity disorder) and direct contact with caretakers.

Finally, we would like to introduce here an issue that has been largely neglected in psychiatry and that we hope to study in a large community sample: that of disgust. While it has been suggested that disgust sensitivity may play a role in the development of animal and blood–injection–injury phobias [4], more research on the relationship of disgust sensitivity to specific phobias and to the expression of disgust in anxiety disorders in general would be quite interesting.

REFERENCES

1. Wakefield J.C., Spitzer R.L. (2002) Why requiring clinical significance does not solve epidemiology's and DSM's validity problem: response to Regier and Narrow. In *Defining Psychopathology in the 21st Century* (Eds J.E. Helzer, J.J. Hudziak), pp. 31–40. American Psychiatric Publishing, Washington, DC.
2. Andrews G., Wilkinson D.D. (2002) The prevention of mental disorders in young people. *Med. J. Australia*, **177**: S97–S100.

3. Karam E.G., Karam A.N., Fayyad J.A., Cordahi C., Mneimneh Z., Melhem N., Zebouni V., Kayali G., Yabroudi P., Rashidi N. et al. (2002) Community group therapy in children and adolescents exposed to war. Presented at the 49th Annual Meeting of the American Association of Child and Adolescent Psychiatry, San Francisco, 22–27 October.
4. Sawchuk C.N., Lohr J.M., Tolin D.F., Lee T.C., Kleinknecht R.A. (2000) Disgust sensitivity and contamination fears in spider and blood–injection–injury phobias. *Behav. Res. Ther.*, **38**: 753–762.

2.10
Phobias: Facts or Fiction?

Rudy Bowen[1] and Murray B. Stein[2]

Phobias, fears and avoidance are a fascinating topic because fears touch on the lives of most people. Even though many studies enable broad agreement about the prevalence of phobias, questions remain about the validity of prevalence rates and the identification of cases by lay interviewers in large studies. In an assessment of Diagnostic Interview Schedule (DIS) diagnoses that were obtained by lay interviewers at one site of the Epidemiological Catchment Area (ECA) study, psychiatrists used the Present State Examination supplemented by additional questions [1]. The agreement was low for phobias, with the lay interviewers finding a 1-month prevalence of 11.2% and the psychiatrists finding 21.3%. Even for cases negative for phobias, the agreement between psychiatrists and lay interviewers about the absence of phobias (82.5%) was the lowest of the eight disorders studied. Quite apart from the rates, the lay interviewers and psychiatrists for the most part identified different individuals as having phobias. Subsequent studies have shown that good agreement can be attained, but these are usually in smaller subgroups of subjects [2].

Disagreements tend to be most marked when subjects have several complaints that place them close to the boundaries of phobic syndromes. People report many fears that are difficult to classify into a few discrete categories [2]. In Canada, it is common in clinical practice to encounter patients with an apparently unreasonable fear of slipping on the ice, as a reason for not leaving the home in winter, but it is not clear whether this is agoraphobia or a specific fear [2]. Minor differences in wording of questions can make large differences to rates. Prevalence of phobias for ethnic

---

[1] *Department of Psychiatry, University of Saskatchewan, 103 Hospital Drive, Saskatoon, S7N 0W8, Canada*
[2] *Department of Psychiatry, University of California, San Diego, 8950 Villa La Jolla Drive, La Jolla, CA 92037, USA*

minority women was higher in one ECA site apparently because they lived in genuinely more dangerous neighbourhoods, so it is sometimes unclear whether avoidance is reasonable or not.

It is also undecided whether phobias are best seen as distinct categories or whether a dimensional view might be more useful for research, but if one takes the latter position, the best approach to dimensions is not apparent. One can measure fear and/or avoidance although some of both are usually required. Questions about avoidance often become hypothetical, if the individual never or rarely encounters the fear. Does someone who fears aardvarks and thinks he would avoid one if he did encounter one, and yet has never encountered an aardvark, have an aardvark phobia? Disability is important since not all of the phobias identified in epidemiological surveys are clinically significant, even if a general question on disability is included in the diagnostic criteria. Other factor(s) such as neuroticism, or fear of anxiety symptoms, or whether the phobia remits spontaneously, or the person learns to overcome it on his own, may be important in determining disability.

Furthermore, even the choice of an appropriate measurement instrument is a dilemma. The 9-point avoidance scale used in the 13 specific situation Fear Questionnaire (15 questions total) has been widely used, because despite its known limitations there is no adequate replacement [3,4]. The alternative solution would be to measure the number of fears, but there is no acknowledged ideal number, as illustrated in the many versions of the Fear Survey Schedule (FSS) [5].

On the question of comorbidity, it not easy even for experienced clinicians to elicit, in a reasonable amount of time, all of the phobic behaviours in different psychiatric conditions such as the fears of being seen in public in body dysmorphic disorder, avoidance of situations associated with obsessing, avoidance of complex stimuli in the autism spectrum disorders, difficulty in interacting with people and consequent avoidance in depression, fears of expressing some emotions, interoceptive fears, and the huge problem of avoidance "ascribed to medical causes without adequate evidence" [6]. A few examples of these are gastrointestinal symptoms, total allergy syndromes, fatigue and pain syndromes.

We agree that panic and phobias are common problems that are often limiting and disabling, and that they constitute a public health problem. Public policy such as teaching in schools about coping may play a role. When seat-belt use was made mandatory in the Canadian province of Saskatchewan, there were dozens of requests from physicians for medical exemptions for patients. These people were apparently anxious about wearing seatbelts, and believed that they had medical complaints that prevented them from complying with the law, and they sought medical intervention for the condition. Presumably some of them would have met diagnostic criteria for a seatbelt or a situational phobia. It was soon recognized that there were practically no medical reasons for exemptions and this was publicized, so no exemptions were granted [7]. Presumably, these people continue to drive with seatbelts because compliance among Saskatchewan drivers is high. This example suggests that avoidance and disability attached to phobias are highly contextual, and subject to social (and, apparently, legal) influences. These factors make it all the more difficult to accurately gauge the prevalence and impairment associated with phobias.

We concur with the conclusion that effective treatments are available and that better use could be made of existing resources, but how and when to introduce effective treatments for people with several comorbid conditions is not well researched. We would add the proviso that more funding for targeted research on phobias is needed and particularly for research on the implementation of treatment.

REFERENCES

1. Anthony J.C., Folstein M., Romanowski A.J., Von Korff M.R., Nestad G.R., Chahal R., Merchant A., Brown C.H., Shapiro S.K., Kramer M. et al. (1985) Comparison of the lay Diagnostic Interview Schedule and a standardized psychiatric diagnosis: experience in eastern Baltimore. *Arch. Gen. Psychiatry*, **42**: 667–675.
2. Wittchen H.-U., Reed V., Kessler R.C. (1998) The relationship of agoraphobia and panic in a community sample of adolescents and young adults. *Arch. Gen. Psychiatry*, **55**: 1017–1024.
3. Marks I.M., Mathews A.M. (1979) Brief standard self-rating for phobic patients. *Behav. Res. Ther.*, **17**: 263–267.
4. Shear M.K., Maser J.D. (1994) Standardized assessment for panic disorder research. *Arch. Gen. Psychiatry*, **51**: 346–354.
5. Wolpe J., Lang P.J. (1964) A fear survey schedule for use in behaviour therapy. *Behav. Res. Ther.*, **2**: 27–30.
6. Walker E.A., Katon W.J., Jemelka R.P., Roy-Bryne P.P. (1992) Comorbidity of gastrointestinal complaints, depression, and anxiety in the Epidemiologic Catchment Area (ECA) Study. *Am. J. Med.*, **92** (Suppl. 1A): 26S–30S.
7. Christian M.S. (1979) Exemption from compulsory wearing of seat belts—medical indications. *Br. Med. J.*, **26**: 1411–1412.

2.11
Epidemiology of Phobias: The Pathway to Early Intervention in Anxiety Disorders

Michael Van Ameringen[1,2], Beth Pipe[2] and Catherine Mancini[1,2]

Comparison of epidemiological data for most psychiatric disorders is a complicated endeavour, and Gavin Andrews has accurately identified problems inherent to epidemiological reviews, such as variance in instruments, classification of psychiatric disorders (i.e. DSM-III versus DSM-IV versus ICD-10), variations in sampling method, sample size and characteristics, as well as the time frame for symptom duration (i.e. 1 month, 1 year, lifetime). Nevertheless, the global prevalence rates for the panic/phobic group of disorders in a 12-month period is 8%, strongly supporting the argument that anxiety disorders, including panic and phobic disorders, are quite prevalent in the general population. Compiling the sociodemographic data presented is an additional challenge, as there is very little data specific to panic disorder and phobias. Gavin Andrews ameliorated this problem by using data from several anxiety disorders prevalence studies. This was a reasonable solution, given that 80% of anxiety disorders patients suffer from panic or phobias. When examining the question of what type of people suffer from panic and phobias, consistently identified risk factors included being female, of young age, and having low education and socioeconomic status. Interestingly, this population is characteristically less likely to access treatment.

In clinical practice, comorbidity [1,2] is the rule rather than the exception, be it a comorbid mood disorder, substance abuse disorder or a co-occurring anxiety disorder. According to the reviewed literature, the combination of an anxiety disorder with a comorbid mood disorder appears to contribute the most disability as well as utilization of health services [2]. This is very consistent with what is typically seen in psychiatric tertiary care settings. However, with or without comorbidity, the presence of an anxiety disorder seems to be a strong determinant of disability and days off work, ranking just below that of mood disorders [3]. As seen in clinical samples, both panic disorder with agoraphobia and social phobia comorbid with depression may have considerably more associated impairment than the presence of either condition alone [4]. The age of onset of social phobia seems to be a strong predictor of comorbidity, with an early age of onset more likely to have comorbid depression [5].

---

[1] *Department of Psychiatry and Behavioural Neurosciences, McMaster University, 1200 Main St. West, Hamilton, ON, L8N 3Z5, Canada*
[2] *Anxiety Disorders Clinic, McMaster University Medical Centre, Hamilton, ON, Canada*

Social phobia is discussed in a special section of Andrews' review, with the case being made that the generalized form of the disorder (that is, fearfulness of a range of social and performance situations) is more persistent, impairing and comorbid as compared to those social phobics with primarily public speaking fears [6]. In fact, the latter group are rarely seen in clinical settings. When these individuals seek treatment in primary care, they are more likely to be recognized as having a psychiatric illness if they exhibit associated depressive symptomatology with their social phobia. There is a low level of identification of the anxiety disorder in these cases [5]. Due to the strong relationship between social phobia and the subsequent development of mood disorders, Kessler *et al.* [7] suggest that about 10% of depression could be prevented with early identification and treatment of social phobia. Given that social phobics tend to develop depressive episodes that are frequent and severe, early intervention in social phobia could reduce the point prevalence of seriously impairing mood disorders by as much as one quarter. It has been suggested that physicians should incorporate a more dimensional approach to diagnosis, where symptoms that appear to be key or common features of anxiety disorders are measured. This approach may serve to identify symptom profiles that predict response to treatment or symptoms that are treatment resistant [8].

In spite of many empirically derived treatments (both pharmacological and cognitive-behavioural) for the panic and phobic disorders, few individuals seek treatment. For those who actually seek treatment, the majority do not receive treatment that is adequate or appropriate [9]. Gavin Andrews' review highlights the fact that panic and phobic disorders are an international public health problem with a significant contribution to the burden of disease. His review cries out for a call to action for international prevention programmes aimed at those at high risk for developing these disorders, early identification and treatment of new onset cases, and improved education of educators and healthcare providers.

REFERENCES

1. Van Ameringen M., Mancini C., Styan G., Donison D. (1991) The relationship of social phobia with other psychiatric illness. *J. Affect. Disord.*, **21**: 93–99.
2. Schneier F., Johnson J., Hornig C.D., Liebowitz M.R., Weissman M.M. (1992) Social phobia: comorbidity and morbidity in an epidemiological sample. *Arch. Gen. Psychiatry*, **49**: 282–288.
3. Stein M.B., Kean Y.M. (2000) Disability and quality of life in social phobia: epidemiologic findings. *Am. J. Psychiatry*, **157**: 1606–1613.

4. Quilty L.C., Van Ameringen M., Mancini C., Oakman J., Farvolden P. (2003) Quality of life and the anxiety disorders. *J. Anxiety Disord.*, **17**: 405–426.
5. Lecrubier Y., Weiller E. (1997) Comorbidities in social phobia. *Int. Clin. Psychopharmacol.*, **12** (Suppl. 6): S17–S21.
6. Stein M.B., Chavira D.A. (1998) Subtypes of social phobia and comorbidity with depression and other anxiety disorders. *J. Affect. Disord.*, **50**: S11–S16.
7. Kessler R.C., Stang P., Wittchen H.-U., Stein M.B., Walters E.E. (1999) Lifetime co-morbidities between social phobia and mood disorders in the US National Comorbidity Survey. *Psychol. Med.*, **29**: 555–567.
8. Brown T.A., Barlow D.H. (1992) Comorbidity among anxiety disorders: implications for treatment and DSM-IV. *J. Consult. Clin. Psychol.*, **60**: 835–844.
9. Katzelnick D.J., Kobak K.A., DeLeire T., Henk H.J., Greist J.H., Davidson J.R.T., Schneier F.R., Stein M.B., Helstad C.P. (2001) Impact of generalized social anxiety disorder in managed care. *Am. J. Psychiatry*, **158**: 1999–2007.

CHAPTER 3

Pharmacotherapy of Phobias: A Review

Dan J. Stein

MRC Unit on Anxiety Disorders, University of Stellenbosch, Cape Town, South Africa and University of Florida, Gainesville

Bavanisha Vythilingum and Soraya Seedat

MRC Unit on Anxiety Disorders, University of Stellenbosch, Cape Town, South Africa

INTRODUCTION

This chapter reviews the pharmacotherapy of social phobia (or social anxiety disorder), agoraphobia and simple phobia. Although the pharmacotherapy of social phobia is a relatively new area of study, a series of randomized controlled trials (RCTs) have now been undertaken [1–4]. Clinicians today have a number of effective medications at their disposal for the treatment of this disorder, and the bulk of this chapter will focus on this area.

The pharmacotherapy of other phobias, however, remains a relatively underdeveloped area. While many RCTs of medication for the treatment of panic disorder with or without agoraphobia have been undertaken, little pharmacotherapy research has been done on patients who meet diagnostic criteria for agoraphobia without panic disorder. Similarly, there are relatively few studies of the pharmacotherapy of specific phobia. Nevertheless, some interesting work has been undertaken, and will also be summarized here.

PHARMACOTHERAPY OF SOCIAL PHOBIA

Targets of pharmacotherapy in social phobia include social anxiety, avoidant behaviours, autonomic and physiological symptoms, comorbid

---

Phobias. Edited by Mario Maj, Hagop S. Akiskal, Juan José López-Ibor and Ahmed Okasha.
©2004 John Wiley & Sons Ltd: ISBN 0-470-85833-8

mood and anxiety disorders, and associated impairments in function and quality of life [5]. In clinical settings the generalized subtype of social phobia is common, although some patients may require treatment only for more limited performance anxiety. Major depression is a particularly frequent sequela of social phobia, so that medications with antidepressant effects are often required.

Social phobia symptoms often date back to adolescence, with impairments seen in a range of different areas; while medication can certainly reduce disability in patients with social phobia, the role of other interventions such as psychotherapy should not be neglected. Conversely, apparently enduring personality traits may simply reflect social phobia itself, and therefore respond to pharmacotherapy [6–8].

A range of different medications have been studied in social phobia. We will cover antidepressants (monoamine oxidase inhibitors (MAOIs), reversible inhibitors of monoamine oxidase A (RIMAs), selegiline, tricyclic antidepressants (TCAs), selective serotonin reuptake inhibitors (SSRIs), serotonin antagonists and reuptake inhibitors, serotonin and noradrenaline reuptake inhibitors, and bupropion), benzodiazepines, azapirones, odansetron, anticonvulsants, antipsychotics and beta-blockers in turn. Although many useful open-label trials have been undertaken, the focus here will be on RCTs.

Monoamine Oxidase Inhibitors (MAOIs)

Early open-label trials with the MAOIs phenelzine [9] and tranylcypromine [10,11] suggested that these agents were effective for social phobia. In the case of tranylcypromine, response was maintained over one year of treatment. The efficacy of phenelzine was then studied in a series of controlled trials, beginning with mixed samples of patients with anxiety disorders including social phobia [12–15], and then later focused primarily on social phobia.

Thus, in an 8-week trial of phenelzine, atenolol and placebo in social phobia, phenelzine (mean dose 76 mg/day) had a response rate of 64%, significantly better than the response rate of atenolol (30%) and placebo (23%) [16,17]. Both social and performance anxiety decreased, and both social and work function improved. Phenelzine was clearly effective in generalized social phobia, but the sample of performance anxiety patients was too small for definitive conclusions to be reached. During an additional 8 weeks of treatment in responders, gains were maintained but, in a subsequent discontinuation phase, a third of those switched to placebo relapsed.

Similarly, in a 12-week trial of phenelzine, alprazolam, group cognitive-behavioural therapy (CBT) or pill placebo, in which all subjects were also given exposure instructions (i.e. there was not a no-treatment arm), phenelzine (mean dose 55 mg/day) had a response rate of 69%, in comparison to the placebo response rate of 20%. Sample sizes were small and no statistical differences across groups were found in primary efficacy measures; nevertheless, findings tended to favour phenelzine, with this agent showing superiority to alprazolam and placebo on a disability scale [18]. Patients treated with phenelzine also tended to maintain response 2 months after treatment discontinuation, arguably reflecting the enduring value of combined exposure instructions.

Subsequent studies have further supported the impressive efficacy of phenelzine in social phobia. In an 8-week comparison of phenelzine, moclobemide and placebo, phenelzine (mean dose 68 mg/day) had a response rate of 85%, moclobemide of 65%, and placebo of 15% [7]. Phenelzine was, however, less well tolerated than both moclobemide and placebo. Active treatments had significantly better effects on measures of disability, and there was further improvement in response to medication during treatment to week 16, with relapse of patients switched to placebo during week 16 to 24.

Furthermore, in a 12-week study of phenelzine, group CBT, educational-supportive group therapy and pill placebo, phenelzine had a response rate of 65% in comparison to the placebo response of 33% [19]. Both phenelzine and group CBT were superior to the control conditions, with some evidence that phenelzine had a faster and more robust effect than CBT. Patients with generalized and non-generalized social phobia improved to the same extent. The superior efficacy of the active interventions was maintained during long-term treatment, but phenelzine patients showed a trend toward greater relapse during treatment-free follow-up [20].

Research on MAOIs in social phobia has been crucially important in suggesting that monoaminergic neurotransmitters play a role in the neurobiology of this disorder [21], and in emphasizing that social phobia deserves the attention of psychopharmacologists. Nevertheless, despite the high response rates of phenelzine in RCTs, MAOIs are associated with a range of practical problems in the clinical context. These include the need for a tyramine-free diet, the potential for dangerous drug–drug interactions, and a relatively poor adverse effect profile. The use of these agents is therefore currently restricted to the treatment of refractory patients [22,23].

Reversible Inhibitors of Monoamine Oxidase A (RIMAs)

The RIMA moclobemide does not require the use of a tyramine-free diet, may be taken together with a range of other medications, and has a relatively good adverse event profile. Indeed, in contrast to a number of new generation antidepressants, moclobemide is not associated with significant sexual dysfunction or weight gain.

Nevertheless, data on the efficacy of moclobemide in social phobia are inconsistent. An early study suggested that moclobemide (mean dose 581 mg/day) had comparable efficacy to phenelzine, but was better tolerated [7]. Moclobemide appeared to have a slower onset than phenelzine, but response continued to improve until 16 weeks, with relapse noted during subsequent withdrawal. A large multicentre placebo-controlled fixed-dose 12-week study found that moclobemide 300 mg/day, and especially 600 mg/day, was more effective than placebo, but response rates were modest (47% in the 600 mg/day group versus 34% in the placebo group) [24].

Furthermore, in an 8-week study there was a low response rate to both moclobemide (mean dose 728 mg/day) and placebo (17.5% versus 13.5%) [25]. An 8-week extension phase offered to treatment responders also did not demonstrate a drug–placebo difference. In addition, in a large multicentre dose-finding study, there was no clear efficacy of different doses of moclobemide (75–900 mg) over placebo [26]. Nevertheless, there was some evidence of a dose–response relationship, and of the superior efficacy of moclobemide in more severe patients [27].

In a 6-month study of moclobemide, CBT and their combination, there was significant improvement in all groups, although the combination treatment was the most effective intervention. The authors suggested that moclobemide was the best treatment for immediate reduction of symptoms, but that CBT was important for later reductions in avoidant behaviour [28].

Open-label data from Versiani *et al.* have pointed to the value of long-term (4-year) treatment. There was an 88% relapse after discontinuation at the end of 2 years of treatment, but during an additional 2 years of treatment those patients who had deteriorated became responders again. When moclobemide was discontinued after 4 years, two out of three patients remained almost asymptomatic without treatment [29,30].

More recently, moclobemide was shown to be effective in a 12-week placebo-controlled study of social phobia patients with and without comorbid anxiety disorders [31]. Interestingly, a predictor analysis showed that the presence of a comorbid anxiety disorder was predictive of response. Subjects were offered an additional 6 months of treatment: during this time moclobemide-treated subjects continued to improve, whereas some of the placebo patients relapsed, so widening the gap between medication and placebo. Moclobemide was effective in patients with and without comorbid disorders, as well as in different subtypes of social phobia (generalized and performance). Importantly, in the maintenance phase adverse events were similar in the medication and placebo groups.

Brofaromine is a RIMA and serotonin reuptake inhibitor. Trials of this agent in social phobia were also promising [32–34], with response rates for active medication (ranging from 50% to 78%), significantly superior to those for placebo (ranging from 0% to 23%). The trials in which a higher dose (150 mg/day) was used had the higher medication response rates. Some of these trials included extension phases [32,33]; for example, in a 9-month maintenance study, the brofaromine group improved further, whereas 60% of placebo responders who were continued on placebo relapsed [33]. Unfortunately, brofaromine is not commercially available.

Moclobemide is also not available in a number of regions, including the United States. Given the inconsistent data and consequently relatively low effect size [2], some experts would not include this medication as a first-line intervention for social phobia [23]. On the other hand, given that a head-to-head study showed comparable responses of moclobemide to another new generation antidepressant (citalopram) [35], and given its good tolerability, a potential role for moclobemide as a first-line intervention cannot be entirely ruled out.

Selegiline

In an open trial of selegiline (10 mg/day), a selective inhibitor of monoamine oxidase B, in a small group of social phobia patients, there was only a 33% response rate [36]. This does not, however, rule out the possibility that this agent might be effective at higher, nonselective doses.

Tricyclic Antidepressants (TCAs)

Despite the proven efficacy of TCAs in major depression, reports of efficacy in social phobia have been inconsistent [37,38]. Data from an early RCT with mixed phobias [39] and from an unpublished RCT have not supported the efficacy of imipramine [40]. Lack of efficacy is further supported by findings that atypical depression, including symptoms of interpersonal sensitivity, responds better to MAOIs than to TCAs [41]. Interestingly, comorbid depression in social phobia is often characterized by atypical features.

Clomipramine is a predominantly serotonergic antidepressant, and therefore may have a somewhat different pharmacotherapeutic profile from other TCAs and be useful in social phobia [42–44]. Nevertheless, given the lack of placebo-controlled data, and the relatively poor adverse effect profile of the TCAs, this agent has not been recommended in consensus guidelines as a first-line agent for the treatment of this condition [22,23]. An anecdotal report suggests that clomipramine non-responders may respond to a MAOI [10].

Selective Serotonin Reuptake Inhibitors (SSRIs)

SSRIs are the most studied class of medications in the pharmacotherapy of social phobia. Early reports suggested efficacy of these agents in preliminary open-label studies [2]. Further, many of the currently available SSRIs—escitalopram [45], fluoxetine [46], fluvoxamine [47,48], paroxetine [49–54] and sertraline [55–57]—have been studied in one or more placebo-controlled trials.

Paroxetine was the first medication to receive US Food and Drug Administration (FDA) approval for the treatment of social phobia. Several large multicentre 12-week studies, in which most patients had generalized social phobia, demonstrated response rates to paroxetine (ranging from 55% to 70%) that were significantly greater than those seen after placebo (ranging from 8% to 32%) [50–52,54]. In the fixed-dose study, there was no additional advantage in raising paroxetine beyond 20 mg/day, although the authors noted that response rates in the flexible dose studies were higher than in the fixed-dose study, suggesting that upward titration of dosage should be individualized. Notably, paroxetine led to remission significantly more often than placebo [58]. Furthermore, medication was useful not only in improving social anxiety symptoms, but also in reducing disability.

Similar findings of efficacy are apparent in the studies of sertraline and fluvoxamine. The work by Blomhoff *et al.* on sertraline was particularly interesting insofar as it was undertaken in a primary care setting, and insofar as it found that there was no significant difference in outcome between exposure and non-exposure treated subjects [57]. Thus, while the bulk of the evidence supporting the use of pharmacotherapy for social phobia has emerged from efficacy trials in academic centres, there is at least some evidence for the effectiveness of SSRIs in more typical clinical contexts.

One of the interesting features of the earliest controlled SSRI trial in social phobia, on fluvoxamine, was that around a quarter of patients had non-generalized social phobia, suggesting that this subtype was also medication responsive [47]. Arguably, in SSRI trials as a whole, too few patients with non-generalized social phobia have been studied to reach definitive conclusions about the value of SSRIs in this subtype of the disorder. Nevertheless, an analysis of the paroxetine data set provides some support for the conclusion that SSRIs are effective not only in more generalized but also in less generalized social phobia [59].

Another of the smaller controlled SSRI studies is interesting in that it focused on patients with comorbid alcohol use disorders [53]. Despite high rates of comorbid substance use in social phobia, such patients have invariably been excluded from RCTs. There is some evidence from open-label work that comorbid alcohol use is a negative predictor of outcome [10]. However, in an 8-week study of paroxetine versus placebo, patients with social phobia and comorbid alcohol use disorders showed significantly more improvement on medication [53].

The only published negative trial of an SSRI in social phobia is that of fluoxetine [46]. This trial had a relatively high placebo response rate, perhaps accounting for the failure to differentiate medication. Certainly, the earliest evidence that SSRIs might be effective for social phobia was provided by a number of small open-label trials that reported that fluoxetine was useful in this condition [60–62].

Taken together, then, the SSRIs have proven effective not only in improving social phobia symptoms but also in reducing associated disability. In terms of response rate, around twice as many patients respond to SSRIs as to placebo [2]. On the Liebowitz Social Anxiety Scale (LSAS), which remains the most widely used symptom severity scale in social phobia, the majority of trials demonstrate a large effect size, larger than that reported with moclobemide [2].

Furthermore, these agents have the advantage of being reasonably well tolerated, with adverse events in social phobia similar to those previously seen in studies of depression. Although there are no comparative studies of SSRIs versus older antidepressants in social phobia, there is good evidence from the literature on other disorders that SSRIs are better tolerated than a number of the TCAs [63]. Finally, although few studies of social phobia have specifically included patients with comorbid depression, given the efficacy of SSRIs in depression, it is likely that such patients would also respond to treatment with these agents.

Based on these considerations, expert consensus recommendations have listed SSRIs as first-line medication interventions for social phobia [22,23]. In the RCTs of SSRIs, social phobia symptoms begin to decrease early after treatment, although differentation from placebo may take some weeks. A predictor analysis of the paroxetine trials found that the only predictor of response was duration of treatment, and examination of the data showed that non-responders at week 8 could still become responders by week 12 [64]. There are few fixed-dose studies of the SSRIs, and little evidence of a dose–response relationship; nevertheless, in clinical practice, higher doses may be tried in non-responders.

There are now also several long-term data sets on SSRIs in social phobia. Fluvoxamine patients continued to show improvement during the 24 weeks of treatment [47]. Sertraline studies showing efficacy were conducted over 24 [57] and 20 [56] weeks. At the end of the latter study, a 24-week relapse prevention study was undertaken; relapse rates in the sertraline continuation group (4%) were significantly lower than those in the sertraline-switch group (36%) [65].

Similarly, an early paroxetine placebo-controlled discontinuation study suggested the value of paroxetine in preventing relapse, although sample sizes were too small to reach statistical significance [66]. In a large multicentre study, after a 12-week open-label paroxetine study, a 24-week relapse prevention study demonstrated that paroxetine-treated patients continued to show improvement, and that placebo-treated patients were significantly more likely to relapse [67]. Prevalence of adverse events in the maintenance phase was lower than in the acute phase, and fewer patients in the paroxetine group than in the placebo group withdrew because of side effects.

There is also evidence that some of the SSRIs are effective in childhood and adolescent social phobia. Several open trials have been undertaken with promising results [68]. A combined psychoeducation and citalopam trial, for example, reported that 10 of 12 children and adolescents with generalized social anxiety responded by week 12 [69]. An RCT of fluoxetine versus placebo in selective mutism, a condition that has significant overlap with social phobia, showed some evidence for efficacy of this agent [70]. In addition, in a recent trial, fluvoxamine was more effective than placebo in paediatric patients with a number of different anxiety disorders, including social phobia [71].

Serotonin Antagonists and Reuptake Inhibitors

Nefazodone proved effective in open-label studies of social phobia [72,73]. Nevertheless, given the lack of controlled data and recent awareness that nefazodone may be associated with significant hepatic toxicity, this agent cannot be considered as a first-line intervention for this disorder.

Serotonin and Noradrenaline Reuptake Inhibitors

Although the supporting RCTs have not to date been published, venlafaxine was recently registered by the FDA for the treatment of social phobia. There are also uncontrolled data suggesting that venlafaxine may be useful in patients with social phobia who have not responded to one or more of the SSRIs [74,75]. In depression, it is certainly the case that patients who have not responded to one SSRI respond to another, or that patients who have not responded to one class of medication respond to a different one [76,77]. The venlafaxine data is important in encouraging similar work to take place in social phobia.

Bupropion

There is evidence from open-label treatment that buproprion [78] and bupropion-SR (mean 366 mg/day) [79] may be useful in social phobia. Nevertheless, there is also conflicting data [80]. Given the increased awareness of the importance of dopaminergic neurocircuitry in mediating social phobia [21], this agent deserves controlled investigation.

Benzodiazepines

Early work on barbiturate-assisted desensitization for social phobia was not promising [81]. A number of early open-label trials suggested, however, the efficacy of the high-potency benzodiazepine clonazepam in this condition [82]. After a 6-month open trial, a 5-month extension study with placebo controlled tapering suggested maintained efficacy and declining dosage during long-term clonazepam treatment, increased relapse during switch to placebo, and a lack of significant problems during slow taper [83,84].

Clonazepam was subsequently shown to be effective in a 10-week RCT, at the end of which response rate (mean dose 2.4 mg/day) was 78%, versus a response rate on placebo of 20% [85]. Clonazepam also had a better response than placebo on the work and social subscales of the Sheehan Disability Scale. Interestingly, follow-up 2 years later showed maintained gains, with predictors of response including less severe symptoms at baseline and treatment with clonazepam [86]. In addition, clonazepam and group CBT were comparable in a 12-week study, although there was greater improvement on clonazepam on several measures by week 12 [87].

There are also a number of open-label reports of the efficacy of alprazolam in social phobia [82]. As noted earlier, in a 12-week trial of phenelzine, alprazolam, group CBT, or pill placebo, together with exposure instructions, there were no statistical differences across the relatively small groups in primary efficacy measures [18]. In this study, the alprazolam mean dose was 4.2 mg/day, and response rate was 38%, in comparison to the placebo response rate of 20%. At assessment of alprazolam responders 2 months later, despite the exposure instructions, symptoms had returned in most cases.

A 16-week study of bromazepam versus placebo showed that this benzodiazepine was also effective in social phobia [88]. Response rate on bromazepam (mean dose 21 mg/day) was 83%, and on placebo was 20%. Nevertheless, unwanted adverse effects in the bromazepam group were frequent, especially cognitive disturbance and sedation.

Indeed, significant problems with the benzodiazepines include potential cognitive impairment and withdrawal symptoms. Longer-acting benzodiazepines such as clonazepam may have less interdose rebound symptomatology during maintenance therapy and fewer withdrawal reactions on discontinuation. Nevertheless, these agents are ineffective for depression, which is a common comorbid disorder in social phobia. Thus, many have concluded that SSRIs should replace benzodiazepines as first-line agents in social phobia [22,23]. Adverse effects of benzodiazepines (e.g. sedation) are also to be taken into account when considering the prescription of these agents for performance anxiety [89].

Azapirones

Open-label studies suggested that buspirone might be useful in treating social phobia. Schneier et al., for example, reported that buspirone responders were receiving higher doses than non-responders (56.9 mg versus 38.3 mg/day) [90]. In a 12-week RCT of relatively low-dose buspirone (30 mg/day), this agent was not found to be more effective than placebo [91]. Furthermore, an RCT in performance anxiety found that CBT was more effective than buspirone (mean dose 32 mg/day) or placebo [92].

In an open-label study, van Ameringen et al. [93] found that buspirone was useful in social phobia patients with a partial response to SSRIs. Given that controlled studies of buspirone augmentation of antidepressants have proven inconsistent in other anxiety disorders, further work is needed to ascertain whether this and other strategies that act to optimize serotonergic neurotransmission [44] are indeed useful in social phobia.

Odansetron

Odansetron, a 5-HT_3 antagonist, was studied in a multicentre RCT for social phobia [94]. There was some evidence that, at a dose of 0.5 mg/day, it was more effective than placebo. However, the effect size was reportedly small, and this agent has not subsequently been studied.

Anticonvulsants

Gabapentin, a compound that has GABAergic actions, has been suggested to be effective in a 14-week RCT of social phobia [95]. Response rates were moderate—32% in the gabapentin group versus 14% in the placebo group. The majority of responders were being treated at maximally allowed gabapentin doses (3600 mg/day), suggesting that higher doses may be needed for efficacy. There is ongoing work on a related compound, pregabalin.

Work on these agents is interesting insofar as there is theoretical data for suggesting that both monoaminergic systems and the GABAergic system are involved in underpinning anxiety symptoms. Given the problematic adverse event profile of the benzodiazepines, it is possible that safer GABAergic medications may ultimately take their place as first-line agents for the treatment of social phobia. Theoretically, a combination of agents that exert effects via different mechanisms may be particularly useful, although there is currently no data from controlled trials to support combined pharmacotherapy in social phobia.

Antipsychotics

An 8-week study of 12 social phobia patients found that olanzapine (5–20 mg/day) was superior to placebo [96]. There is also data, however, that antipsychotic agents can increase social anxiety symptoms [97]. Thus, additional data is needed before this class of medication can be recommended for use in the treatment of social phobia.

Adrenergic Agents

An early open-label trial suggested that the beta-blocker atenolol (50–100 mg/day) might be useful for both generalized and performance symptoms of social phobia [98]. Atenolol (mean dose 95 mg/day) did not, however, prove superior to placebo in a placebo-controlled study [17]. There was a suggestion that atenolol was useful in performance anxiety, but the sample size was too small to allow definitive conclusions. Trials of behaviour therapy versus atenolol [99] and of social skills training with atenolol versus placebo [100] also failed to show efficacy for this agent.

A series of controlled studies have, however, suggested the efficacy of beta-blockers in non-clinical populations with performance anxiety [101–109]. Propranolol 10–40 mg, taken 45–60 minutes before a performance, has been recommended. Theoretically, non-selective beta-blockers (e.g. propranolol), affecting $beta_1$ receptors in the heart and $beta_2$ receptors mediating tremor, may be more effective than selective beta-blockers (e.g. atenolol), although this question has not been empirically studied [110]. There are also case reports that clonidine (0.1 mg twice daily) may be useful for the autonomic symptoms of social phobia [111].

Nevertheless, given the lack of positive RCTs of adrenergic agents in social phobia *per se*, the finding that patients with both more generalized and less generalized symptoms respond to treatment [31,47,59], and the evidence that autonomic symptoms in social phobia respond to a range of medications, including the SSRIs [5,112], the role of these medications is currently limited to selected cases of performance anxiety. Augmentation with pindolol (15 mg/day), a beta-blocker and 5-HT$_{1A}$ antagonist, was ineffective in an RCT for patients with generalized social phobia who failed to respond to SSRIs [113].

PHARMACOTHERAPY OF AGORAPHOBIA

Soon after the introduction of the TCA imipramine into clinical practice, Klein and Fink reported that hospitalized patients with agoraphobia who had failed to respond to psychotherapy and phenothiazines responded to imipramine and supportive psychotherapy [114]. At the same time, Dally and colleagues first reported that "phobic anxiety" responded to the MAOIs [115,116]. These findings were confirmed in a series of seminal controlled studies [12–15,117–119].

From this work, it emerged that antidepressants such as imipramine were significantly more effective than placebo for treating patients who experienced spontaneous panic [120], but were ineffective for the treatment of phobic patients without such spontaneous panic attacks [39]. Accordingly, studies of the pharmacotherapy of agoraphobia have invariably taken place within the context of studies of panic disorder, which is frequently accompanied by agoraphobia.

Panic disorder responds to a range of antidepressants (including TCAs and SSRIs) as well as to high-potency benzodiazepines [23,121]. More recently, a range of other agents, such as anticonvulsants, have also been studied [121,122]. Although there is some work suggesting that SSRIs are particularly effective [123,124], a recent meta-analysis has reported no differences in efficacy between different antipanic agents [125]. Conversely, early suggestions that effects of antidepressants in panic disorder are mediated primarily by mood reduction have received little support.

Pharmacotherapy studies in panic disorder have invariably included patients with agoraphobia symptoms, and have routinely demonstrated that both panic and avoidance symptoms respond to medication. In Klein et al.'s classic observations, onset of the illness was characterized by spontaneous panic followed by anticipatory anxiety and only then by phobic avoidance. Conversely, during pharmacotherapy with antidepressants, there was first a decrease in panic symptoms, followed by a secondary improvement in anticipatory anxiety and phobic avoidance [39].

Low doses of antidepressants are initially used in panic disorder, in order to avoid early symptom exacerbation and adverse effects. However, in a number of studies, patients with agoraphobia have been found to ultimately require higher doses of medication, whether this be imipramine [126], clomipramine [127] or alprazolam [128]. Perhaps agoraphobia is a marker of a more severe condition, with somewhat different psychobiological dysfunctions, and requiring more robust pharmacological and psychological intervention.

Indeed, although epidemiological surveys suggest the existence of agoraphobia without panic disorder, this disorder is uncommonly seen in clinical practice. Based on the literature on panic disorder and agoraphobia, clinicians might well consider treatment with an antidepressant to ensure blockade of possible panic symptoms. Cognitive-behavioural techniques may, however, also be crucial in encouraging patients to decrease avoidance. Nevertheless, more research is needed on the optimal treatment of this population of patients [129].

PHARMACOTHERAPY OF SPECIFIC PHOBIA

Specific phobia is typically conceptualized using a cognitive-behavioural model, with the treatment of choice involving exposure therapy. Furthermore, early influential work suggested that phobias without spontaneous panic were not responsive to imipramine [39]. As the neurobiology of fear conditioning becomes increasingly understood [130], determining whether specific phobia responds to pharmacological intervention again becomes particularly relevant.

A range of other early reports of medication for phobias are now difficult to interpret given the absence of diagnostic criteria, but there is also evidence suggesting the value of certain drugs, such as phenelzine [13], for specific phobia. SSRIs have also been suggested effective [131], and a recent small but controlled trial suggested that paroxetine was more effective than placebo in specific phobia [132]. This finding is one that deserves replication in an extended sample.

Early reports also focused on the possibility of using barbiturates during behavioural desensitization [81,133]. Later reports indicated that benzodiazepines may increase behavioural performance [134] or decrease anxiety [135] during exposure to phobic stimuli. Nevertheless, there is also evidence that these agents can interfere with exposure instructions for phobias [136,137]. An RCT in which a kava-kava extract proved superior to placebo in anxiety disorders included subjects with specific phobia, but further work is needed before the results can be generalized.

A trial of a beta$_1$-blocker (atenolol), a beta$_2$-blocker and placebo suggested a moderate but significant effect of atenolol in alleviating somatic symptoms of flight phobia [138]. However, in other controlled work, beta-blockade did not relieve subjective anxiety on exposure to flying or other phobic stimuli [134,139,140]. Furthermore, there is preliminary evidence that these agents can interfere with behavioural therapy for specific phobia. These agents have not commonly been recommended for the treatment of this condition.

PHARMACOTHERAPY OF OTHER PHOBIAS

Although social phobia, agoraphobia and specific phobias are the most commonly seen phobias, a range of other syndromes characterized by situational fear and avoidance have been described in the literature, and may also be responsive to pharmacotherapy. Nevertheless, in many cases it may be preferable to reassign such patients to a more commonly used diagnosis.

"School phobia", for example, likely comprises a heterogenous group of conditions including separation anxiety disorder and social phobia. Nevertheless, early open-label studies of benzodiazepines and placebo-controlled work on TCAs reported that these agents were effective for "school phobia", although not all findings were consistent [68]. More recent work has underlined the possible efficacy of SSRIs in both separation anxiety disorder and social phobia of children [71].

Taijin-kyofusho (TKS), or anthropophobia, is a disorder described in the East. Although characterized by social anxiety, fear of offending others is more prominent than fear of embarrassing oneself [141]. Many patients with TKS also meet diagnostic criteria for social phobia, although there is also a subgroup of patients with poor insight. There is preliminary evidence that TKS responds to clomipramine or fluvoxamine [142].

"Illness phobia" is another diagnostic label that can today be replaced by DSM-IV diagnoses such as obsessive–compulsive disorder (OCD) or hypochondriasis. There is growing evidence that patients with hypochondriasis, like those with OCD, respond to serotonin reuptake inhibitors [143]. Various other agents may also be useful, but have not been as well studied [143]. Choking phobia, often acquired after an episode of choking on food, is arguably reminiscent of suffocation fears in panic disorder, and may respond to antipanic medication.

The term "dysmorphophobia" has been replaced in the nomenclature by "body dysmorphic disorder". There is increasing evidence that, like OCD, this disorder responds more robustly to serotonergic than to noradrenergic antidepressants [144]. Given the efficacy of the SSRIs in this disorder, they are currently considered a first-line pharmacotherapy [145].

"Dental phobia" is another category that may be relatively diverse, and in which careful diagnostic assessment is required. Such patients may, for example, meet criteria for specific phobia or for generalized anxiety disorder. Nevertheless, it has been reported that patients with "dental phobia" demonstrate a decrease in symptoms after administration of nitrous oxide [146].

Patients who meet criteria for social phobia, excepting the exclusion criterion of presence of physical illness as a focus of social concern, may also respond to standard social phobia medications [147].

SUMMARY

Consistent Evidence

Although social phobia is a relatively new area of psychopharmacological investigation, there is now good evidence for the efficacy and tolerability of a number of the SSRIs over both the short term and long term for the treatment of this disorder. Expert consensus has therefore highlighted these agents as first-line pharmacotherapy agents in this condition.

The evidence is also consistent that the SSRIs not only reduce social phobia symptoms, but that they reduce associated disability. While additional work is needed to determine the pharmacoeconomic implications of this finding, despite the chronicity and morbidity of social phobia, current work on the mediators and moderators of pharmacotherapy suggests that this has broad-spectrum effects [8] in a broad range of patients [64].

This evidence is important in persuading primary care practitioners to diagnose and treat social phobia appropriately, and in the psychoeducation of patients who consider themselves merely "shy" but are considering treatment options. Perhaps the universality of the experience of social anxiety has contributed to its relative underdiagnosis and undertreatment. It is important that this situation be reversed. Better understanding of the neurobiology of social phobia and medication response will likely contribute to this task [21,148].

Panic disorder with agoraphobia responds to a number of different classes of medications, including the TCAs and benzodiazepines. In view of their efficacy, tolerability and safety, expert consensus has again recommended that the SSRIs are a first-line intervention for this disorder [23,121]. SSRIs should be initiated at relatively low dosages when treating panic disorder with agoraphobia.

Incomplete Evidence

For social phobia, additional work is needed to replicate evidence of the efficacy of SSRIs in childhood and adolescent social phobia, to demonstrate their efficacy in patients with comorbid depression, and to clarify whether they are effective in non-generalized social phobia. Additional work is also needed to determine their effectiveness in routine clinical settings, perhaps using a broader range of measures—e.g. physiological symptoms [5,112], fearful cognitions [85] and quality of life—than are usually studied.

A range of other promising agents (e.g. pregabalin) deserve further study. Specific agents may also be required for patients with comorbid substance use disorders [53,149]. Although a meta-analysis supports the relatively larger effect sizes of SSRIs compared to moclobemide [2], head-to-head studies of newer medications for social phobia are needed to determine their relative efficacy and tolerability. An open-label, rater-blinded study found that citalopram and moclobemide had similar response rates in social phobia [35]; further such work is needed.

Limited evidence suggests that a considerable proportion of non-responders to SSRIs at week 8 may respond by week 12 [64], but that the dose–response curve of these agents is relatively flat [54]. There is growing evidence that long-term treatment with these agents is needed in order to prevent early relapse, with expert consensus advising that medication be continued for at least a year [22]. Nevertheless, to date there have been few dose finding studies of SSRIs in social phobia, and relatively few long-term pharmacotherapy studies.

Avoidant personality traits in patients with social phobia may respond to pharmacotherapy, but relatively little is known about the pharmacotherapy of a range of putative social phobia spectrum disorders (e.g. pathological shyness, taijin-kyofusho, olfactory reference syndrome) [142,150].

Agoraphobia without panic disorder and specific phobia are thought to respond to cognitive-behavioural therapy, but there is relatively little data on the use of pharmacological interventions for these disorders. Specific phobia does not seem to respond to imipramine, but there is limited data from one small study that SSRIs may be useful in its treatment.

Areas Still Open to Research

The optimal approach to social phobia patients who have failed to respond to an SSRI remains unclear. The literature on depression suggests switching to a different SSRI or different class, and there is anecdotal support from the social phobia literature for this conclusion [10,74,75]. There is also open-label data on the possible value of certain augmentation strategies [93]. Although in clinical practice augmentation strategies are often reserved for partial responders, there is little information addressing the question of when to switch and when to augment. Some authors have suggested the use of sympathetic block for severe resistant social phobia. Additional research is, however, needed.

It has been suggested that early robust intervention for social phobia may prevent the onset of the comorbid depression that so frequently complicates this condition in later years. Certainly it seems reasonable to initiate treatment of adolescent social phobia early and robustly. Similar considerations might conceivably also apply to children with behavioural inhibition and social avoidance, who are at risk of developing social phobia. It would be useful to have empirical data to demonstrate the long-term advantages of these kinds of approaches.

Another area for future research is that of the placebo response in social phobia [151]. Placebo response in the large multicentre pharmacotherapy trials for this disorder has been moderately high, and relatively little is known about its predictors or neurobiological basis. Interestingly, there is evidence that whereas medication responders show some continued improvement during long-term treatment, continuation of placebo in placebo-responders may result in relapse [31,33,65].

The question of how to optimize pharmacotherapy and psychotherapy combination [28,57,92,100] and sequencing in social phobia to reduce symptoms in the short term and prevent relapse after treatment discontinuation deserves additional study. One hypothesis that emerges from previous work [18,20,152,153], for example, is that medications have faster onset, but that the effects of CBT endure longer. Another hypothesis is that certain medications (e.g. benzodiazepines) may counter the positive effects of exposure [18].

Additional RCTs are needed to establish whether SSRIs and other medications are effective in agoraphobia without panic and in specific phobia, and to determine whether the addition of medications can optimize psychotherapeutic intervention in these disorders.

ACKNOWLEDGEMENTS

The authors are supported by the Medical Research Council of South Africa.

REFERENCES

1. Fedoroff I.C., Taylor S. (2001) Psychological and pharmacological treatments of social phobia: a meta-analysis. *J. Clin. Psychopharmacol.*, **21**: 311–324.
2. van der Linden G.J.H., Stein D.J., van Balkom A.J.L.M. (2000) The efficacy of the selective serotonin reuptake inhibitors for social anxiety disorder (social phobia): a meta-analysis of randomized controlled trials. *Int. Clin. Psychopharmacol.*, **15** (Suppl. 2): 15–24.

3. Gould R.A., Buckminister S., Pollack M.H., Otto M.W., Yap L. (1997) Cognitive-behavioral and pharmacological treatments of social phobia. *Clin. Psychol. Sci. Pract.*, **4**: 291–306.
4. Blanco C., Schneier F.R., Schmidt A.B., Blanco-Jerez C.R., Marshall R.D., Sanchez-Lacay A., Liebowitz M.R. (2003) Pharmacological treatment of social anxiety disorder: a meta-analysis. *Depress. Anxiety*, **18**: 29–40.
5. Davidson J.R.T. (1998) Pharmacotherapy of social anxiety disorder. *J. Clin. Psychiatry*, **59** (Suppl. 17): 47–51.
6. Deltito J.A., Stam M. (1989) Psychopharmacological treatment of avoidant personality disorder. *Compr. Psychiatry*, **30**: 498–504.
7. Versiani M., Nardi A.E., Mundim F.D., Alves A.B., Liebowitz M.R., Amrein R. (1992) Pharmacotherapy of social phobia: a controlled study with moclobemide and phenelzine. *Br. J. Psychiatry*, **161**: 353–360.
8. Fahlen T. (1995) Personality traits in social phobia, II: Changes during drug treatment. *J. Clin. Psychiatry*, **56**: 569–573.
9. Liebowitz M.R., Fyer A.J., Gorman J.M., Campeas R., Levin A. (1986) Phenelzine in social phobia. *J. Clin. Psychopharmacol.*, **6**: 93–98.
10. Versiani M., Mundim F.D., Nardi A.E., Liebowitz M.R. (1988) Tranylcypromine in social phobia. *J. Clin. Psychopharmacol.*, **8**: 279–283.
11. Versiani M., Nardi A.E., Mundim F.D. (1989) Fobia social. *J. Brasil. Psiquiatria*, **38**: 251–263.
12. Tyrer P., Candy J., Kelly D. (1973) A study of the clinical effects of phenelzine and placebo in the treatment of phobic anxiety. *Psychopharmacologia*, **32**: 237–254.
13. Solyom L., Heseltine G.F., McClure D.J., Solyom C., Ledwidge B., Steinberg G. (1973) Behaviour therapy versus drug therapy in the treatment of phobic neurosis. *Can. Psychiatr. Assoc. J.*, **18**: 25–32.
14. Solyom C., Solyom L., La Pierre Y., Pecknold J., Morton L. (1981) Phenelzine and exposure in the treatment of phobias. *Biol. Psychiatry*, **16**: 239–247.
15. Mountjoy C.Q., Roth M., Garside R.F., Leitch I.M. (1977) A clinical trial of phenelzine in anxiety depressive and phobic neuroses. *Br. J. Psychiatry*, **131**: 486–492.
16. Liebowitz M.R., Gorman J.M., Fyer A.J., Campeas R., Levin A.P., Sandberg D., Hollander E., Papp L., Goetz D. (1988) Pharmacotherapy of social phobia: an interim report of a placebo-controlled comparison of phenelzine and atenolol. *J. Clin. Psychiatry*, **49**: 252–257.
17. Liebowitz M.R., Schneier F., Campeas R., Hollander E., Hatterer J., Fyer A., Gorman J., Papp L., Davies S., Gully R. et al. (1992) Phenelzine vs atenolol in social phobia: a placebo-controlled comparison. *Arch. Gen. Psychiatry*, **49**: 290–300.
18. Gelernter C.S., Uhde T.W., Cimbolic P., Arnkoff D.B., Vittone B.J., Tancer M.E., Bartko J.J. (1991) Cognitive-behavioral and pharmacological treatments of social phobia: a controlled study. *Arch. Gen. Psychiatry*, **48**: 938–945.
19. Heimberg R.G., Liebowitz M.R., Hope D.A., Schneier F.R., Holt C.S., Welkowitz L.A., Juster H.R., Campeas R., Bruch M.A., Cloitre M. et al. (1988) Cognitive behavioral group therapy vs phenelzine therapy for social phobia: 12-week outcome. *Arch. Gen. Psychiatry*, **55**: 1133–1141.
20. Liebowitz M.R., Heimberg R.G., Schneier F.R., Hope D.A., Davies S., Holt C.S., Goetz D., Juster H.R., Lin S.H., Bruch M.A. et al. (1999) Cognitive-behavioral group therapy versus phenelzine in social phobia: long-term outcome. *Depress. Anxiety*, **10**: 89–98.

21. Stein D.J., Westenberg H., Liebowitz M.R. (2002) Social anxiety disorder and generalized anxiety disorder: serotonergic and dopaminergic neurocircuitry. *J. Clin. Psychiatry*, **63** (Suppl. 6): 12–19.
22. Ballenger J.C., Davidson J.A., Lecrubier Y., Nutt D.J., Bobes J., Beidel D.C., Ono Y., Westenberg H.G. (1998) Consensus statement on social anxiety disorder from the international consensus group on depression and anxiety. *J. Clin. Psychiatry*, **59** (Suppl. 8): 54–60.
23. Bandelow B., Zohar J., Hollander E., Kasper S., Moller H.-J., WFSBP Task Force on Treatment Guidelines for Anxiety Obsessive–Compulsive and Posttraumatic Stress Disorders (2002) World Federation of Societies of Biological Psychiatry (WFSBP) guidelines for the pharmacological treatment of anxiety, obsessive–compulsive and posttraumatic stress disorders. *World J. Biol. Psychiatry*, **3**: 171–199.
24. Katschnig K., Stein M.B., Buller R., International Multicenter Clinical Trial Group on Moclobemide for Social Phobia (1997) Moclobemide in social phobia: a double-blind, placebo-controlled clinical study. *Eur. Arch. Psychiatry Clin. Neurosci.*, **247**: 71–80.
25. Schneier F.R., Goetz D., Campeas R., Fallon B., Marshall R., Liebowitz M.R. (1998) Placebo-controlled trial of moclobemide in social phobia. *Br. J. Psychiatry*, **172**: 70–77.
26. Noyes R.J., Moroz G., Davidson J.R., Liebowitz M.R., Davidson A., Siegel J., Bell J., Cain J.W., Curlik S.M., Kent T.A. et al. (1997) Moclobemide in social phobia: a controlled dose–response trial. *J. Clin. Psychopharmacol.*, **17**: 247–254.
27. Nutt D., Montgomery S.A. (1996) Moclobemide in the treatment of social phobia. *Int. Clin. Psychopharmacol.*, **11** (Suppl. 3): 77–82.
28. Prasko J., Kosova J., Paskova B., Praskova H., Klaschka J., Seifertova D., Sipek J. (1999) Pharmacotherapy and/or cognitive-behavioral therapy in the treatment of social phobia—controlled study. *Psychiatrie*, **3**: 13–18.
29. Versiani M., Nardi A.E., Mundim F.D., Pinto S., Saboya E., Kovacs R. (1996) The long-term treatment of social phobia with moclobemide. *Int. Clin. Psychopharmacol.*, **11** (Suppl. 3): 83–88.
30. Versiani M., Amrein R., Montgomery S.A. (1997) Social phobia: long-term treatment outcome and prediction of response—a moclobemide study. *Int. Clin. Psychopharmacol.*, **12**: 239–254.
31. Stein D.J., Cameron A., Amrein R., Montgomery S.A. (2002) Moclobemide is effective and well tolerated in the long-term pharmacotherapy of social anxiety disorder with or without comorbid anxiety disorder. *Int. Clin. Psychopharmacol.*, **17**: 161–170.
32. van Vliet I.M., den Boer J.A., Westenberg H.G. (1992) Psychopharmacological treatment of social phobia: clinical and biochemical effects of brofaromine, a selective MAO-A inhibitor. *Eur. Neuropsychopharmacol.*, **2**: 21–29.
33. Fahlen T., Nilsson H.L., Borg K., Humble M., Pauli U. (1995) Social phobia: the clinical efficacy and tolerability of the monoamine oxidase-A and serotonin uptake inhibitor brofaromine: a double-blind placebo-controlled study. *Acta Psychiatr. Scand.*, **92**: 351–358.
34. Lott M., Greist J.H., Jefferson J.W., Kobak K.A., Katzelnick D.J., Katz R., Schaettle S.C. (1997) Brofaromine for social phobia: a multicenter, placebo-controlled, double-blind study. *J. Clin. Psychopharmacol.*, **17**: 255–260.
35. Atmaca M., Kuloglu M., Tezcan E., Unal A. (2002) Efficacy of citalopram and moclobemide in patients with social phobia: some preliminary findings. *Hum. Psychopharmacol.*, **17**: 401–405.

36. Simpson H.B., Schneier F.R., Marshall R.D., Campeas R.B., Vermes D., Silvestre J., Davies S., Liebowitz M.R. (1998) Low dose selegiline (L-Deprenyl) in social phobia. *Depress. Anxiety*, **7**: 126–129.
37. Benca R., Matuzas W., Al-Sadir J. (1986) Social phobia, MVP, and response to imipramine. *J. Clin. Psychopharmacol.*, **6**: 50–51.
38. Simpson H.B., Schneier F.R., Campeas R., Marshall R.D., Fallon B.A., Davies S., Klein D.F., Liebowitz M.R. (1998) Imipramine in the treatment of social phobia. *J. Clin. Psychopharmacol.*, **18**: 132–135.
39. Zitrin C.M., Klein D.F., Woerner M.G., Ross D.C. (1983) Treatment of phobias. I. Comparison of imipramine hydrochloride and placebo. *Arch. Gen. Psychiatry*, **40**: 125–138.
40. Emmanuel N.P., Jonson M., Villareal G. (1998) Imipramine in the treatment of social phobia. Presented at the 36th Annual Meeting of the American College of Neuropsychopharmacology, Kamuela, 8–12 December.
41. Liebowitz M.R., Quitkin F.M., Stewart J.W., McGrath P.J., Harrison W.M., Markowitz J.S., Rabkin J.G., Tricamo E., Goetz D., Klein D. (1988) Antidepressant specificity in atypical depression. *Arch. Gen. Psychiatry*, **45**: 129–137.
42. Allsopp L.F., Cooper G.L., Poole P.H. (1984) Clomipramine and diazepam in the treatment of agoraphobia and social phobia in general practice. *Curr. Med. Res. Opin.*, **9**: 64–70.
43. Pecknold J.C., McClure D.J., Appeltauer L., Allan T., Wrzesinski L. (1982) Does tryptophan potentiate clomipramine in the treatment of agoraphobic and social phobic patients? *Br. J. Psychiatry*, **140**: 484–490.
44. Beaumont G. (1997) A large open multicenter trial of clomipramine (Anafranil) in the management of phobic disorders. *J. Int. Med. Res.*, **5**: 116–123.
45. Kasper S., Loft H., Smith J.R. (2002) Escitalopram is efficacious and well tolerated in the treatment of social anxiety disorder. Presented at the Annual Meeting of the American Psychiatric Association, Philadelphia, 18–23 May.
46. Kobak K.A., Greist J.H., Jefferson J.W., Katzelnick D.J. (2002) Fluoxetine in social phobia: a double-blind, placebo-controlled pilot study. *J. Clin. Psychopharmacol.*, **22**: 275–262.
47. van Vliet I.M., den Boer J.A., Westenberg H.G.M. (1994) Psychopharmacological treatment of social phobia; a double blind placebo controlled study with fluvoxamine. *Psychopharmacology*, **115**: 128–134.
48. Stein M.B., Fyer A.J., Davidson J.R.T., Pollack M.H., Wita B. (1999) Fluvoxamine treatment of social phobia (social anxiety disorder): a double-blind, placebo-controlled study. *Am. J. Psychiatry*, **156**: 756–760.
49. Allgulander C. (1999) Paroxetine in social anxiety disorder: a randomised placebo-controlled study. *Acta Psychiatr. Scand.*, **100**: 193–198.
50. Baldwin D., Bobes J., Stein D.J., Scharwachter I., Faure M. (1999) Paroxetine in social phobia/social anxiety disorder: randomised, double-blind, placebo-controlled study. *Br. J. Psychiatry*, **175**: 120–126.
51. Stein M.B., Liebowitz M.R., Lydiard R.B., Pitts C.D., Bushnell W., Gergel I. (1998) Paroxetine treatment of generalized social phobia (social anxiety disorder): a randomized controlled trial. *JAMA*, **280**: 708–713.
52. Lydiard R.B., Bobes J. (2000) Therapeutic advances: paroxetine for the treatment of social anxiety disorder. *Depress. Anxiety*, **11**: 99–104.
53. Randall C.L., Johnson M.R., Thevos A.K., Sonne S.C., Thomas S.E., Willard S.L., Brady K.T., Davidson J.R.T. (2001) Paroxetine for social anxiety and alcohol use in dual-diagnosed patients. *Depress. Anxiety*, **14**: 255–262.

54. Liebowitz M.R., Stein M.B., Tancer M., Carpenter D., Oakes R., Pitts C.D. (2002) A randomized, double-blind, fixed-dose comparison of paroxetine and placebo in the treatment of generalized social anxiety disorder. *J. Clin. Psychiatry*, **63**: 66–74.
55. Katzelnick D.J., Kobak K.A., Greist J.H., Jefferson J.W., Mantle J.M., Serlin R.C. (1995) Sertraline for social phobia: placebo-controlled crossover study. *Am. J. Psychiatry*, **152**: 1368–1371.
56. van Ameringen M.A., Lane R.M., Walker J.R., Bowen R.C., Chokka P.R., Goldner E.M., Johnston D.G., Lavallee Y.J., Nandy S., Pecknold J.C. et al. (2001) Sertraline treatment of generalised social phobia: a 20-week, double-blind, placebo-controlled study. *Am. J. Psychiatry*, **158**: 275–281.
57. Blomhoff S., Haug T.T., Hellström K., Holme I., Humble M., Madsbu H.P., Wold J.E. (2001) Randomised controlled general practice trial of sertraline, exposure therapy and combined treatment in generalised social phobia. *Br. J. Psychiatry*, **179**: 23–30.
58. Stein D.J., Hunter B., Rolfe T., Oakes R. (2002) Paroxetine in social anxiety disorder: a remission analysis. Presented at the Congress of the European College of Neuropsychopharmacology, Barcelona, 5–9 October.
59. Stein D.J., Stein M.B., Goodwin W., Hunter B. (2001) The selective serotonin reuptake inhibitor paroxetine is effective in more generalized and less generalized social anxiety disorder. *Psychopharmacology*, **158**: 267–272.
60. Black B., Uhde T.W., Tancer M.E. (1992) Fluoxetine for the treatment of social phobia. *J. Clin. Psychopharmacol.*, **12**: 293–295.
61. Schneier F.R., Chin S.J., Hollander E., Liebowitz M.R. (1992) Fluoxetine in social phobia. *J. Clin. Psychopharmacol.*, **12**: 62–64.
62. van Ameringen M., Mancini C., Streiner D.L. (1992) Fluoxetine efficacy in social phobia. *J. Clin. Psychiatry*, **54**: 27–32.
63. Anderson I.M. (2000) Selective serotonin reuptake inhibitors versus tricyclic antidepressants: a meta-analysis of efficacy and tolerability. *J. Affect. Disord.*, **58**: 19–36.
64. Stein D.J., Stein M.B., Pitts C.D., Kumar R., Hunter B. (2002) Predictors of response to pharmacotherapy in social anxiety disorder: an analysis of 3 placebo-controlled paroxetine trials. *J. Clin. Psychiatry*, **63**: 152–155.
65. Walker J.R., van Ameringen M., Swinson R., Bowen R.C., Chokka P.R., Goldner E., Johnston D.C., Lavallie Y.J., Nandy S., Pecknold J.C. et al. (2000) Prevention of relapse in generalized social phobia: results of a 24-week study in responders to 20 weeks of sertraline treatment. *J. Clin. Psychopharmacol.*, **20**: 636–644.
66. Stein M.B., Chartier M.J., Hazen A.L., Kroft C.D., Chale R.A., Cote D., Walker J.R. (1996) Paroxetine in the treatment of generalized social phobia: open-label treatment and double-blind placebo-controlled discontinuation. *J. Clin. Psychopharmacol.*, **16**: 218–222.
67. Stein D.J., Versiani M., Hair T., Kumar R. (2002) Efficacy of paroxetine for relapse prevention in social anxiety disorder: a 24-week study. *Arch. Gen. Psychiatry*, **59**: 1111–1118.
68. Hawkridge S., Stein D.J. (1998) Risk-benefit assessment of drug therapies for anxiety disorders in children and adolescents. *Drug Safety*, **19**: 283–297.
69. Chavira D.A., Stein M.B. (2003) Combined psychoeducation and treatment with selective serotonin reuptake inhibitors for youth with generalized social anxiety disorder. *J. Child Adolesc. Psychopharmacol.*, **12**: 47–54.

70. Black B., Uhde T.W. (1994) Treatment of elective mutism with fluoxetine: a double-blind, placebo-controlled study. *J. Am. Acad. Child Adolesc. Psychiatry*, **33**: 1000–1006.
71. Research Unit on Pediatric Psychopharmacology Anxiety Study Group (2001) Fluvoxamine for the treatment of anxiety disorders in children and adolescents. *N. Engl. J. Med.*, **34**: 1279–1285.
72. Worthington J.J., Zucker B.F., Fones C.S., Otto M.W., Pollack M.H. (1998) Nefazodone for social phobia: a clinical case series. *Depress. Anxiety*, **8**: 131–133.
73. van Ameringen M., Mancini C., Oakman J.M. (1999) Nefazodone in social phobia. *J. Clin. Psychiatry*, **60**: 96–100.
74. Kelsey J.E. (1995) Venlafaxine in social phobia. *Psychopharmacol. Bull.*, **31**: 767–771.
75. Altamura A.C., Pioli R., Vitto M., Mannu P. (1999) Venlafaxine in social phobia: a study in selective serotonin reuptake non-responders. *Int. Clin. Psychopharmacol.*, **14**: 239–245.
76. Thase M.E., Rush J., Howland R.H., Kornstein S.G., Kocsis J., Gelenberg A.J., Schatzberg A.F., Koran L.M., Keller M.B., Russell J.M. et al. (2002) Double-blind switch study of imipramine or sertraline treatment of antidepressant-resistant chronic depression. *Arch. Gen. Psychiatry*, **59**: 233–239.
77. Marangell L.B. (2001) Switching antidepressants for treatment-resistant major depression. *J. Clin. Psychiatry*, **62** (Suppl. 18): 12–17.
78. Emmanuel N.P., Lydiard R.B., Ballenger J.C. (1991) Treatment of social phobia with bupropion. *J. Clin. Psychiatry*, **11**: 276–277.
79. Emmanuel N.P., Brawman-Mintzer O., Morton W.A., Book S.W., Johnson M.R., Lorderbaum J.P., Ballenger J.C., Lydiard R.B. (2000) Bupropion-SR in treatment of social phobia. *Depress. Anxiety*, **12**: 111–113.
80. Potts N.L.S., Davidson J.R.T. (1995) Pharmacological treatments: literature review. In *Social Phobia: Diagnosis, Assessment, and Treatment* (Eds R. Heimberg, M.R. Liebowitz, D.A. Hope, F.R. Schneier), pp. 334–365. Guilford Press, New York.
81. Silverstone J.T., Salkind M.R. (1973) Controlled evaluation of intravenous drugs in the specific desensitization of phobias. *Can. Psychiatr. Assoc. J.*, **18**: 47–53.
82. Davidson J.R., Tupler L.A., Potts N.L. (1994) Treatment of social phobia with benzodiazepines. *J. Clin. Psychiatry*, **55** (Suppl. 6): 28–32.
83. Davidson J.R.T., Ford S.M., Smith R.D., Potts N.L. (1991) Long-term treatment of social phobia with clonazepam. *J. Clin. Psychopharmacol.*, **52** (Suppl. 11): 16–20.
84. Connor K.M., Davidson J.R.T, Potts N.L.S., Tupler L.A., Miner C.M., Malik M.L., Book S.W., Colket J.T., Ferrell F.T. (1998) Discontinuation of clonazepam in the treatment of social phobia. *J. Clin. Psychopharmacol.*, **18**: 373–378.
85. Davidson J.R.T., Potts N., Richichi E., Krishnan R., Ford S.M., Smith R., Wilson W.H. (1993) Treatment of social phobia with clonazepam and placebo. *J. Clin. Psychopharmacol.*, **13**: 423–428.
86. Sutherland S.M., Tupler L.A., Colket J.T., Davidson J.R. (1996) A 2-year follow-up of social phobia: status after a brief medication trial. *J. Nerv. Ment. Dis.*, **184**: 731–738.
87. Otto M., Pollack M.H., Gould R.A., Worthington J.J., McArdle E.T., Rosenbaum J.F. (2000) A comparison of the efficacy of clonazepam and cognitive-behavioral group therapy for the treatment of social phobia. *J. Anxiety Disord.*, **14**: 345–348.

88. Versiani M., Nardi A.E., Figueira I., Mendlowicz M., Marques C. (1997) Double-blind placebo-controlled trial with bromazepam in social phobia. *J. Brasil Psiquiatria*, **46**: 167–171.
89. James I., Savage I. (1984) Beneficial effect of nadolol on anxiety-induced disturbances of performance in musicians: a comparison with diazepam and placebo. *Am. Heart J.*, **108**: 1150–1155.
90. Schneier F.R., Saoud J., Campeas R., Falloon B., Hollander E., Coplan J., Liebowitz M.R. (1993) Buspirone in social phobia. *J. Clin. Psychopharmacol.*, **13**: 251–256.
91. van Vliet I.M., den Boer J.A., Westenberg H.G., Pian K.L. (1997) Clinical effects of buspirone in social phobia: a double-blind placebo-controlled study. *J. Clin. Psychiatry*, **58**: 164–168.
92. Clark D.B., Agras W.S. (1991) The assessment and treatment of performance anxiety in musicians. *Am. J. Psychiatry*, **148**: 598–605.
93. van Ameringen M., Mancini C., Wilson C. (1996) Buspirone augmentation of selective serotonin reuptake inhibitors (SSRIs) in social phobia. *J. Affect. Dis.*, **39**: 115–121.
94. Bell J., DeVeaugh-Geiss J. (1994) Multicenter trial of a 5-HT$_3$ antagonist, ondansetron, in social phobia. Presented at the 33rd Annual Meeting of the American College of Neuropsychopharmacology, San Juan, 12–16 December.
95. Pande A.C., Davidson J.R., Jefferson J.W., Janney C.A., Katzelnick D.J., Weisler R.H., Greist J.H., Sutherland S.M. (1999) Treatment of social phobia with gabapentin: a placebo-controlled study. *J. Clin. Psychopharmacol.*, **19**: 341–348.
96. Barnett S.D., Kramer M.L., Casat C.D., Connor K.M., Davidson J.R. (2002) Efficacy of olanzapine in social anxiety disorder: a pilot study. *J. Psychopharmacol.*, **16**: 365–368.
97. Pallanti S., Quercioli L., Rossi A., Pazzagli A. (1999) The emergence of social phobia during clozapine treatment and its response to fluoxetine augmentation. *J. Clin. Psychiatry*, **60**: 819–823.
98. Gorman J.M., Liebowitz M.R., Fyer A.J., Campeas R., Klein D.F. (1985) Treatment of social phobia with atenolol. *J. Clin. Psychopharmacol.*, **5**: 298–301.
99. Turner S., Beidel D.C., Jacob R.G. (1994) Social phobia: a comparison of behaviour therapy and atenolol. *J. Consult. Clin. Psychol.*, **62**: 350–358.
100. Falloon I.R., Llody G.G., Harpin R.E. (1981) The treatment of social phobia. Real-life rehearsal with nonprofessional therapists. *J. Nerv. Ment. Dis.*, **169**: 180–184.
101. Brantigan C.O., Brantigan T.A., Joseph N. (1982) Effects of beta-blockade and beta-stimulation on stage fright. *Am. J. Med.*, **72**: 88–94.
102. Drew P.J.T, Barnes J.N., Evans S.J.W. (1983) The effects of acute B-adrenoceptor blockade on examination performance. *Br. J. Psychiatry*, **19**: 782–786.
103. Gates G.A., Saegert J., Wilson N., Johnson L., Shepard A., Hearne E.M. (1985) Effect of beta-blockage on singing performance. *Ann. Otol. Rhinol. Laryngol.*, **94**: 570–574.
104. Hartley L.R., Ungapen S., Davie I., Spencer D.J. (1983) The effect of beta adrenergic blockade on speaker's performance and memory. *Br. J. Psychiatry*, **142**: 512–517.
105. James I.M., Griffith D.N.W, Pearson R.M., Newby P. (1977) Effect of oxprenolol on stage-fright in musicians. *Lancet*, **ii**: 952–954.

106. Siitonen L., Janne J. (1976) Effect of beta-blockade during bowling competition. *Ann. Clin. Res.*, **8**: 393–398.
107. Liden S., Gottfries C.G. (1974) Beta-blocking agents in the treatment of catecholamine-induced symptoms in musicians. *Lancet*, **2**: 529.
108. Neftel K.A., Adler R.H., Kappeli L., Rossi M., Kaser H.E., Bruggesser H.H., Vorkauf H. (1982) Stage fright in musicians: a model illustrating the effect of beta blockers. *Psychosom. Med.*, **44**: 461–469.
109. James I.M., Burgoyne W., Savage I.T. (1983) Effect of pindolol on stress-related disturbances of musical performance: preliminary communication. *J. Roy. Soc. Med.*, **76**: 194–196.
110. Schneier F.R. (1995) Clinical assessment strategies for social phobia. *Psychiatr. Ann.*, **25**: 550–553.
111. Goldstein S. (1987) Treatment of social phobia with clonidine. *Biol. Psychiatry*, **22**: 369–372.
112. Davidson J.R., Foa E.B., Connor K.M., Churchill L.E. (2002) Hyperhidrosis in social phobia. *Prog. Neuropsychopharmacol. Biol. Psychiatry*, **26**: 1327–1331.
113. Stein M.B., Sareen J., Hami S., Chao J. (2001) Pindolol potentiation of paroxetine for generalized social phobia: a double-blind, placebo-controlled, crossover study. *Am. J. Psychiatry*, **158**: 1725–1727.
114. Klein D.F., Fink M. (1962) Psychiatric reaction patterns to imipramine. *Am. J. Psychiatry*, **119**: 432–438.
115. West E.D., Dally P.J. (1959) Effects of iproniazid in depressive syndromes. *Br. Med. J.*, **1**: 1491–1494.
116. Sargant W., Dally P. (1962) Treatment of anxiety states by antidepressant drugs. *Br. Med. J.*, **1**: 6–9.
117. Klein D.F. (1964) Delineation of two drug-responsive anxiety syndromes. *Psychopharmacologia*, **5**: 397–408.
118. Lipsedge M.S., Hajioff J., Huggins P., Napier L., Pearce J., Pike D.J., Rich M. (1973) The management of severe agoraphobia: a comparison of iproniazid and systematic desensitization. *Psychopharmacologia*, **32**: 67–80.
119. Sheehan D.V., Ballenger J., Jacobsen G. (1980) Treatment of endogenous anxiety with phobic, hysterical, and hypochondriacal symptoms. *Arch. Gen. Psychiatry*, **37**: 51–59.
120. Zitrin C.M., Klein D.F., Woerner M.G. (1980) Treatment of agoraphobia with group exposure in vivo and imipramine. *Arch. Gen. Psychiatry*, **37**: 63–72.
121. Ballenger J.C., Davidson J.R.T, Lecrubier Y., Nutt D.J., Bobes J., Beidel D.C., Ono Y., Westenberg H.G. (1998) Consensus statement on panic disorder from the International Consensus Group on Depression and Anxiety. *J. Clin. Psychiatry*, **59** (Suppl. 8): 47–54.
122. Pande A.C., Pollack M.H., Crockatt J., Greiner M., Chouinard G., Lydiard R.B., Taylor C.B., Dager S.R., Shiovitz T. (2000) Placebo-controlled study of gabapentin treatment of panic disorder. *J. Clin. Psychopharmacol.*, **20**: 467–471.
123. Boyer W. (1995) Serotonin uptake inhibitors are superior to imipramine and alprazolam in alleviating panic attacks: a meta-analysis. *Int. Clin. Psychopharmacol.*, **10**: 45–49.
124. Evans L., Kenardy J., Schneider P., Hoey H. (1986) Effect of a selective serotonin reuptake inhibitor in agoraphobia with panic attacks: a double-blind comparison of zimeldine, imipramine and placebo. *Acta Psychiatr. Scand.*, **73**: 49–53.
125. Otto M.W., Tuby K.S., Gould R.A., McLean R.Y., Pollack M.H. (2001) An effect–size analysis of the relative efficacy and tolerability of serotonin

selective reuptake inhibitors for panic disorder. *Am. J. Psychiatry*, **158**: 1989–1992.
126. Mavissakalian M.R., Perel J.M. (1995) Imipramine treatment of panic disorder with agoraphobia: dose ranging and plasma level-response relationships. *Am. J. Psychiatry*, **152**: 673–682.
127. Gloger S., Grunhaus L., Gladic D., O'Ryan F., Cohen L., Codner S. (1989) Panic attacks and agoraphobia: low dose clomipramine treatment. *J. Clin. Psychopharmacol.*, **9**: 28–32.
128. Lesser I.M., Lydiard R.B., Antal E., Rubin R.T., Ballenger J.C., DuPont R. (1992) Alprazolam plasma concentrations and treatment response in panic disorder and agoraphobia. *Am. J. Psychiatry*, **142**: 1556–1662.
129. Wardle J., Hayward P., Higgitt A., Stabl M., Blizard R., Gray J. (1994) Effects of concurrent diazepam treatment on the outcome of exposure therapy in agoraphobia. *Behav. Res. Ther.*, **32**: 203–215.
130. Le Doux J. (1998) Fear and the brain: where have we been, and where are we going? *Biol. Psychiatry*, **44**: 1229–1238.
131. Abene M.V., Hamilton J.D. (1998) Resolution of fear of flying with fluoxetine treatment. *J. Anxiety Disord.*, **12**: 599–603.
132. Benjamin J., Ben-Zion I.Z., Karbofsky E., Dannon P. (2000) Double-blind placebo-controlled pilot study of paroxetine for specific phobia. *Psychopharmacology*, **149**: 194–196.
133. Mawson A.B. (1970) Methohexitone-assisted desensitisation in treatment of phobias. *Lancet*, **i**: 1084–1086.
134. Berndt M.W., Silverstone T., Singleton W. (1980) Behavioral and subjective effects of beta-adrenergic blockade in phobic subjects. *Br. J. Psychiatry*, **137**: 452–457.
135. Sartory G., MacDonald R., Gray J.A. (1990) Effects of diazepam on approach, self-reported fear and psychophysiological responses in snake phobias. *Behav. Res. Ther.*, **28**: 273–282.
136. Marks I.M., Viswanathan R., Lipsedge M.S., Gardner R. (1972) Enhanced relief of phobias by flooding during waning diazepam effect. *Br. J. Psychiatry*, **121**: 493–505.
137. Wilhelm F.H., Roth W.T. (1997) Acute and delayed effects of alprazolam on flight phobics during exposure. *Behav. Res. Ther.*, **35**: 831–841.
138. Ekeberg O., Kjeldsen S.E., Greenwood D.T., Enger E. (1990) Effects of selective beta-adrenoceptor blockade on anxiety associated with flight phobia. *J. Psychopharmacol.*, **4**: 35–41.
139. Campos P.E., Solyom L., Koelink A. (1984) The effects of timolol maleate on subjective and physiological components of air travel phobia. *Can. J. Psychiatry*, **29**: 570–574.
140. Fagerstrom K.O., Hugdahl K., Lundstrom N. (1985) Effect of beta-receptor blockade on anxiety with reference to the three-systems model of phobic behavior. *Neuropsychobiology*, **13**: 187–193.
141. Stein D.J., Matsunaga H. (2001) Cross-cultural aspects of social anxiety disorder. *Psychiatr. Clin. North Am.*, **24**: 773–782.
142. Matsunaga H., Kiriike N., Matsui T., Iwasaki Y., Stein D.J. (2001) Taijin kyofusho: a form of social anxiety disorder that responds to serotonin reuptake inhibitors? *Int. J. Neuropsychopharmacol.*, **4**: 231–237.
143. Fallon B.A., Schneier F.R., Marshall R., Campeas R., Vermes D., Goetz D., Liebowitz M.R. (1996) The pharmacotherapy of hypochondriasis. *Psychopharmacol. Bull.*, **32**: 607–611.

144. Hollander E., Allen A., Kwon J., Aronowitz B., Schmeidler J., Wong C., Simeon D. (1999) Clomipramine vs desipramine crossover trial in body dysmorphic disorder: selective efficacy of a serotonin reuptake inhibitor in imagined ugliness. *Arch. Gen. Psychiatry*, **56**: 1033–1039.
145. Phillips K.A. (1998) Body dysmorphic disorder: clinical aspects and treatment strategies. *Bull. Menninger Clin.*, **62A4**: 33–48.
146. Goodall E., File S.E., Sanders F.L., Skelly A.M. (1994) Self-ratings by phobic patients during dental treatment: greater improvement with nitrous oxide than midazolam. *Hum. Psychopharmacol.*, **9**: 203–220.
147. Oberlander E.L., Schneier F.R., Liebowitz M.R. (1994) Physical disability and social phobia. *J. Clin. Psychopharmacol.*, **14**: 136–143.
148. Furmark T., Tillfors M., Marteinsdottir I., Fischer H., Pissiota A., Langstrom B., Fredrikson M. (2002) Common changes in cerebral blood flow in patients with social phobia treated with citalopram or cognitive-behavioral therapy. *Arch. Gen. Psychiatry*, **59**: 425–433.
149. Camacho A., Stein M.B. (2002) Modafinil for social phobia and amphetamine dependence. *Am. J. Psychiatry*, **159**: 1947–1948.
150. Stein D.J., Le Roux L., Bouwer C., van Heerden B. (2003) Is olfactory reference syndrome on the obsessive–compulsive spectrum? Two cases and a discussion. *J. Neuropsychiatry Clin. Neurosci.*, **10**: 96–99.
151. Oosterbaan D.B., van Balkom A.J., Spinhoven P., van Dyck R. (2001) The placebo response in social phobia. *J. Psychopharmacol.*, **15**: 199–203.
152. Turner S.M., Beidel D.C., Cooley-Quille M.R. (1995) Two-year follow-up of social phobias treated with social effectiveness therapy. *Behav. Res. Ther.*, **33**: 553–555.
153. Heimberg R.G., Salzman D.G., Holt C.S., Blendell K.A. (1993) Cognitive behavioural group treatment for social phobia: effectiveness at five-year follow-up. *Cogn. Ther. Res.*, **17**: 325–339.

Commentaries

3.1
Placing the Pharmacotherapy of Phobic Disorders in a New Neuroscience Context
Jack M. Gorman[1]

The treatment of anxiety disorders has certainly undergone curious transformations. Originally, Freud developed his first notions of the etiology of phobias by treating a boy, Little Hans. Hans was afraid to leave home, fearing he would be attacked by a horse. Apparently, Freud never actually met the patient, but conducted the therapy through Hans' father. Freud gleaned that Hans was suffering from an unconscious conflict, in this case an unresolved oedipal crisis, and its resolution rendered Hans cured. Later, Freud significantly refined his ideas in the seminal book *Signals, Inhibition and Anxiety*, but the basic concept, that anxiety results from unresolved unconscious conflict, essentially remained intact.

From this concept came the notion of "symptom substitution". According to psychoanalytic theory, any attempt to avert a phobia without reaching its root cause will only succeed superficially; another symptom will of necessity arise to protect the patient from the unacceptable implications of unconscious conflicts. Behaviourists seized upon the theory of symptom substitution to argue against the psychoanalytic formulation: "symptom substitution" is simply an erroneous concept; when a patient is relieved of a phobia by a desensitization procedure the phobia is gone, and the patient remains symptom free. Gradually, particularly in the UK but later in the US as well, psychologists embraced the new behavioural and later cognitive-behavioural methods as the *sine qua non* for the treatment of phobic disorders.

As Stein *et al.* comprehensively affirm, the use of medications to treat phobias is now the major modality employed by psychiatrists. This is in part due to the successes we have realized with pharmacotherapy; most patients respond and get better. It is also due to convenience: for the physician, prescribing medication is much simpler than conducting psychotherapy, even one as compact as cognitive-behavioural therapy

---

[1] *Department of Psychiatry, Mount Sinai School of Medicine, One Gustave L. Levy Place, New York, NY 10029, USA*

(CBT). Although long-term medication management is actually more expensive than a single course of CBT, patients rarely stay on medications very long and therefore national health and managed care organizations believe that pharmacotherapy is the cheaper approach if they agree to pay for the treatment of phobias at all.

For the treatment of social phobia, Stein et al. note that monoamine oxidase inhibitors work well and that selective serotonin reuptake inhibitors (SSRIs) are the medications of choice. Three antidepressants are now approved in the US for the treatment of social phobia: paroxetine, sertraline and venlafaxine. The authors do not emphasize one irony, however: the biggest effect size for social phobia therapy comes from the Davidson et al. study [1] in which the benzodiazepine clonazepam was effective in 78% of patients compared to only 20% who received placebo. Despite the constant warnings of the dangers of benzodiazepines, at two-year follow-up most of the patients were still doing well and the medication was both well-tolerated and rarely misused. It is absolutely true that benzodiazepines have serious drawbacks, but it must be acknowledged that the adverse side effect burdens of antidepressants are not trivial either. Admittedly, the Davidson et al. study has not been replicated and needs to be, but it is worthwhile for clinicians and academics to take note of the evident success of clonazepam therapy for a phobic disorder.

We still have no idea how long to treat patients with any phobic disorder, including social anxiety disorder. As Stein et al. note, a number of SSRI studies indicate that patients with social phobia seem to remain well as long as they continue to take their medication. Is there ever a point, however, at which the patient can discontinue medication and the relapse rate remain acceptably low? We generally recommend that patients remain on medication for six months to a year after response, but these recommendations are not empirically based. Clearly, this is one area that urgently needs an answer.

Pregabalin is certainly an interesting medication, but it turns out to have absolutely no effect on the GABA system. Rather, it binds potently to the alpha-2-delta voltage gated calcium channel, thereby reducing calcium influx into the neuron [2]. One result is a decrease in the release of several neurotransmitters thought to be key in the generation of pathological anxiety, including glutamate, noradrenaline and substance P.

The issue of agoraphobia without panic disorder is interesting and it is useful that Stein et al. have addressed it. Many still insist that the diagnosis does not exist in the community [3]. Nevertheless, epidemiological studies continue to find it in large numbers and therefore it is essential that we begin to develop algorithms for its treatment.

We have little data to confirm or deny the therapeutic efficacy of psychoanalytic treatment for phobic disorders. Nevertheless, all of a sudden neuroscientists and psychoanalysts seem to be speaking something of a common language. The unconscious conflicts of the analysts are now described as hippocampally-based implicit memories and contextual fears by neuroscientists [4]. Although the latter do not talk about Oedipus, neuroscience has placed the idea that unconscious memories can drive pathological behaviours as central to modern theories of the biology of emotion.

Furthermore, there is an enormous empirical literature on the efficacy of CBT for phobias. The results are at least as impressive as those of medication approaches and many studies indicate that the effect of CBT is more durable [5]. One wonders if there could ever be a book on treatments of common general medical conditions that separated behavioural and pharmacological therapies for hypertension. My guess is that both would appear in the same chapter in such a book, because the physician needs to remember that the first approach to most cases of high blood pressure is behavioural: weight reduction, salt restriction, exercise and stress management. Medications are only given when these approaches fail.

Stein et al. have provided us with an excellent survey of the literature supporting the use of medication in the treatment of phobias. This information now needs to be evaluated in the context of all the modalities that have been proven to work.

REFERENCES

1. Davidson J.R.T., Potts N., Richichi E., Krishnan R., Ford S.M., Smith R., Wilson W.H. (1993) Treatment of social phobia with clonazepam and placebo. *J. Clin. Psychopharmacol.*, **13**: 423–428.
2. Pande A.C., Crockatt J.G., Feltner D.E., Janney C.A., Smith W.T., Weisler R., Londborg P.D., Bielski R.J., Zimbroff D.L., Davidson J.R. et al. (2003) Pregabalin in generalized anxiety disorder: a placebo-controlled trial. *Am. J. Psychiatry*, **160**: 533–540.
3. Horwath E., Lish J.D., Johnson J., Hornig C.D., Weissman M.M. (1993) Agoraphobia without panic: clinical reappraisal of an epidemiologic finding. *Am. J. Psychiatry*, **150**: 1496–1501.
4. LeDoux J. (1998) *The Emotional Brain*. Touchstone Books, New York.
5. Barlow D.H., Gorman J.M., Shear M.K., Woods S.W. (2000) Cognitive-behavioral therapy, imipramine, or their combination for panic disorder: a randomized controlled trial. *JAMA*, **283**: 2529–2536.

3.2
Psychobiology and Pharmacotherapy of Phobias
Rudolf Hoehn-Saric[1]

Large, industry-driven drug studies demonstrate the efficacy and safety of a medication. They provide valuable general information but, by necessity, neglect important theoretical and practical aspects of treatment. One can conclude from these studies that benzodiazepines are valuable in attenuating acute phobic symptoms, while antidepressants that inhibit synaptic serotonin reuptake (serotonin reuptake inhibitors, SRIs) or reduce its deactivation (monoamine oxidase inhibitors, MAOIs) are the medications of choice for long-term treatment. Few of these studies deal with the interactions between the psychobiological mechanisms of phobias and the pharmacodynamic properties of the medications. These interactions, however, are important for the understanding of the effects of therapy.

The psychobiology of phobias is complex. Twin studies suggest a genetic predisposition for the development of phobias but also emphasize the formative role of the environment in their acquisition [1]. Recent animal studies have clarified important biological mechanisms of fear acquisition and extinction. Acquisition and extinction are active processes, and fears have to be unlearned through the same mechanisms as they have been acquired [2]. These findings explain why extinction necessitates exposure to the phobic situation in an anxiety-reduced environment, a fact that was known to Kraepelin [3] and to Freud [4]. Moreover, phobias differ in their psychopathology. As long as they remain encapsulated, specific phobias or non-generalized social phobias rarely cause anxiety. However, if an individual becomes regularly exposed to the feared situation, for instance, when a snake phobic person moves to a region in which snakes are common, the circumscribed fear may generalize into an anxiety state [5]. In generalized social phobia the exposure is unavoidable and, therefore, is constantly reinforced. Patients who already suffer heightened anxiety, particularly panic attacks, are more likely to acquire phobias and are more resistant to their extinction [6]. Moreover, agoraphobics who develop their fears in response to panic attacks perceive, in contrast to most other phobics, a clear relationship between cause and effect.

How do medications reduce phobias? Benzodiazepines have a calming effect and are useful in reducing acute anxiety or as a prophylactic in anticipation of fear-inducing situations, such as fear of flying. However,

---

[1] *Johns Hopkins Hospital, 115 Meyer Building, Baltimore, MD 21287, USA*

their regular use is problematic because of their addiction potential. They also seem to interfere with the process of extinction, biologically by reducing long-term potentiation necessary for unlearning the fear [2], as well as psychologically, by lowering one's willingness to endure anxiety when exposed unmedicated to the feared situation [7]. Antidepressants reduce phobic anxiety and improve patient's functions through several mechanisms. Antidepressants with norepinephrine or serotonin reuptake inhibitory properties block panic attack and, therefore, eliminate the initial cause of agoraphobia. They probably also reduce to some degree the panic-like surge of anxiety in other phobias when a person is exposed to the phobic situation. However, when studying agoraphobic patients with panic attacks, Mavissakalian et al. found imipramine but not norepinephrine plasma levels related to improvement of agoraphobia [8]. Imipramine has norepinephrine and serotonin reuptake inhibitory properties, while desipramine predominantly inhibits norepinephrine reuptake. We also found imipramine but not desipramine blood levels associated with anxiety reduction in patients with generalized anxiety disorder [9]. In a recent imaging study, we observed in patients with generalized anxiety disorder that anxiety reduction with the SRI citalopram reduced excessive brain activation to specific symptom provocation as well as to non-specific stimuli [10]. It appears that SRIs reduce the general level of anxiety by lowering a patient's disproportionate sensitivity to external and internal stimuli. In addition, SRIs may induce an emotional indifference toward the stimuli, possibly by attenuating frontal lobe activity [11]. For these reasons, SRIs appear to be more effective than other antidepressants in reducing psychic, including phobic, anxiety. With less anxiety, patients can confront feared situations, which leads to a gradual desensitization. The observation that phobic patients continue to improve over 12 weeks and longer suggests a gradual unlearning process.

The long-term effectiveness of therapy depends on biological and psychological factors. We need to explore the effects of new drugs but in addition address, in smaller hypothesis-driven studies, questions that are frequently ignored in larger studies. For instance, why do some but not other patients respond to certain medications or treatments? Pharmacogenetic studies may provide some answers. Can we develop drugs that enhance learning, leading to faster desensitization? What are the effects of drugs on patients who improve only partially? Why do some but not other patients relapse after discontinuation of medications? In these patients, does generalized anxiety re-emerge after discontinuation of medications, which reactivates phobic fears? To what degree does the desensitization of phobias, including residual phobias in drug-treated patients, depend on patients' motivation to overcome fears and on their personality traits? These are some questions than need to be explored.

REFERENCES

1. Kendler K.S., Neale M.C., Kessler R.C., Heath A.C., Eaves L.J. (1992) The genetic epidemiology of phobias in women: the interrelationship of agoraphobia, social phobia, situational phobia, and simple phobia. *Arch. Gen. Psychiatry*, **49**: 273–281.
2. Davis M. (1992) The role of the amygdala in conditioned fear. In *The Amygdala* (Ed. J.P. Aggleton), pp. 255–305. Wiley-Liss, New York.
3. Kraepelin E. (1914) *Psychiatrie*, 8th edn. Barth, Leipzig.
4. Freud S. (1919) Turnings in the world of psychoanalytic therapy. In *Collected Papers*, vol. 2, pp. 399–400. Hogarth Press, London.
5. Marks I. (1987) *Fears, Phobias and Rituals*. Oxford University Press, New York.
6. Lader M.H., Gelder M.G., Marks I.M. (1967) Palmar skin conductance measures as predictors of response to desensitization. *J. Psychosom. Res.*, **11**: 283–290.
7. Laughren T.P., Dias A.M., Keene C., Greenblatt D.J. (1986) Can chronically anxious patients learn to cope without medications? *McLean Hosp. J.*, **11**: 72–78.
8. Mavissakalian M., Perel J.M., Michelson L. (1984) The relationship of plasma imipramine and N-desmethylimipramine to improvement in agoraphobia. *J. Clin. Psychopharmacol.*, **4**: 36–39.
9. McLeod D.R., Hoehn-Saric R., Porges S.W., Kowalski P.A., Clark C.M. (2000) Therapeutic effects of imipramine are counteracted by its metabolite, desipramine, in patients with generalized anxiety disorder. *J. Clin. Psychopharmacol.*, **20**: 615–621.
10. Hoehn-Saric R., Schlund M.W., Wong S.H.Y. (submitted) Effect of citalopram on patients with generalized anxiety disorder: an imaging study.
11. Hoehn-Saric R., Lipsey J.R., McLeod D.R. (1990) Apathy and indifference in patients on fluvoxamine and fluoxetine. *J. Clin. Psychopharmacol.*, **10**: 343–345.

3.3
The Neuropsychology of Defence: Implications for Syndromes and Pharmacotherapy

Neil McNaughton[1]

Social phobia, agoraphobia and simple phobia are all normally termed "phobia", i.e. fear. Yet all are DSM "anxiety disorders". This confound is clear in the "pharmacotherapy of phobias" when Stein *et al.* refer to "social phobia (or social anxiety disorder)". I argue that the "pharmacotherapy of phobias" will be clearer if we apply neuroscientific theory [1]. From a basic science perspective, fear and anxiety are functionally, neurally and pharmacologically distinct. On this view, simple phobia is correctly named. However, much of the phenomenology of social phobia is best

---

[1] *Department of Psychology, University of Otago, P.O. Box 56, Dunedin, New Zealand*

thought of as social anxiety. Agoraphobia itself should strictly be renamed "agoranxiety". But, to confuse the issue, its treatment normally targets panic, a primarily phobic entity, rather than agoraphobia itself.

Entities that are functionally, neurologically and pharmacologically distinct in the laboratory are, nonetheless, frequently comorbid in the clinic. This occurs for two reasons. First, one clinical entity can, over time, result in another. Recurring panic can give rise to agoraphobia; chronic anxiety can give rise to depression. Second, genetics, personality and stress, as predisposing factors to morbidity, operate on pituitary–adrenal and monoamine systems that modulate the entire defence system. The occurrence of a specific disorder (or chronic stress) can "kindle" sensitivity to neurotic disorders in general [2–4].

Despite comorbidity, the neurotic syndromes can be located [1] in a two-dimensional view of defensive systems (Table 3.3.1). The first dimension is that of defensive direction. Anxiety (and anxiolytic drug action) involve systems controlling approach into threatening situations (i.e. approach–avoidance conflict) and assessment of risk. Fear (and panicolytic drug action) involve systems controlling avoidance of, and escape from, threatening situations [5,6]. The second dimension is that of defensive distance: the level of perceived threat. This defines a functional and neural hierarchy [7]. Stress, personality factors and more generally effective drugs operate via monoamine systems that innervate all of the relevant structures. Syndrome-specific variation in drug effects (and variations in effectiveness between patients) arises from variation in receptor and uptake system subtypes from region to region (Table 3.3.2).

To see a pattern in the actions of clinically effective compounds, one must ignore exceptional effects of individual members of a class. The antidepressant and panicolytic actions of the benzodiazepine alprazolam are atypical of benzodiazepines. It should also be noted that novel anxiolytics such as buspirone and tricyclic drugs such as imipramine have anxiolytic and antidepressant actions that proceed independently. When we group drugs, then, we can view any common anxiolytic action as due to changes in one neural system and any common antidepressant action as due to changes in another neural system. Likewise the relative specificity of monoamine oxidase inhibitors for atypical depression (in which many symptoms overlap anxiety disorders but are resistant to anxiolytic drugs) argues for this being a third distinct neural entity. Following this procedure, we can see a pattern of distinct neural entities underlying the partially overlapping effects of drugs.

In Table 3.3.2, then, benzodiazepines mark out a distinct entity of generalized anxiety, distinct for all other neurotic disorders, except social anxiety. Novel anxiolytics have an additional antidepressant action but, importantly, show that panic is neurally quite distinct from anxiety proper,

TABLE 3.3.1 A two-dimensional view of defence systems. Specific syndromes result from specific dysfunction of specific neural areas as indicated

Defensive avoidance		Defensive approach	
Anterior cingulate	Obsessive–compulsive disorder	Posterior cingulate	Complex avoidance
Amygdala	Phobic avoidance	Hippocampal system	Anxious avoidance
Amygdala	Phobic arousal	Amygdala	Anxious arousal
Hypothalamus	Phobic escape		
Periaqueductal grey	Panic		

TABLE 3.3.2 Various classes of drugs effective in treating neurotic disorders and their relative effects on different neurotic syndromes

	Classical anxiolytics	Novel anxiolytics	IMI	CMI	MAOIs	SSRIs
Generalized anxiety	↓	↓	↓	↓	0?	↓
Social anxiety	↓	↓?	0	↓?	↓	↓
Unipolar depression	0	↓	↓	↓	↓	↓
Obsessions/compulsions	0	↓?	↓?	↓↓	↓?	↓↓
Panic attacks	0*	0	↓	↓↓***	↓	↓
Atypical depression	0		↓?		↓	↓?****
Simple phobia	0**		0		↓?	↓?

IMI, imipramine; CMI, clomipramine; MAOIs, monoamine oxidase inhibitors; SSRIs, selective serotonin reuptake inhibitors; 0, no effect; ↓, reduction; ↓↓, extensive reduction; ↓?, small or discrepant reduction
*excluding alprazolam (e.g. [12]); **Sartory et al. [11] report decreased *anxiety*, that is, reported aversion during *approach* and a possible reduction in approach distance, but previous studies show no effect on phobic avoidance; *** [13]; **** [14]. For details see McNaughton [10] and Stein et al. (this volume)

while the effects of imipramine show that antidepressant action does not imply effects on social anxiety. Both pharmacologically, and because it involves entry into a dangerous situation, we should, therefore, talk about social anxiety rather than social phobia. Likewise, because of its pharmacological specificity, and because compulsions involve avoidance of danger, we should see obsessive–compulsive disorder as a form of phobia. Simply in terms of pharmacological pattern one might wish to link panic with obsession. However, there is good reason to see obsession as linked to the cingulate cortex [8] and panic as linked to the periaqueductal grey [9] and this would suggest that the apparent differences in their pharmacological sensitivities are real. The insensitivity to anxiolytic drugs of avoidance behaviour in simple phobia is as would be expected from Table 3.3.1. However, animal studies would place its neural control intermediate between panic and obsessive–compulsive disorder. Stein *et al.* report some positive results with serotonergic drugs on simple phobia, as might be expected. But the data of Table 3.3.2 suggest that clomipramine could be particularly effective.

In conclusion, then, careful review of the clinical literature (especially in relation to diagnostic criteria used in different studies) as carried out by Stein *et al.* is important. But it may also be considerably aided, and anomalous results more easily detected, when the data are placed in the context of neural theories of drug action and of the disorders being treated.

REFERENCES

1. Gray J.A., McNaughton N. (2000) *The Neuropsychology of Anxiety: An Enquiry into the Functions of the Septo-Hippocampal System*, vol. 2. Oxford University Press, Oxford.
2. Adamec R.E., Blundell J., Collins A. (2002) Neural plasticity and stress induced changes in defense in the rat. *Neurosci. Biobehav. Rev.*, **25**: 721–744.
3. Adamec R., Shallow T. (1993) Lasting effects on rodent anxiety of a single exposure to a cat. *Physiol. Behav.*, **54**: 101–109.
4. Adamec R., Kent P., Anisman P., Shallow T., Merali Z. (1998) Neural plasticity, neuropeptides and anxiety in animals—implications for understanding and treating affective disorder following traumatic stress in humans. *Neurosci. Biobehav. Rev.*, **23**: 301–318.
5. Blanchard R.J., Blanchard D.C. (1990) *An Ethoexperimental Analysis of Defense, Fear and Anxiety*. Otago University Press, Dunedin.
6. Blanchard R.J., Griebel G., Henrie J.A., Blanchard D.C. (1997) Differentiation of anxiolytic and panicolytic drugs by effects on rat and mouse defense test batteries. *Neurosci. Biobehav. Rev.*, **21**: 783–789.
7. Graeff F.G. (1994) Neuroanatomy and neurotransmitter regulation of defensive behaviors and related emotions in mammals. *Brazil J. Med. Biol. Res.*, **27**: 811–829.
8. Rapoport J.L. (1989) The biology of obsessions and compulsions. *Sci. Am.*, **260**: 83–89.
9. Deakin J.F.W., Graeff F.G. (1991) 5-HT and mechanisms of defence. *J. Psychopharmacol.*, **5**: 305–315.
10. McNaughton N. (2002) Aminergic transmitter systems. In *Textbook of Biological Psychiatry* (Eds H. D'haenen, J.A. Den Boer, H. Westenberg, P. Willner), pp. 895–914. John Wiley & Sons, Chichester.

11. Sartory G., MacDonald R., Gray J.A. (1990) Effects of diazepam on approach, self-reported fear and psychophysiological responses in snake phobics. *Behav. Res. Ther.*, **28**: 273–282.
12. Sanderson W.C., Wetzler S., Asnis G.M. (1994) Alprazolam blockade of CO_2-provoked panic in patients with panic disorder. *Am. J. Psychiatry*, **151**: 1220–1222.
13. Gentil V., Lotufo-Neto F., Andrade L., Cordás T., Bernik M., Ramos R., Maciel L., Miyakawa E., Gorenstein C. (1993) Clomipramine, a better reference drug for panic/agoraphobia. I. Effectiveness comparison with imipramine. *J. Psychopharmacol.*, **7**: 316–324.
14. McGrath P.J., Stewart J.W., Janal M.N., Petkova E., Quitkin F.M., Klein D.F. (2000) A placebo-controlled study of fluoxetine versus imipramine in the acute treatment of atypical depression. *Am. J. Psychiatry*, **157**: 344–350.

3.4
Social Phobia: Not Neglected, Just Misunderstood
David S. Baldwin[1]

In Autumn 1998 a press briefing for UK journalists organized by a major pharmaceutical company began with the statement "shyness is to social phobia, what sadness is to depression". This maxim has proved both helpful and unhelpful.

Social phobia can no longer be described as the "neglected anxiety disorder". The last decade has seen considerable advances in our understanding of the epidemiology, pathophysiology and management of this typically chronic and burdensome medical condition. Without doubt, this knowledge and the widespread availability of evidence-based treatments such as the prescription of selective serotonin reuptake inhibitors and the use of cognitive therapy have together improved the lot of countless individuals—people whose lives would otherwise have been blighted by the inhibiting influence of social phobia on academic achievement, employment opportunities and interpersonal relationships. Through giving clear and readily understandable accounts of the nature of social phobia and how doctors can help people with that condition, responsible journalists have played a major role in public education, and must be applauded for their efforts. By developing effective and acceptable treatments, offering the prospect of symptom relief and improved quality of life, the considerable and dogged efforts of pharmaceutical companies should be acknowledged and respected.

---

[1] *Department of Psychiatry, University of Southampton, Royal South Hants Hospital, Southampton, SO14 0YG, UK*

But not everything has gone well. Some drugs have been hyped, and some press coverage has been unbalanced. Doctors have been accused of "medicalizing shyness". People with minor or self-limiting social distress have been encouraged to present for often needless treatment at specialist "shyness clinics". By contrast, severely afflicted potential patients with considerable and persistent disability do not present, having received alarmist messages about the risks of treatment. Social phobia is so much more than mere shyness, and effective patient-centred treatment is much more than just reaching for a prescription pad.

Dan Stein and colleagues have provided a clear and comprehensive account of the efficacy of a range of treatment approaches for social phobia and the other phobic disorders. They rightly emphasize the findings of randomized controlled trials, and highlight continuing uncertainties about the relative efficacy and tolerability of the differing classes of psychotropic drugs, and the comparative efficacy of psychological and pharmacological treatments. Progress in this area is so rapid that their review will need updating very soon, once the results of double-blind treatment studies with serotonin-noradrenaline reuptake inhibitor (SNRI) antidepressants and novel anticonvulsant drugs appear in peer-reviewed scientific publications. For example, Japanese colleagues have demonstrated that milnacipran treatment can be helpful in patients with taijin-kyofusho [1], and large multicentre studies have confirmed that venlafaxine, another SNRI, has efficacy in both the acute and continuation treatment of patients with DSM-IV generalized social anxiety disorder [2]. In addition, the anticonvulsant drug pregabalin has been found efficacious in short-term treatment [3].

A meeting of the European College of Neuropsychopharmacology in March 2003 sought to clarify some uncertainties relating to the assessment of efficacy of potential new treatments in social anxiety disorder, with the remit of providing clear guidance on preferable trial design in a forthcoming consensus statement. Many issues were discussed, including the methods for diagnostic assessment, the requisite level of symptom severity at baseline, the acceptable level of psychiatric comorbidity, and the description of response and remission. Particular attention was focused on the duration of acute treatment studies and the best method for demonstrating the maintenance of acute treatment effects over the longer term. It seems likely that regulatory authorities will require more than the simple demonstration of a reduction in symptom severity when assessing potential new drugs for social phobia; another key outcome is the diminution of symptom-related disability. This clarification should help reduce some of the current concern about the disorder and its treatment, without hindering the development of new and hopefully improved treatments.

Much of the cynicism about social phobia arises as much from a failure to appreciate the considerable and enduring burden of the condition, as from concern about the marketing activities of some pharmaceutical companies. Further epidemiological research into the costs of social phobia, and into the cost-effectiveness and long-term acceptability of prolonged treatment, would be welcome. Closer collaboration between academic centres and adequate support from grant-giving bodies is essential. We cannot rely on the industry to conduct such major work.

REFERENCES

1. Nagata T., Oshima J., Wada A., Yamada H., Iketani T., Kiriike N. (2003) Open trial of milnacipran for Taijin-Kyofusho in Japanese patients with social anxiety disorder. *Int. J. Psychiatry Clin. Pract.*, **7**: 107–112.
2. Liebowitz M., Mangano R. (2002) Efficacy of venlafaxine XR in generalised social anxiety disorder. *Int. J. Neuropsychopharmacol.*, **5** (Suppl. 1): S211.
3. Feltner D.E., Pollack M.H., Davidson J.R., Stein M.B., Futterer R., Jefferson J.W., Lydiard R.B., DuBoff E., Robinson P., Phelps M. et al. (2000) A placebo-controlled study of pregabalin in the treatment of social phobia: outcome and predictors of response. *Eur. Neuropsychopharmacol.*, **10** (Suppl. 3): S344.

3.5
Research in Pharmacotherapy of Social Anxiety Disorder
Siegfried Kasper and Dietmar Winkler[1]

Although there is a large database already available for the pharmacotherapy of social phobia, there is still a need for further studies to be conducted. Recently, efforts have been undertaken to develop guidelines for the investigation of this disorder by European health authorities. One question involved in future studies regards the selection of populations, e.g. generalized versus non-generalized social phobia, since there is some evidence that the more severe group of generalized social phobia has a higher likelihood to present a placebo/drug difference. However, Stein *et al.* correctly mention that too few patients with non-generalized social phobia have been studied to reach definite conclusions on the value of pharmacotherapy in this subtype. Interestingly, considering generalized

---

[1] *Department of General Psychiatry, University of Vienna, Währinger Gürtel 18-20, A-1090 Vienna, Austria*

social phobia, there usually is a higher rate of comorbidity with other psychiatric diseases, most often with major depression or anxiety disorder, but also secondary alcohol or substance abuse. This is specifically important if a known antidepressant drug is being tested in social phobia. It should be recommended to exclude comorbid major depression in order to establish that the studied compound is directly working in social phobia and the effect is not secondary to its antidepressant properties.

Although standardized criteria are available for the diagnosis of social phobia based on ICD-10 and DSM-IV-TR, it would be wise to establish the diagnosis in future trials by structured or semi-structured interviews. Based on these, it should be clear that the patient should fear a predefined number of social situations, e.g. four situations, in order to study a more severe form of the disease, therefore being able to detect placebo/drug differences.

Commonly used scales in social phobia include the Liebowitz Social Anxiety Scale (LSAS) [1] and the Brief Social Phobia Scale [2]. Both of these scales are able to distinguish and quantify the fear and avoidance components separately, which is of clinical importance. Looking at the literature, however, it is not entirely clear what cut-offs of these scales should be used.

Social phobia has recently more often been named in the literature as social anxiety disorder and the abbreviation SAD was used. Since over the past 20 years there have been a large number of publications (over 1000) on seasonal affective disorder, which is also abbreviated as SAD, we recommend that the abbreviation SAD is not used for social phobia, as this would otherwise confuse the field of research substantially. Since social anxiety disorder, however, seems to be an acceptable terminology and an acronym is always necessary for easier communication, we would propose the abbreviation SOAD, which is also easy to use in different languages.

REFERENCES

1. Liebowitz M.R. (1987) Social phobia. *Mod. Prob. Pharmacopsychiatry*, **22**: 141–173.
2. Davidson J.R., Miner C.M., De-Veaugh-Geiss J., Tupler L.A., Colket J.T., Potts N.L. (1997) The Brief Social Phobia Scale: a psychometric evaluation. *Psychol. Med.*, **27**: 161–166.

3.6
Pharmacotherapy for Phobic Disorders: Where Do We Go from Here?
Mark H. Pollack[1]

Like all good scholarly reviews, the paper by Stein and colleagues examining the pharmacotherapy of the phobias examines what is already known, while raising at least as many questions as it answers. As our knowledge on the underlying neurophysiological substrate of the anxiety disorders grows [1], it seems clearer that both pharmacological and psychosocial therapies for the treatment of anxiety may exert their beneficial effects by accessing the same underlying neurobiological systems. However, although there is a substantial degree of overlap in the spectrum of efficacy of the pharmacological agents and psychosocial therapies, there is also some evidence of specificity and differences. For instance, tricyclic antidepressants are effective for panic disorder but apparently not for social phobia; similarly, specific phobias respond to cognitive-behavioural therapy (CBT) but apparently not to tricyclics. These observations may help better tease out differences and commonalities in the underlying pathophysiology of the anxiety disorders and lead to the development of more targeted and efficacious treatments.

Whether different components of each anxiety disorder respond differentially to diverse treatment modalities within and between therapeutic classes also requires additional study. Although it was initially believed that medications like imipramine block panic attacks while CBT treats phobic avoidance, accruing evidence suggests that phobic avoidance responds to pharmacotherapy over time, and that CBT can block panic attacks [2]. In social phobia, both pharmacological and cognitive-behavioural therapies have demonstrated equivalent acute and long-term efficacy, although the evidence suggests that the therapeutic effects of CBT persist to a greater degree than those of phenelzine following treatment discontinuation [3,4]. It is clear that a number of pharmacotherapies as well as CBT have demonstrated efficacy for the treatment of social anxiety disorder; however, despite the belief that combining these two effective treatment modalities would be more effective than either intervention alone, there is little empirical data addressing this issue in social phobia. Data from a recently completed multicentre randomized controlled trial in patients with panic disorder, comparing the efficacy of imipramine, CBT and the combination, demonstrated that both modalities were effective and that there was incremental additional benefit for the

---

[1] *Center for Anxiety and Traumatic Stress Related Disorders, Massachusetts General Hospital, 15 Parkman St., Boston, MA 02114, USA*

combination [5]. However, the magnitude of this added effect was not great, and it is not clear from a cost–benefit perspective that routine administration of formal combined therapy is warranted. Thus, extrapolating from this work, a pressing issue in the clinical practice of the anxiety disorders, including social anxiety disorder and other phobic disorders, is the identification of patients who might most benefit from initial treatment with combined therapies and those who may best be started with monotherapy, with combined or augmentation interventions reserved for partial or non-responders. Further, given limitations on the availability of empirically based CBT in most settings, there is a pressing need to devise efficient and effective ways of embedding CBT into the routine administration of pharmacotherapy of social phobia and other phobic disorders. There is a growing consensus that exposure instructions should be included along with the prescription of medication for the treatment of phobic disorders, with the recognition that even minimal encouragement and directions about exposure can have a salutary effect on panic disorder and accompanying phobic disorders [6]. The greater dissemination of exposure-based treatments into pharmacologic practice and the skilful blending of these therapeutic modalities are critical challenges for the field.

Related to these concerns is the understudied area of treatment refractory anxiety disorders. What to do with patients with social anxiety disorder or other phobic disorders who do not respond fully to initial treatment is an issue facing practising clinicians on a regular basis, and yet there is little empirically derived data to offer guidance. Fixed-dose studies do not, in general, show evidence of a clear dose–response relationship for the anxiety disorders. However, identification of patients who may benefit from higher doses earlier in treatment is an important clinical issue deserving of systematic inquiry. Further, there has been little done to date addressing the question of whether partial or non-responders to initial treatment benefit from increased doses of the initial medication, combination therapy or consideration of alternative or augmentative strategies. Research on these areas may provide important answers that will improve our ability to render optimal care to patients affected by these distressing and often disabling conditions.

REFERENCES

1. Gorman J.M., Kent J.M., Sullivan G.M., Coplan J.D. (2002) Neuroanatomical hypothesis of panic disorder, revised. *Am. J. Psychiatry*, **157**: 493–505.
2. Pollack M.H., Marzol P.C. (2000) Course, complications and treatment of panic disorder. *J. Psychopharmacol.*, **14**: 25–30.

3. Heimberg R.G., Liebowitz M.R., Hope D.A., Schneier F.R., Holt C.S., Welkowitz L.A., Juster H.R., Campeas R., Bruch M.A., Cloitre M. et al. (1998) Cognitive behavioral group therapy vs phenelzine therapy for social phobia: 12-week outcome. Arch. Gen. Psychiatry, **55**: 1133–1141.
4. Liebowitz M.R., Heimberg R.G., Schneier F.R., Hope D.A., Davies S., Holt C.S., Goetz D., Juster H.R., Lin S.H., Bruch M.A. et al. (1999) Cognitive-behavioral group therapy versus phenelzine in social phobia: long-term outcome. Depress. Anxiety, **10**: 89–98.
5. Barlow D.H., Gorman J.M., Shear M.K., Woods S.W. (2000) Cognitive-behavioral therapy, imipramine, or their combination for panic disorder: a randomized controlled trial. JAMA, **283**: 2529–2536.
6. Swinson R.P., Soulios C., Cox B.J., Kuch K. (1992) Brief treatment of emergency room patients with panic attacks. Am. J. Psychiatry, **149**: 944–946.

3.7
Progress in Pharmacotherapy for Social Anxiety Disorder and Agoraphobia

Bruce Lydiard[1]

Social phobia or social anxiety disorder (SAD) was accorded official psychiatric diagnostic status less than 20 years ago, but has been described in the medical literature for centuries. Hippocrates described such a patient over 2000 years ago: "He dare not come in company for fear he should be misused, disgraced, overshoot himself in gestures or speeches or be sick; he thinks every man observes him" [1]. The National Comorbidity Survey (NCS) estimated lifetime prevalence of SAD at 13.3% and 12-month prevalence at 7.6%, making it the third most common psychiatric disorder, following only major depression and alcohol abuse/dependence [2]. Despite this high prevalence, SAD remains woefully under-recognized, despite the availability of quick and easy-to-use screening tools [3] which could be easily applied in primary care settings [4].

Two main subtypes of SAD exist. Roughly one-third of sufferers have discrete social fears which focus almost entirely on public speaking, are generally less disabling, and have a better prognosis. The other two-thirds suffer from generalized SAD, a much more severe, potentially disabling, subtype in which all or nearly all interpersonal interactions outside of close friends and family are difficult to impossible [5].

---

[1] *Department of Psychiatry, University of South Carolina, 1 Poston Road, Charleston, SC 29407, USA*

Generalized SAD often begins early in life: 35% of the time SAD occurs in individuals before age 10. Thus, it is a disorder of children as well as adults [6]. Further, as noted by the authors, it represents a risk factor for subsequent development of additional psychiatric disorders, especially depression.

Pharmacological treatment for the discrete versus generalized subtypes should be emphasized. Patients with generalized SAD require constant treatment, preferably with a selective serotonin reuptake inhibitor (SSRI). Those individuals with speaking fears may be able to manage their symptoms acutely by using benzodiazepines or beta-blockers. Though empirical data are lacking for either of these classes, significant clinical experience indicates that they provide satisfactory relief of symptoms related to the feared situation.

The average dosage of SSRIs used in the large clinical trials in which flexible dosing was allowed suggests that patients with SAD may require dosages higher than those with uncomplicated major depression. For example, Stein *et al.* reported that an average of 36.6 mg paroxetine per day was needed [7], while Liebowitz (personal communication, 2003) used 168 mg daily of sertraline. Sertraline has also been shown to prevent relapse over a six-month study period [8].

Very recently, venlafaxine, which is a serotonin-norepinephrine reuptake inhibitor, has been approved for the treatment of generalized SAD after successful multicentre placebo-controlled studies (Wyeth Laboratories, data on file, 2003).

The section on agoraphobia of Stein *et al.*'s review brings up the different theoretical constructs by which agoraphobia is viewed. The American perspective, first elucidated by Donald Klein, places a central role on the appearance of unexpected panic attacks which initiate and maintain the related fearful avoidance called agoraphobia. According to the DSM-IV Text Revision, "the essential features of agoraphobia without history of panic disorder are similar to those of panic disorder with agoraphobia except that the focus of fear is on the occurrence of incapacitating or extremely embarrassing panic-like symptoms or limited symptom attacks rather than full panic attacks". Stein *et al.* mention panic disorder and the data supporting the link between panic and agoraphobia in their review. It seems worthwhile to add here that, from a clinical perspective, control of panic attacks is imperative in ameliorating the anticipatory anxiety and agoraphobia, and that they should be considered a target symptom of importance.

There is general agreement that a broadly based assessment—which includes attention to avoidance, anticipatory anxiety, panic attacks and depression—is necessary to get a good idea of progress, since the ascertainment of panic attacks is necessary but not sufficient for assessing overall outcome.

REFERENCES

1. Burton R. (1845) *The Anatomy of Melancholy*, vol. 1, 11th edn. Thomas Tegg, London.
2. Kessler R.C., McGonagle K.A., Zhao S., Nelson, C.B., Hughes M., Eshleman, S., Wittchen H.U., Kendler K.S. (1994) Lifetime and 12-month prevalence of DSM-III-R psychiatric disorders in the United States. Results from the National Comorbidity Survey. *Arch. Gen. Psychiatry*, **51**: 8–19.
3. Connor K.M., Kobak K.A., Churchil L.E., Katzelnick D., Davidson J.R. (2001) Mini-SPIN: a brief screening assessment for generalized social anxiety disorder. *Depress. Anxiety*, **14**: 137–140.
4. Katzelnick D.J., Greist J.H. (2001) Social anxiety disorder: an unrecognized problem in primary care. *J. Clin. Psychiatry*, **62** (Suppl. 1): 11–15.
5. Kessler R.C., Stein M.B., Berglund P. (1998) Social phobia subtypes in the National Comorbidity Survey. *Am. J. Psychiatry*, **155**: 613–619.
6. Schneier F.R., Johnson J., Hornig C.D., Liebowitz M.R., Weissman M.M. (1992) Social phobia: comorbidity and morbidity in an epidemiologic sample. *Arch. Gen. Psychiatry*, **49**: 282–288.
7. Stein M., Liebowitz M., Lydiard B., Pitts N., Bushnell W., Gergel I. (1998) Paroxetine treatment of generalized social phobia (social anxiety disorder): a randomized, double-blind, placebo-controlled study. *JAMA*, **260**: 708–713.
8. Walker J.R., Van Ameringen M.A., Swinson R., Bowen R.C., Chokka P.R., Goldner E., Johnston D.C., Lavallie Y.J., Nandy S., Pecknold J.C. et al. (2000) Prevention of relapse in generalized social phobia: results of a 24-week study in responders to 20 weeks of sertraline treatment. *J. Clin. Psychopharmacol.*, **20**: 636–644.

3.8
Psychopharmacology Treatment of Phobias and Avoidance Reactions
Carl Salzman[1]

Dan Stein et al. have produced a comprehensive and lucid summary of the current "state-of-the-art" treatments for phobias. The review is based on the DSM diagnostic system, which subcategorizes phobias into social anxiety disorder (a term I prefer to social phobia), agoraphobia and simple phobia. All of these are included in the anxiety-spectrum category and share considerable comorbidity with other anxiety disorders, especially generalized anxiety disorder. Comorbidity among anxiety-spectrum disorders is the rule rather than the exception. Virtually all patients with a form of phobic avoidance disorder—whether it be social, simple, or agoraphobic—suffer from high degrees of anxiety and many also meet diagnostic criteria

---

[1] *Department of Psychiatry, Massachusetts Mental Health Center, 74 Fenwood Road, Boston, MA 02115, USA*

for major depression or dysthymia (or both). Many self-medicate with alcohol or other drugs and thus may suffer from a comorbid substance abuse disorder. Phobic disorders are also not unusual in the elderly, although their appearance for the first time in late life may be due to environmental circumstances rather than inner psychological or neurobiologic dysfunction.

The hallmark of phobic disorders, regardless of subtype, is avoidance behaviour. Those suffering from social anxiety disorder avoid circumstances such as parties, restaurants, stores, or classrooms that place them in the company of large numbers of other individuals. Those with agoraphobia avoid virtually all social interactions, resulting in constricted as well as restricted activity. Patients with simple phobias, like Freud's Little Hans, classically avoid the specific phobic stimulus.

The avoidance behaviour, however, is rarely therapeutic. Phobic individuals not only experience anxiety when confronted with their phobic stimulus, but experience considerable anticipatory anxiety as well. Merely the thought of shopping, flying or speaking publicly is enough to produce overwhelming anxiety symptoms. Anticipatory anxiety, in turn, usually reinforces the phobic avoidance, leading to a chronic repetitive pattern of avoidance—anxiety—more avoidance—more anxiety.

It is likely that humans have been attempting to treat phobic anxiety and its comorbid symptoms for thousands of years. The use of alcohol, perhaps the earliest antianxiety agent, is still widespread (just attend any social gathering or observe fellow travellers at an airport). Prayer, talismans, superstition, as well as various relaxation techniques have all been used with varying success, and some are still widely practised, also with varying success. Perhaps the first major pharmacologic breakthrough came about with the availability of benzodiazepine anxiolytic medication in the 1960s. For the first time it was possible to rapidly and safely treat phobic anxiety without the hazards of alcohol or other potent sedative hypnotic substances. Benzodiazepines rapidly and reliably diminish acute phobic anxiety, enabling individuals to travel, shop, and even dine and speak publicly. Their use, however, is not without hazards. With chronic use, a physiological dependency develops as well as psychological reliance. There may be sedative side effects and mild cognitive impairment (which are worse in the elderly).

Coincident with the appearance of benzodiazepines in the 1960s, a small group of research studies demonstrated the remarkable efficacy of antidepressants to treat phobic anxiety disorders as well. Tricyclics and monoamine oxidase inhibitors were found to be particularly effective for panic anxiety, or panic associated with phobic avoidance behaviours. These early observations paved the way for more recent studies demonstrating the efficacy of the newer serotonergic antidepressants, which are effective in many patients. In recent years, patterns of pharmacotherapy have shifted away from benzodiazepines to the antidepressants for the long-term management of phobic disorders [1].

Antidepressants, new as well as old, are not without their own difficulties. For one thing, they do not work immediately and thus cannot be used for the immediate management of acute anxiety. Second, their own side effects may limit their usefulness. Sexual dysfunction and weight gain, in particular, are a high price to pay for diminished phobic anxiety. What has been emerging clinically, therefore, is a combined use of benzodiazepines and antidepressants for treatment of these potentially disabling disorders. In a typical clinical circumstance, the patient will be started on a benzodiazepine and an antidepressant, and treated with both medications for several weeks or even months until symptoms are satisfactorily resolved and clinical stability has been achieved. At this point, benzodiazepines can be gradually tapered and sometimes even eliminated. In other circumstances, when the antidepressant side effects are not acceptable, the dose of the antidepressant will be reduced and benzodiazepine treatment maintained.

It is likely that new treatments will result in fewer and fewer side effects that limit their usefulness. It is also clear that non-pharmacologic treatments are playing an increasingly important role in the management of phobic disorders [2]. Until the time when we have risk-free treatments, however, the judicious use of psychotropic medications is likely to continue. At present, it appears that benzodiazepines for the acute treatment, antidepressants for the maintenance treatment, and some combination of both for many patients is the state of the art for treatment of these disabling anxiety disorders.

REFERENCES

1. Salzman C., Goldenberg I., Bruce S.E., Keller M.B. (2001) Pharmacologic treatment of anxiety disorders in 1989 versus 1996: results from the Harvard/Brown Anxiety Disorders Research Program. *J. Clin. Psychiatry*, **62**: 149–152.
2. Otto M.W., Pollack M.H., Gould R.A., Worthington J.J. III, McArdle E.T., Rosenbaum J.F. (2000) A comparison of the efficacy of clonazepam and cognitive-behavioral group therapy for the treatment of social phobia. *J. Anxiety Disord.*, **14**: 345–358.

3.9
Crowning Achievement: The Rise of Anti-Phobic Pharmacotherapy
Murray B. Stein[1]

I remember a time (not so long ago, but longer than I care to admit) when a review of the pharmacotherapy of phobias could have been written on the back of an envelope, and summarized in a single word (albeit a hyphenated word): beta-blockers. There is also a legacy of using monoamine oxidase inhibitors (MAOIs) to treat phobic disorders that goes back several decades, but these agents never achieved widespread usage, presumably because of side effects and concerns about safety. This created something of a therapeutic paradox in the state of treatment of phobic disorders, wherein beta-blockers reigned (despite their rather limited scope and magnitude of effect) and MAOIs were relegated to limited use (despite their magnificent efficacy). Tricyclic antidepressants were widely recognized for their efficacy in treating panic disorder (and to a lesser extent, its phobic compatriot, agoraphobia), yet they were unloved by patients due to their relatively poor initial tolerability.

And then came selective serotonin reuptake inhibitors (SSRIs), and the world of phobia pharmacotherapy was forever changed. Fluoxetine, for reasons that are unclear, did not ignite the field of phobias the way it did depressive disorders, but the SSRIs that followed swept through and conquered. Social phobia, in particular, has fared best under the benevolent rule of the SSRIs. Subsequent to the demonstration of their utility for this condition, and the concomitant expenditures by the pharmaceutical industry to increase awareness of social phobia among practitioners and the public, it has gone from being a little mentioned disorder to one that is often in the public eye. Indeed, the lay press has at times been enamoured with the outlandish notion that these powerful medicines are being used to massage ordinary shyness, rather than treat a truly disabling condition. For the most part, this occasional media rhetoric has served to draw additional attention to social phobia and the availability of pharmacotherapeutic options, and the public has been the beneficiary of this information.

Reversible inhibitors of monoamine oxidase type A (RIMAs) were once thought to be the heir-apparent to MAOIs for the treatment of phobic disorders. Although generally well tolerated, expectations ran so high that their modest efficacy (probably no better and no worse than SSRIs, though this has yet to be established) led to lukewarm reviews and modest uptake by practitioners. Their failure to be licensed in the United States did nothing to change these perceptions. Rumours persist that one of the most promising

---
[1] Department of Psychiatry, University of California at San Diego, La Jolla, California, USA

RIMAs of the past, brofaramine [1], may return from self-imposed exile. This would be a welcome event, as our therapeutic armamentarium against phobic disorders is not what it should be, particularly when considering the high rates of partial responders or non-responders to current treatments.

The mechanism of action of SSRIs (and certain other antidepressants, such as venlafaxine extended-release, which at the time of this writing had gained regulatory approval in the United States for the treatment of social phobia) in the treatment of phobic disorders is something of a mystery. Increasing central nervous system availability of serotonin may be important, but this is unproven. Tales have been told of noradrenergically active agents (e.g. desipramine) being ineffective for social phobia, but studies are few and none have included within-study comparisons to serotonergically active agents. Myths also persist about the possible utility of medications with dopaminergic agonist properties, such as bupropion, for treatment of social phobia. Although there continues to accrue evidence that Parkinson's disease, a neuropsychiatric disorder characterized by dopamine deficiency in the basal ganglia, is associated with an increased risk for the development of phobic disorders [2], evidence of anti-phobic properties of dopaminergic agonists is sparse. Indeed, the atypical antipsychotic medications are being heralded as possible anti-phobic medications, further muddying the mechanistic marsh upon which clinicians must tread when trying to explain to our patients how and why our medications work.

Discerning mechanisms of action of anti-phobic medications may not be the Holy Grail for this field, but it is an important objective to be achieved in the coming years. Another important goal will be to develop new treatments for phobic disorders that can be used to help partial responders or non-responders to antidepressants. Here, a return to power of the benzodiazepines may be expected [3], as their utility has too long been overshadowed by concerns about abuse and dependence liability. The potential for misuse of the benzodiazepines is real, but so is the potential benefit to phobic patients, particularly when other treatments have proven ineffective. We await the inevitable and much anticipated coronation of new classes of safer, more effective anti-phobic medications. But while we wait, we must not waver in our determination to apply our entire set of phobia weapons—benzodiazepines included—to the benefit of our patients.

REFERENCES

1. Fahlen T., Nilsson H.L., Borg K., Humble M., Pauli U. (1995) Social phobia: the clinical efficacy and tolerability of the monoamine oxidase-A and serotonin

uptake inhibitor brofaromine: a double-blind placebo-controlled study. *Acta Psychiatr. Scand.*, **92**: 351–358.
2. Pollack M.H., Simon N.M., Worthington J.J., Doyle A.L., Peters P., Toshkov F.S., Otto M.W. (2003) Combined paroxetine and clonazepam treatment strategies compared to paroxetine monotherapy for panic disorder. *J. Psychopharmacol.*, **17**: 276–282.
3. Weisskopf M.G., Chen H., Schwarzschild M.A., Kawachi I., Ascherio A. (2003) Prospective study of phobic anxiety and risk of Parkinson's disease. *Movement Disord.*, **18**: 646–651.

3.10
Comorbidity and Phobias: Diagnostic and Therapeutic Challenges

Joseph Zohar[1]

Comorbidity has been defined as the presence of more than one disorder in a person, for a defined period of time [1]. As the adherence to diagnosis according to operational criteria has been widely accepted, comorbidity has by default become the rule, rather than the exception [2].

Population-based studies probably provide a better estimation of comorbidity rates as compared to studies carried out in primary and secondary care settings, which introduce the artefact of treatment-seeking into the sample. The National Comorbidity Survey (NCS) [3], which documented psychiatric diagnosis of over 8000 individuals in a population-based sample, is an example of a large population-based study.

As phobias are often associated with other axis I disorders, comorbidity may present both diagnostic dilemmas and therapeutic challenges [4].

One common example is comorbidity of social phobia and bipolar disorder. In this situation, the potential therapeutic effect of using medications such as selective serotonin reuptake inhibitors (SSRIs) versus their potential trigger effect presents a therapeutic dilemma. The therapeutic challenge is that agents that effectively treat anxiety disorders are associated with the risk of inducing mania. Therefore, the treating psychiatrist needs to carefully evaluate the potential benefit of treating the anxiety against the potential cost of inducing a manic episode. A possible approach would be to use, when possible, a non-pharmacological intervention, such as a cognitive-behavioural approach, in addition to a mood stabilizer. Encouraging data for the beneficial effect of those interventions suggests that this option should be properly explored. Alternately, it is suggested that the clinician attempts to ensure the patient receives adequate treatment with mood stabilizers before slowly and

---

[1] *Division of Psychiatry, Chaim Sheba Medical Center, Tel-Hashomer, 52621 Israel*

carefully attempting the addition of anti-anxiety compounds with relatively lower risk of mania induction (e.g. SSRIs as compared to tricyclic antidepressants) [4].

Another issue is related to a possible potential diagnostic confusion. For example, the term "germ phobia" was used in the past to diagnose obsessive–compulsive disorder (OCD) with washing rituals. So is it actually phobia for germs or OCD? How can one distinguish specific phobia that the patient is actually preoccupied with from an obsession? After all, in both cases there is excessive worrying related to specific objects or subjects, and the patient is well aware that he is disproportionately tense while facing them and consequently he tries to avoid them as much as he can.

One possible way to distinguish OCD such as "germ phobia" from a simple phobia is by recognizing that in OCD the feared objects are actually not palpable or physically measurable (for instance, radiation, contamination, AIDS, uncleanliness, dust, etc.), while the typical specific phobia is usually related to an object that can actually be touched or would be recognized by other non-phobics as well. In this regard, OCD is a "phobia" of a virtual entity—the patient senses it, but the entity is not concrete and hence it is inescapable, as it could be anywhere at any time.

Another diagnostic and consequently therapeutic challenge is the existing tendency to overlook phobic conditions in the presence of major psychiatric disorders such as schizophrenia, depression, bipolar disorders etc. Several works [5,6] point out the importance of identifying and then treating the phobic conditions. Even though seemingly it might be put forward as a negligible issue, it is often not the case in the eyes of the sufferers. Indeed, in recent research focusing on the issue of anxiety comorbidity in schizophrenic patients, and more specifically phobic comorbidity, it became increasingly clear that unless these phobic conditions are appropriately diagnosed and treated, they seriously interfere with the course and the potential recovery process of those patients [6].

Due to the high prevalence of phobias, comorbidity with other disorders is a frequent phenomenon. A focused effort to establish the proper diagnosis is warranted as reaching the appropriate diagnosis points toward the relevant therapeutic approach.

REFERENCES

1. Wittchen H.U. (1996) Critical issues in the evaluation of comorbidity of psychiatric disorders. *Br. J. Psychiatry*, **168** (Suppl. 30): 9–16.
2. Van Praag H. (1996) Comorbidity (psycho) analysed. *Br. J. Psychiatry*, **168** (Suppl. 30): 129–134.
3. Kessler R.C., McGonagle K.A., Zhao S., Nelson C.B., Hughes M., Eshleman S., Wittchen H.U., Kendler K.S. (1994) Lifetime and 12-month prevalence of

DSM-III-R psychiatric disorders in the United States: results from the National Comorbidity Survey. *Arch. Gen. Psychiatry*, **51**: 8–19.
4. Sasson Y., Chopra M., Harrari E., Amitai K., Zohar J. (2003) Bipolar comorbidity: from diagnostic dilemmas to therapeutic challenge. *Int. J. Neropsychopharmacol.*, **51**: 8–19.
5. Bermanzohn P.C., Porto L., Arlow P.B., Pollack S., Stronger R., Siris S.G. (2000) Hierarchical diagnosis in chronic schizophrenia: a clinical study of co-occurring syndromes. *Schizophr. Bull.*, **26**: 517–525.
6. Cosoff S.J., Hafner R.J. (1998) The prevalence of comorbid anxiety in schizophrenia, schizoaffective disorder and bipolar disorder. *Aust. N. Zeal. J. Psychiatry*, **32**: 67–72.

3.11
Comments on the Pharmacotherapy of Agoraphobia
Matig R. Mavissakalian[1]

The evidence reviewed by Stein *et al.* clearly shows the effectiveness of antidepressants and benzodiazepines in social phobia and presents the more or less promising experience with some other agents. The discussion of the less well developed pharmacotherapy of specific phobias is of heuristic interest rather than practical value because, as the authors clearly state, the availability of very successful and cost-effective behavioural treatments obviates the need for primary, regular pharmacotherapy for these phobias. The effectiveness of antidepressants and benzodiazepines in the treatment of agoraphobia is mentioned as well, but influenced by the vicissitudes of the DSM in the last two decades. The presentation of the evidence leaves a huge void following the early treatment studies with patients suffering from the agoraphobia syndrome, which already in the pre-DSM-III era defined a condition characterized by avoidance of numerous situations motivated by the central fear of panicking. The relabelling of agoraphobia in the DSM-III-R to denote a phobic category with no functional relationship to the fear of panicking has been an unfortunate development, because, as the authors rightly mention, this new "agoraphobia" is rarely, if ever, seen in the clinic and, if anything, would be best conceptualized as a type of specific phobia.

There are good reasons to dispel the discontinuity created by the frequent changes in the DSM and to realize that there is a natural syndromal continuity between agoraphobia and panic disorder [1]. First, the definition

---
[1] *Anxiety Disorders Program, University Hospitals of Cleveland, 11100 Euclid Avenue, Cleveland, OH 44106, USA*

of panic disorder has evolved to assume the essential syndromal character of agoraphobia, with emphasis on the fear of panic and the avoidance/escape mechanisms it motivates, but without the required frequency of panic attacks or even the presence of current active panic attacks for a diagnosis. Second, the development of successful cognitive behavioural treatments based on the exposure/habituation paradigm has established the utility and validity of conceptualizing panic attacks as phobic anxiety. Third, panic attacks improve with exposure treatment that targets solely agoraphobic avoidance and, conversely, pharmacological treatments alone improve agoraphobic avoidance. Fourth, a critical review of combination treatment studies of agoraphobia strongly suggests mutual potentiation between imipramine and exposure treatments, probably mediated through the enhanced process of fear reduction. The same appears to apply in panic disorder without agoraphobia [2]. Finally, antidepressants that are effective in the treatment of panic disorder are also effective in virtually all other anxiety disorders, including obsessive–compulsive disorder, post-traumatic stress disorder and generalized anxiety disorder. It would be parsimonious to invoke common mechanisms such as reduction of fear/apprehensive expectation, rather than claiming separate effects based on diagnostic categories.

Therefore, it would be justified to incorporate the panic disorder literature in the formulation of evidence-based treatment guidelines for (the) agoraphobia (syndrome). A treatment plan would begin by acknowledging the presence of three specific treatment principles with established efficacy of equal value, namely, serotonergic antidepressants, benzodiazepines and exposure-based behavioural treatments, that can and need to be often integrated to deliver the maximum benefit to patients [1]. The following selected updates supplement a previously published article on the rational treatment of panic disorder/agoraphobia with antidepressants [3].

- *Choice of treatment.* Although the selective serotonin reuptake inhibitors (SSRIs) have become first-line treatment in developed countries, there is no firm evidence for superior efficacy compared to imipramine and clomipramine, despite the generally more favourable side effects profile of the SSRIs. When resources are limited and economic considerations a priority, one can obtain optimal results with imipramine (at approximately 2.25 mg/kg/day and plasma concentrations of 110–140 ng/ml) and with even smaller doses (50 mg/day) of clomipramine [3]. Only patients who fail treatment with the tricyclics, because of non-response or intolerance of side effects, can then be switched to an SSRI, with successful outcome in approximately 50% of the switched patients [4]. However, the clinician should keep in mind that the effectiveness of the

same SSRI as the switch treatment may be considerably less compared to its effectiveness as an initial treatment in this disorder [5].
- *Combined treatment.* The delayed action of antidepressants can be overcome by the addition of benzodiazepines in the first month of treatment. This strategy has the advantage of rapid onset without otherwise affecting the final outcome with antidepressants [6]. Exposure treatment has lasting effects, but the observation that relapse after combined treatment and antidepressants alone is similar suggests that exposure may not protect from relapse following discontinuation of antidepressants [2].
- *Targeted maintenance treatment.* The relatively low risk of relapse in the first year following discontinuation of antidepressants found in recent studies creates a clinical dilemma between the nearly absolute prophylaxis provided by maintenance treatment and the realization that this may be unnecessary in over 50% of patients [7]. Targeted maintenance treatment for only those patients who need it is hampered by the lack of reliable predictors of relapse in remitted panic disorder patients, aside from history of previous relapses and perhaps comorbidity especially with depression [8]. A viable alternative approach, given that retreatment of relapsers restores remission virtually every time [9], would be the early detection of relapse while patients are still in remission off the drug. Models of early detection developed in my research appear promising in achieving the optimal treatment goal of long-term remission without unnecessary treatment.

REFERENCES

1. Mavissakalian M. (1993) Combined behavioral/pharmacological treatment of anxiety disorders. In *American Psychiatric Press Annual Review of Psychiatry*, vol. 12 (Eds J.M. Oldham, M.B. Riba, A. Tasman), pp. 565–584. American Psychiatric Press, Washington, DC.
2. Barlow D.H., Gorman J.M., Shear M.K., Woods S.W. (2000) Cognitive-behavioral therapy, imipramine or their combination for panic disorder: a randomized control trial. *JAMA*, **283**: 2529–2536.
3. Mavissakalian M., Ryan M.T. (1998) Rational treatment of panic disorders with antidepressants. *Ann. Clin. Psychiatry*, **10**: 185–195.
4. Mavissakalian M.R. (2002) Switching from imipramine to sertraline in panic disorder. Presented at the Annual Meeting of the American Psychiatric Association, Philadelphia, 18–23 May.
5. Mavissakalian M. (2003) Sertraline in panic disorder: initial treatment versus switch strategy. *J. Clin. Psychopharmacol.*, **23**: 646–651.
6. Goddard A.W., Brouette T., Almai A., Jetty P., Woods S., Charney D. (2001) Early coadministration of clonazepam with sertraline for panic disorder. *Arch. Gen. Psychiatry*, **58**: 681–686.

7. Mavissakalian M., Perel J.M. (1999) Long-term maintenance and discontinuation of imipramine therapy in panic disorder with agoraphobia. *Arch. Gen. Psychiatry*, **56**: 821–827.
8. Mavissakalian M., Perel J. (2002) Duration of imipramine therapy and relapse in panic disorder with agoraphobia. *J. Clin. Psychopharmacol.*, **22**: 294–299.
9. Mavissakalian M., Perel J.M, de Groot C. (1993) Imipramine treatment of panic disorder with agoraphobia: the second time around. *J. Psychiatr. Res.*, **27**: 61–68.

3.12
Pharmacotherapy of Phobias: A Long-Term Endeavour

Marcio Versiani[1]

A number of medications have proven efficacy in the treatment of social phobia (or social anxiety disorder). Selective serotonin reuptake inhibitors (SSRIs), particularly paroxetine and sertraline, emerged as the first-line treatment, given the amount of evidence related to efficacy and their benign tolerability and safety profiles.

Evidence for the efficacy of benzodiazepines (clonazepam and bromazepam) in the treatment of social phobia has also been shown. Their use in large samples of patients has been problematic, though, due to dependence, extreme difficulty to withdraw the medication after medium- or long-term treatment, sedation, cognitive disturbance and behavioural disinhibition [1]. Benzodiazepines should, therefore, be reserved for refractory cases, as third-line treatment and employed with caution, for short periods of time.

Many well-controlled studies have demonstrated the efficacy of classical monoamine oxidase inhibitors (MAOIs) such as phenelzine, and one open long-term study has pointed to the high efficacy of tranylcypromine in the treatment of social phobia. Extreme caution should surround the use of classical MAOIs in clinical practice, though. The risk of hypertensive crises, potentially fatal or leading to irreversible and serious neurological sequelae, induced by drug or food interactions, but also "endogenous" (without any apparent reason), renders these drugs too dangerous for such a condition as social phobia, with very rare exceptions, such as an extremely severe case, completely refractory to other treatments and under close monitoring [1].

Social phobia is a chronic, unremitting condition that commences early, in childhood or initial adolescence. When the clinician sees a case, he will be dealing with an illness history of decades. The chronicity coupled with ingrained avoidance behaviours probably underlies the partial response

---

[1] *Department of Psychiatry, Federal University of Rio de Janeiro, R. Visconde de Piraja 407 s. 805, Rio de Janeiro, 22410-003, Brazil*

seen in most patients in short-term clinical trials with drugs. The mean reduction in the total score of the Liebowitz Social Anxiety Scale (LSAS) in 8- to 12-week drug trials has been almost invariably inferior to 50%, meaning that a lot remains for remission to be achieved [2].

Long-term pharmacotherapy trials in social phobia, although still few in number, do provide evidence for greater degrees of improvement as the drug treatment progresses over months. Sustained remission, measured by very low total scores of the LSAS, is seen after one year or more of continuous drug treatment in approximately half of the initially treated patients, in open studies [1,3,4]. These observations need confirmation in long-term placebo-controlled drug studies.

Another indication of the need for long-term pharmacotherapy in social phobia stems from the high relapse rate seen after 6 months or even 2 years of treatment [4,5].

The long-term pharmacotherapy of social phobia poses problems for patients that should be dealt with by their doctors. The symptoms of social phobia are not continuous like those of, e.g., major depression. Patients when not exposed to phobic situations or free from anticipatory anxiety may be quite asymptomatic, "normal" indeed, and may become more sensitive to the unwanted effects of medications, such as weight gain, sexual inhibition or gastrointestinal disturbances. One may try to reduce the maintenance dose of the drug for better tolerability, but if signs of relapse appear the effective dose should be reinstated [1].

The absolute majority of drug trials for the treatment of agoraphobia have included patients with panic disorder (with or without agoraphobia). Also, in most of these studies the primary variable for the assessment of efficacy has been the frequency of panic attacks, thought to be the major target for drug effects. The rationale is that by blocking panic attacks the drug results in the amelioration of agoraphobia, as a consequence or in a secondary way [6].

The relationship between panic attacks and the development of agoraphobia does not seem to be that simple, though, and studies have yielded conflicting findings [7,8]. Some patients develop agoraphobia early, after few panic attacks, others later after many attacks and others do not develop agoraphobia at all. Other factors, e.g. comorbidity and personality features, seem to be important in the development of agoraphobia. In a few studies, such as one with paroxetine [9], the drug was effective in treating agoraphobia resistant to psychotherapy. Findings such as this highlight the need for pharmacotherapy studies aimed at agoraphobia *per se*.

Agoraphobia with a history or presence of panic attacks, the condition that has been studied in clinical trials, is a chronic disorder with a continuous course in the majority of cases. Although scarce, long-term treatment studies with drugs support the need for chronic treatment for more than a year for relapse prevention [6,8].

REFERENCES

1. Versiani M. (submitted) The long-term drug treatment and follow-up of over 250 patients with social anxiety disorder (social phobia) over 10 years.
2. Versiani M. (2000) A review of 19 double-blind placebo-controlled studies in social anxiety disorder (social phobia). *World J. Biol. Psychiatry*, **1**: 27–33.
3. Liebowitz M.R. (1999) Update on the diagnosis and treatment of social anxiety disorder. *J. Clin. Psychiatry*, **60** (Suppl. 18): 22–26.
4. Versiani M., Amrein R., Montgomery S.A. (1997) Social phobia: long-term treatment outcome and prediction of response—a moclobemide study. *Int. Clin. Psychopharmacol.*, **12**: 239–254.
5. Stein D.J., Versiani M., Hair T., Kumar R. (2002) Efficacy of paroxetine for relapse prevention in social anxiety disorder: a 24-week study. *Arch. Gen. Psychiatry*, **59**: 1111–1118.
6. Keller M.B. (2002) Raising the expectations of long-term treatment strategies in anxiety disorders. *Psychopharmacol. Bull.*, **36** (Suppl. 2): 166–174.
7. Katerndahl D.A. (2000) Predictors of the development of phobic avoidance. *J. Clin. Psychiatry*, **61**: 618–623.
8. Katschnig H., Amering M. (1998) The long-term course of panic disorder and its predictors. *J. Clin. Psychopharmacol.*, **18** (Suppl. 2): 6S–11S.
9. Kampman M., Keijsers G.P., Hoogduin C.A., Hendriks G.J. (2002) A randomized, double-blind, placebo-controlled study of the effects of adjunctive paroxetine in panic disorder patients unsuccessfully treated with cognitive-behavioral therapy alone. *J. Clin. Psychiatry*, **63**: 772–777.

3.13
Behavioural Toxicity of Pharmacotherapeutic Agents Used in Social Phobia

Ian Hindmarch and Leanne Trick[1]

Stein et al. have identified a wide range of different medications which have been found to be useful therapeutic agents for the management of social phobia. All psychoactive drugs, by definition, change behaviour. While appropriate behavioural changes (a reduction in social anxiety and reduction in avoidance behaviours) would be regarded as positive evidence of clinical efficacy, impairment of cognitive and psychomotor functions, which reduce the patient's overall quality of life, would be seen as

---

[1] *Human Psychopharmacology Research Unit, Medical Research Centre, University of Surrey, Egerton Road, Guildford, Surrey GU2 7XP, UK*

unwanted side effects. Behavioural toxicity refers not only to the extent to which these side effects raise the likelihood of a patient having an accident or cognitive failure while receiving pharmacotherapy, but also to the magnitude of countertherapeutic effects (e.g. somnolence, sleep disturbance, memory loss, loss of balance etc.) produced by a particular medication.

As behavioural toxicity is an intrinsic property of the pharmacotherapeutic agent, it is assessed in those subjects who are not impaired or suffering from a clinical condition or disorder that, in itself, could change performance on the relevant psychometric.

Behavioural toxicity measures are derived from psychometric assessments of the effects of drugs on psychomotor and cognitive function. These include tests of memory, sensory speed, mental arithmetic, information processing capacity, mental speed, vigilance, divided attention, reaction time, balance, motor control, motor coordination, manual dexterity, car driving ability etc.

In isolation, a singular assessment of the pharmacodynamics of a particular compound reveals little in absolute terms about the behavioural toxicity of that drug. However, if a database is constructed from the totality of information available from reports in peer-reviewed journals, then a reliance can be made on the results of such a "meta-analysis".

The present summary reviews the data contained in 90 studies from peer-reviewed literature featuring the drugs found by Stein *et al.* to have a proven utility in the management of social phobia. To be included in the analysis, the results had to be from cross-over studies with placebo controls and where the sensitivity of the psychometrics employed was confirmed by the results from an internal positive control (verum).

No acceptable data were found for phenelzine, tranylcypromine, selequine and escitalopram. These drugs are, therefore, removed from further consideration.

Data presented in Table 3.13.1 refer to the number of objective psychometrics used in the various studies to assess a particular drug. We include the number of instances in which a statistically significant impairment of cognitive and/or psychomotor function is reported, as well as the total number of tests performed on that particular compound. The number of instances where the results showed no significant impairment from placebo can be deduced from the difference of the two values.

In order to compare a discrete clinical entity with the totality of drugs in the database, i.e. the extent to which a particular drug produces behavioural toxicity (impairment of the various psychometrics) when compared to *all* other drugs in the database, a proportional impairment ratio (PIR) is calculated for each substance.

TABLE 3.13.1 Proportional Impairment Ratios (PIR): behavioural toxicity of drugs used in the management of social phobia

Drug	No. Studies	No. Tests	No. Tests Impaired	PIR
Fluvoxamine	8	168	0	0.00
Buprorion	4	42	0	0.00
Gabapentin	2	164	1	0.03
Fluoxetine	6	90	3	0.15
Clomipramine	2	63	4	0.29
Moclobemide	7	136	10	0.33
Buspirone	11	156	24	0.70
Olanzapine	2	82	16	0.90
Venlafaxine	2	36	8	1.00
Paroxetine	4	26	6	1.10
Atenolol	9	217	53	1.10
Nefazadone	2	62	19	1.40
Sertraline	4	190	64	1.60
Clonazepam	3	76	26	1.60
Alprazolam	24	781	236	2.20

The calculation of the PIR is adapted from that used in pharmacovigilance [1] and has been previously used successfully in rating the sedative potential of antihistamines [2]. The greater the PIR, the greater the behavioural toxicity. If the PIR value is less than unity (1.00), then that particular drug is less behaviourally toxic than the other members of the group. Unity represents parity with the group and a PIR greater than 1.0 represents a proportionally greater behavioural toxicity than the group (e.g. fluvoxamine and buprorion have no measurable behavioural toxicity, moclobemide possesses a third of the behavioural toxicity of the group as a whole, venlafaxine is as behaviourally toxic as the average for the group, and alprazolam is twice as behaviourally toxic as the average).

There are many reasons as to why a particular drug may benefit an individual patient, but the use of a PIR can identify those substances, other things being equal, which may prove countertherapeutic or increase the chance of accident or cognitive failure.

While PIRs may not necessarily be the principal guide for prescribing a particular substance, there is sufficient cause for concern regarding the impact of psychoactive drugs on a patient's safety and quality of life to seriously consider such ratings of a drug's intrinsic behavioural toxicity when using pharmacotherapy to manage patients suffering from social phobias.

REFERENCES

1. Stather R. (1998) Update on collecting ADRs and new methods of signal generation. *Reactions*, **718**: 3–5.
2. Shamsi Z., Hindmarch I. (2000) Sedation and antihistamines: a review of inter-drug differences using proportional impairment ratios. *Hum. Psychopharmacol. Clin. Exper.*, **15**: S3–S30.

3.14
Medication Treatment of Phobias: Theories Hide Effectiveness
James C. Ballenger[1]

Stein et al. have done a masterful job with the difficult assignment to review the medication treatment of phobias. They summarize the rich literature on the various medications which are effective in social phobia, a syndrome that is better described as social anxiety disorder, i.e. anxiety specifically about being in social situations which patients secondarily phobically avoid. We now know from controlled trials that both sertraline and venlafaxine are effective in this syndrome. Whether venlafaxine will prove to be more effective than the other antidepressants in social anxiety disorder, as it appears to be in depression, is an important research issue.

The medication treatment of agoraphobia without panic disorder is difficult to discuss, because it almost never appears in that form in treatment settings and therefore there are almost no valid studies. Agoraphobia without a history of panic disorder appears largely in epidemiologic surveys but, when studied clinically, many patients actually have subthreshold or full panic disorder.

Finally, studies of simple phobia are sparse, because predominant theories have literally inhibited exploration of this area. Recent studies suggest that patients with this disorder are in fact responsive to traditional anti-anxiety medications such as selective serotonin reuptake inhibitors (SSRIs). This is an important finding, because simple phobias are actually the most common mental disorders. Although most are not clinically significant, many do involve significant avoidance (phobic) behaviours which are personally and occupationally disabling. Perhaps the most common is flying phobia, which can significantly hamper some individuals. Similarly, some individuals who fear single objects like spiders and snakes

---

[1] *Department of Psychiatry, University of South Carolina, 67 President St., Charleston, SC 29425, USA*

can have significant interference with their lives if they live in areas where exposure to them is likely. Also, certain apparently single/simple phobias like using a public toilet or writing a cheque in public are often pieces of a broader syndrome like social anxiety disorder. Similarly, cultural issues can obscure the true nature of some anxious, phobic behaviour. In Japan, taijin-kyofusho is often considered to be a different syndrome from social anxiety disorder. However, in my meetings with Japanese psychiatrists on this issue, it seems quite clear that it is only superficially different and in fact is the same disorder. Early evidence suggests it is in fact SSRI responsive.

It is clear that medications work, but how well? There is the "rule of thirds" here as in many things. In recent trials, usually a third have an excellent response, one third a partial response, and about a third little to no response. The emerging consensus is that we certainly should be treating to remission, i.e. complete or almost complete resolution of symptoms and any functional impairment [1,2]. Remission is what each patient wants, and this is the goal which should guide clinician treatment choices. Clinicians need to continue aggressive treatment until remission is either achieved or realistically seems unattainable. There are increasing data in the anxiety field that treatment beyond the acute phase (6 to 12 weeks) leads to increasing numbers of patients who actually experience a remission. In generalized anxiety disorder, approximately a third of patients reach remission in 6 to 12 weeks, whereas treatment for 6 months generally doubles the number [3]. This requires clinicians to change how they think about partial remission. Whereas most patients and clinicians conclude that a treatment for 6 to 8 weeks is sufficient to determine optimal response, many partial responders will become complete responders if treated for 6 months. We should probably continue treatment in partial responders, rather than switch to another agent.

Stein *et al.* also touch on an absolutely critical question, i.e. whether treating anxiety disorders which begin in childhood, such as social anxiety and panic disorder, could block the full evolution of the adult syndrome and its consequences. Could the low educational and vocational entertainment, lower rates of marriage, and high rates of substance abuse and depression in social anxiety disorder be prevented by effective treatment of these children? This is a critical question with a disorder that ultimately affects 13% of the population. However, our general unwillingness to treat children with medications has slowed the exploration of this important question.

Stein *et al.* also touch on the issue that although cognitive-behavioural therapy has been demonstrated to be effective in carefully controlled trials, it remains unclear which patients should be treated with psychotherapy alone or in combination with medications. In many instances, combination treatment has been demonstrated to have greater efficacy, although this has not been a consistent finding. The larger problem is that cognitive-behavioural therapy is simply unavailable in most cities. However, the delivery of this treatment by manuals or computer programs is under development and is a promising approach to this critical problem.

REFERENCES

1. Ballenger J.C. (1999) Clinical guidelines for establishing remission in patients with depression and anxiety. *J. Clin. Psychiatry*, **60** (Suppl. 22): 29–34.
2. Ballenger J.C. (2001) Treatment of anxiety disorders to remission. *J. Clin. Psychiatry*, **62** (Suppl. 12): 5–9.
3. Ballenger J.C., Tylee A. (2003) *Anxiety*. Mosby, London.

CHAPTER

4

Psychotherapeutic Interventions for Phobias: A Review

David H. Barlow, David A. Moscovitch and Jamie A. Micco
*Center for Anxiety and Related Disorders at Boston University,
648 Beacon Street, Boston, MA 02215-2002, USA*

INTRODUCTION

There have been considerable advancements in the development of empirically supported treatments for phobias over the past three decades. Prior to the advent of exposure-based treatments for agoraphobia, social phobia and specific phobia, relatively little was known about the application of psychotherapeutic interventions to relieve the suffering of individuals who were diagnosed with these disorders. Below, we will provide a critical, comprehensive review of the treatment outcome literature for each of these disorders. We will also describe patient and other treatment variables that may influence therapy response and relapse rates. Finally, we will summarize the empirical literature as it currently stands and provide directions for future research.

AGORAPHOBIA AND PANIC

Individuals with panic disorder and agoraphobia experience significant interference in social, occupational and physical aspects of their lives [1,2]. This interference signifies the importance of researching and disseminating the most effective treatments for these individuals. Since the development of agoraphobia is nearly always preceded by full-blown or limited-symptom panic attacks [3,4], it is often necessary to address panic in the

---

Phobias. Edited by Mario Maj, Hagop S. Akiskal, Juan José López-Ibor and Ahmed Okasha.
©2004 John Wiley & Sons Ltd: ISBN 0-470-85833-8

treatment of agoraphobia. Over the past several decades, however, it has been traditional to separate treatments for agoraphobia and panic disorder into two categories: (a) treatments for agoraphobia and other avoidance behaviours; and (b) treatments targeting panic attacks and anxiety focused on panic [5]. The review of psychosocial treatments presented here will follow this tradition, beginning with treatments for agoraphobia.

Agoraphobia

Initial treatments for agoraphobia were developed in the 1960s and 1970s. These mainly consisted of systematic desensitization, with little attention given to panic attacks [6]. Systematic desensitization involves imaginal exposure to the feared situation, simultaneously accompanied by muscle relaxation. This technique was used primarily because it was thought that actual exposure to feared situations would be too overwhelming for agoraphobic patients. However, studies evaluating the use of systematic desensitization for treatment of agoraphobia have found the technique to be ineffective [7,8]. Around the same time, some researchers began successfully treating people with agoraphobia using *in vivo* exposure [9], whereby patients were encouraged to venture away from "safe places" and enter their feared situations. Since then, *in vivo* exposure has become the most widely studied psychotherapy for agoraphobia.

Basic Components of In Vivo Exposure

In vivo exposure begins with the construction of a hierarchy of situations that the agoraphobic individual fears and avoids, arranged from least to most frightening. Common items on a fear and avoidance hierarchy include "driving alone on the highway", "eating at a crowded restaurant", "shopping at the mall" and "riding on the subway". Patients are then encouraged to repeatedly and systematically enter the situations on their hierarchy and remain in the situations for as long as possible, often with the use of coping strategies learned in session. Although the presence of the therapist during *in vivo* exposure may be necessary for it to be effective with severely agoraphobic individuals [10], those with mild to moderate levels of agoraphobia are usually able to engage in exposures on their own or with a friend or family member serving as a supportive coach [5].

Efficacy of In Vivo Exposure

Research has consistently supported the efficacy of *in vivo* exposure for treating agoraphobia. By the mid-1980s, studies revealed that 60–70% of agoraphobic patients who completed *in vivo* exposure treatment showed significant clinical improvement, with follow-up assessments indicating that treatment gains were maintained for four or more years [11–17]. These results were replicated in several controlled studies, which used no-treatment or placebo control groups [18–20].

In vivo exposure for agoraphobia has been the subject of more recent research as well. Fava *et al.* [21] completed a long-term follow-up study of 90 patients who received 12 sessions of graduated, self-paced exposure treatment, conducted biweekly over a 6-month period. At post-treatment assessment, 87% were panic-free and "much improved" on global clinical measures. The authors used survival analysis to predict the probability that treatment responders would remain in remission, and they determined that 96% of treatment responders remained panic-free through the first two years, 77% through five years, and 67% through seven years. Predictors of relapse in this study included the presence of residual agoraphobia and comorbid personality disorders; this finding emphasizes the importance of thoroughly treating all vestiges of avoidance before termination.

A number of studies have shown that other cognitive-behavioural techniques combined with *in vivo* exposure are no more effective for the treatment of agoraphobia than *in vivo* exposure alone [22–24]. On the other hand, one study by Michelson *et al.* [25] showed that the addition of cognitive therapy to situational exposure can be significantly beneficial to people with agoraphobia and panic, especially when compared to exposure treatment plus relaxation training. Other controlled studies have shown that relaxation or breathing exercises confer no treatment advantage over *in vivo* exposure [26–28]. A study by Schmidt *et al.* [28] suggested that patients with panic disorder and agoraphobia receiving breathing retraining tended to have *lower* end-state functioning at follow-up when compared to patients not receiving breathing retraining. These findings suggest that breathing retraining and relaxation training may put patients with panic and agoraphobia at risk for relapse, perhaps because the exercises teach patients to minimize and distract from physical sensations during situational exposure, with breathing and relaxation becoming "safety behaviours" [5].

Combined In Vivo Exposure and Pharmacotherapy

A number of studies have studied the efficacy of *in vivo* exposure combined with tricyclic antidepressants, with most studies showing that the combined treatment is superior at the post-treatment assessment [29–31]. However, at the follow-up assessments, after the tricyclic antidepressant is discontinued, the benefits of the combined treatment tend to disappear [32–34]. Similarly, Marks et al. [35] found that alprazolam plus *in vivo* exposure was equally effective as either treatment alone at post-treatment, but those who had received the combined treatment showed significantly higher rates of relapse at six-month follow-up, after the alprazolam had been discontinued. More recent studies have examined the addition of selective serotonin reuptake inhibitors (SSRIs) to *in vivo* exposure for agoraphobia. De Beurs et al. [36] found that the addition of fluvoxamine to situational exposure reduced avoidance significantly more than exposure alone at post-treatment. However, at two-year follow-up, the treatment gains were equivalent for both groups [37]. These studies indicate that although the addition of pharmacotherapy confers a short-term treatment advantage over situational exposure alone, this advantage disappears in the long term, after the medication has been discontinued.

Methods of In Vivo Exposure Delivery

After the efficacy of *in vivo* exposure for agoraphobia and panic was established, researchers turned their attention to discovering the most effective methods of delivering *in vivo* exposure to patients. First, massed exposures, or exposures conducted during long, frequent sessions, have been compared to spaced exposures, or shorter exposure sessions conducted weekly or biweekly. While earlier studies found that massed exposures lead to greater attrition [38,39] and relapse rates [15,40], Chambless [41] found no detrimental outcomes associated with massed exposure in a study comparing massed to spaced exposures. Another study [42] also found that massed exposures resulted in superior treatment effects when compared to spaced exposures. Recent research based on modern learning theory has shown that expanding-spaced schedules of exposures, with exposures initially massed and then gradually spaced out toward the end of treatment, are effective in treating specific phobias [43,44]. Expanding-spaced exposures appear to be promising for the treatment of agoraphobia as well [45], although further research is needed to determine its efficacy.

Exposures conducted in a gradual fashion have been compared to intensive exposures, where the patient immediately enters his or her most difficult situations. Using massed exposures over a ten-day period to treat severely agoraphobic patients, Feigenbaum [46] compared ungraded to graded exposures and found that both were equally effective at post-treatment and eight-month follow-up. At five-year follow-up, however, ungraded exposures proved to be more effective. The long-term efficacy of ungraded exposures was replicated in another follow-up study [47]. In Boston, we are testing an intensive form of cognitive-behavioural therapy for people with panic disorder with moderate to severe agoraphobia, called sensation-focused intensive therapy (S-FIT), which emphasizes the experience of panic-like physical sensations integrated with *in vivo* exposure practices [48]. S-FIT is conducted over eight days, with two of the days devoted to therapist-assisted massed and ungraded exposures and symptom-induction exercises, and an additional two days of independent exposure. Preliminary results based on 23 subjects show that 87% are "much" or "very much" improved on self-reports and clinician-rated measures at post-treatment, with treatment gains maintained at follow-up [49]. Thus, ungraded exposures appear to be as effective as, if not more effective than, graded exposures in the treatment of agoraphobia.

Using computers, telephones and self-help manuals, researchers have examined more cost-effective methods of delivering *in vivo* exposure to people with agoraphobia. In one study, patients participated in a ten-week exposure treatment with three conditions: therapist-directed, self-directed and computer-directed. Results showed that all three conditions were effective, with no significant differences between conditions in treatment outcome [50]. Another study compared telephone-administered exposure treatment for moderate to severe agoraphobia to a waiting list control group and found that the treatment group showed significantly better improvement than the waiting list group at post-treatment, with gains maintained at three- and six-month follow-ups [51]. This study is in contrast to a previous finding that bibliotherapy is ineffective for treating patients with more severe agoraphobia [10]. Thus, severity of agoraphobia may predict the efficacy of treatments with minimal therapist contact.

In conclusion, *in vivo* exposure for agoraphobia can be administered in a number of formats: massed versus spaced, graduated versus intense, and therapist-administered versus computer- or telephone-administered. The literature reviewed above suggests that these methods of exposure delivery are fairly comparable, with the advantages of using massed, intense exposures found in some follow-up studies. The choice of which method to use appears to depend on patient variables, such as patient motivation and willingness to engage independently in difficult exposures, degree of patient avoidance, and availability of financial resources and access to behavioural therapists.

Panic Disorder

The majority of treatment studies for panic disorder with and without agoraphobia have been developed since the publication of DSM-III, with most studies focusing on cognitive-behavioural treatments that tend to include psychoeducation, cognitive restructuring, exposure and coping skills components. Most of these panic treatment studies have included individuals with no more than mild to moderate levels of agoraphobia.

Panic Control Treatment (PCT)

Panic control treatment (PCT) is a cognitive-behavioural therapy for panic disorder originally developed by Barlow and Craske [52] in the mid-1980s. PCT consists of: (a) interoceptive exposure, which involves symptom-induction exercises (such as hyperventilating or breathing through a straw) that expose patients to physical symptoms resembling those associated with panic attacks; (b) cognitive restructuring, which teaches patients about common misconceptions about panic attacks, particularly the emotional belief that panic attacks are dangerous, and ways of challenging these emotional automatic thoughts; and (c) breathing retraining, which was originally included to correct the tendency of patients with panic to chronically hyperventilate. However, as reviewed above, Schmidt et al. [28] showed that breathing retraining does not appear to add to the efficacy of PCT, and indeed may be detrimental to the maintenance of treatment gains.

PCT has been found to be superior at post-treatment and follow-up when compared to progressive muscle relaxation and waiting list controls [53,54]. There is support for the superiority of PCT over benzodiazepenes as well. In a study by Klosko et al. [55], patients received PCT, alprazolam or placebo, or were placed in a waiting list condition. At post-treatment, 87% of patients receiving PCT were panic-free, compared to 50% of those receiving alprazolam, 36% receiving placebo and 33% of those in the waiting list condition.

Results from a large multi-site study comparing monotherapies for panic (PCT and imipramine) to combined therapy have recently become available [56]. In this study, 312 individuals with panic disorder with no more than mild agoraphobia were randomly assigned to one of five treatment conditions: PCT alone, imipramine alone, placebo alone, PCT plus imipramine, and PCT plus placebo. Patients received weekly treatment for three months, and then responders to the acute treatment were seen monthly for six months of maintenance treatment. Patients then completed a follow-up assessment six months after the completion of the maintenance treatment when treatments were discontinued. At the end of the acute treatment phase, all of the treatment conditions were superior to placebo alone, and PCT plus imipramine was not superior to PCT plus placebo, indicating that the combined treatment conferred no additional treatment benefit. At the end of the maintenance treatment phase, these findings continued in effect with the one change that combined treatment was now somewhat better than PCT plus placebo. However, at follow-up, significantly more patients in the imipramine and PCT plus imipramine groups had relapsed than in the PCT alone and PCT plus placebo groups. These results show that the treatment response to PCT is more durable than the response to medication, although further research is necessary to determine if PCT and medication can be combined in other ways, such as sequential combination, that result in an advantage to patients with panic disorder.

Cognitive-Behavioural Therapy and Other Treatments

In addition to PCT, a number of other cognitive-behavioural treatments (CBTs) for panic disorder are available, including Clark's [57,58] cognitive therapy for panic, with a main emphasis on cognitive restructuring of misinterpretations of bodily sensations. Otherwise, CBT approaches to panic disorder are relatively similar. The use of CBT (including PCT) for panic disorder has been supported by more than 25 controlled clinical trials. One meta-analysis revealed that CBT has the largest effect size and smallest attrition rate compared to pharmacotherapy and combined treatments [59]. However, because many studies of panic disorder treatments tend not to include patients with higher levels of agoraphobia, these studies may be overestimating the efficacy of CBT. Indeed, panic patients show less improvement in samples with higher degrees of agoraphobia: 50% of patients with more severe agoraphobia in controlled cognitive-behavioural treatment studies for panic disorder with agoraphobia (PDA) show significant improvement at post-treatment, while 59% show improvement at follow-up [6]. These improvement rates are clearly lower than those reported for patients with mild to moderate agoraphobia.

As with agoraphobia treatments, briefer, more cost-effective versions of CBT for panic disorder have also been supported, including bibliotherapy [60], self-directed CBT using the Internet [61] and treatments with reduced therapist contact [62].

Two non-CBT psychotherapies have also recently been developed for the treatment of panic disorder: emotion-focused therapy (EFT) and panic-focused psychodynamic psychotherapy (PFPP). EFT [63], which focuses on the interpersonal triggers of panic attacks, was found to be less effective than CBT and imipramine and no more effective than pill placebo in the treatment of panic disorder [64]. Milrod *et al.* [65] recently conducted an open pilot study examining the effects of a brief psychodynamic therapy (PFPP), conducted twice weekly for twelve weeks, for PDA. At the end of treatment, 16 out of 21 patients experienced remission of panic and agoraphobia across a number of measures, and these gains were maintained at six-month follow-up. This pilot study shows that PFPP may prove to be a promising alternative to CBT in the treatment of panic and agoraphobia, although PFPP awaits controlled study.

Predictors of Treatment Outcome

Comorbid personality disorders may negatively affect PDA treatment outcome [66,67]. For example, Marchand et al. [68] found that patients with any comorbid personality disorder showed less improvement after treatment than panic-disordered patients without a personality disorder. In contrast, other studies have found no difference in response to CBT for panic disorder between patients with and without personality disorders [69]. Hofmann et al. [70] found that individual CBT and imipramine were as effective in reducing symptoms of panic disorder in individuals with personality disorder characteristics as in those without personality disorder characteristics. Features of a personality disorder did not predict panic disorder treatment outcome [70]. Surprisingly, initial depression seems to have no negative effect on panic treatment outcome, regardless of whether depression is a principal or secondary diagnosis [71–73]. Depressed patients with PDA engage in as many self-directed exposures as non-depressed patients, albeit with greater subjective ratings of anxiety [74].

Treatment outcome may also be affected by demographic and cultural variables. Attrition from the multi-site panic treatment study described above [56] was predicted by lower education, which in turn was dependent on lower income [75]. This finding suggests that patients who are unable to make panic treatment the priority in their lives because of financial constraints will have poorer treatment outcome. There are contradictory findings about the effect of race on panic treatment outcome, with most studies comparing African Americans to European Americans. Some studies show that African Americans fare worse in treatment than European Americans [76,77]. On the other hand, other researchers [78] have found no differences in treatment outcome between African Americans and European Americans. More research is crucial in order to understand how race/ethnicity affects treatment outcome of panic disorder and agoraphobia.

Summary and Future Directions

In vivo exposure appears to be the most efficacious treatment for agoraphobia with and without a history of panic disorder, and there is empirical evidence that it is equally effective alone as when it is combined with pharmacotherapy. More recent research on *in vivo* exposure has focused on its mode of delivery, with massed, intensive exposures proving effective for patients who are willing to tolerate them. Cost-effective versions of situational exposure for agoraphobia are also promising. In the treatment of panic disorder, PCT and other forms of CBT appear to be superior to other psychosocial treatments, such as EFT and relaxation training. CBT has been shown to have greater durability than medication in the treatment of panic disorder, particularly in the multi-site panic treatment study reviewed above.

Future research needs to eliminate the artificial distinction between panic disorder and agoraphobia by including more patients with moderate to severe agoraphobia in treatment outcome studies and integrating these approaches more effectively. An example of such an integrated treatment is the S-FIT [47] described above, which targets both fear of panic-like physical sensations and situational avoidance. Studying integrated treatment approaches will provide a more realistic estimate of the efficacy of CBT and PCT in the general panic-disordered population. Similarly, more work must be done to determine the effectiveness of *in vivo* exposure and CBT by studying the treatments at community mental health centres; effectiveness studies would also enable a more thorough examination of the effect of ethnicity, culture and socioeconomic status on treatment outcome. Wade *et al.* [79] have begun this endeavour, training therapists to use CBT at a large community health centre, whose panic-disordered population is more agoraphobic and less formally educated than most patient samples in controlled studies. The study found treatment outcomes that were comparable to controlled studies, and a one-year follow-up study confirmed the durability of these results [80]. These promising results await replication. Finally, in the era of managed care, cost-effective treatments are becoming increasingly important. Consequently, more research must be performed to determine the long-term benefits of the abbreviated and self-directed forms of treatment for agoraphobia and panic.

SOCIAL PHOBIA

A number of well-controlled studies have established the efficacy of cognitive-behavioural, exposure-based procedures for treating social phobia. The major CBT components that have been applied to the treatment of social phobia include: (a) social skills training; (b) relaxation training; (c) exposure; and (d) cognitive restructuring. Researchers are still debating which therapeutic "ingredients" are most essential for positive treatment outcome in social phobia.

Social Skills Training

The rationale for using social skills training in the treatment of social phobia is based on the assumption that socially phobic patients do not possess the social skills necessary to succeed in the social arena. Individuals with social phobia do tend to report perceived deficits in social skills [81]. However, such deficits may not be apparent to objective observers, lending credence to the suggestion that socially phobic patients may underestimate their own social performance and perceive behavioural deficits when none actually exist [82]. Even when behavioural shortcomings (e.g. poor eye contact, poor conversation skills) do exist, it is unclear whether they reflect deficits in social knowledge *per se*, or whether they represent avoidance strategies that are employed intentionally by individuals with social phobia in an attempt to reduce anxiety and avert an imagined social catastrophe [82].

Although several studies have investigated social skills training as a treatment option, methodological limitations have hampered efforts to determine whether it contributes significantly to positive treatment outcomes [83]. The only well-controlled study involving social skills training [84] concluded that patients who received 15 weeks of such training fared no better than waiting list controls. However, there is some evidence suggesting that combining social skills training with other techniques, such as exposure or cognitive restructuring, leads to positive outcomes [85]. Yet, as Heimberg [86] notes, the techniques that are often used in social skills training, such as therapist modelling and feedback, behavioural practice exercises and homework assignments, may be therapeutic because they inherently contain elements of exposure and cognitive restructuring, and not necessarily because they lead to an expansion or improvement in the patient's repertoire of social skills *per se*.

Relaxation Training

In relaxation training procedures, patients learn strategies to identify and reduce physiological arousal and tension. There is little evidence to support the use of isolated relaxation techniques, such as progressive muscle relaxation, in the treatment of social phobia [87,88]. On the other hand, "applied" relaxation techniques, in which patients learn to use relaxation strategies when entering anxiety-producing social situations, may hold some promise in the treatment of social phobia [89]. Although establishing the efficacy of such procedures requires further investigation [85], it is likely, as with social skills training, that the benefits of applied relaxation treatments are derived more from the patient's exposure to feared situations than the application of relaxation strategies.

In Vivo Exposure and Cognitive Restructuring

Real or imagined exposure to feared situations to facilitate the processing and modification of emotional and behavioural responses is a central component of most CBTs for anxiety disorders [5]. In the context of social phobia, designing appropriate *in vivo* exposures requires careful collaboration with patients. Exposures, which typically involve simulating social role plays, often with the help of confederates, should be tailored to the specific social fears of individual patients. Exposure is often guided by a *fear and avoidance hierarchy*, a list of feared and avoided situations that are rank-ordered by subjective severity ratings assigned by the patient. Implementing the fear and avoidance hierarchy into treatment with socially phobic patients follows a process that is similar to that with patients who have agoraphobia, as described above. As patients progress up the hierarchy, they are encouraged to repeatedly confront situations of increasing difficulty, and remain in each situation until their anxiety response peaks and, eventually, habituates. Patients are instructed to experience each situation fully, and are prevented from using any overt or covert avoidance strategies or "safety behaviours" that may undermine the exposure procedure.

Cognitive restructuring is a therapeutic process which teaches patients how to identify and challenge maladaptive, negative cognitions triggered by social situations. Patients with social phobia perceive social situations as being "dangerous" in some way. On the basis of this belief, individuals with social phobia tend to make biased predictions about their ability to achieve positive outcomes in these situations. They may believe that they will behave in an "unacceptable" social manner, that others will be critical and rejecting of them, or that, in the course of social interaction, they will be overwhelmed and disabled by their physical symptoms of anxiety. In the context of cognitive therapy, exposures are framed as behavioural experiments that are designed to test these negative predictions. On the basis of the information collected during exposures, patients are encouraged to re-evaluate the accuracy of their negative predictions and substitute, in their place, a more realistic, rational and balanced outlook.

A substantial and growing body of literature supports the use of exposure, with or without explicit cognitive intervention, for the treatment of social phobia [90]. Four meta-analytic reviews have been conducted to examine the aggregate of studies comparing CBTs with control conditions [91–94]. The results of these meta-analyses suggest that exposure therapy, either alone or in combination with cognitive restructuring or applied relaxation, produces significantly greater treatment effects than waiting list or placebo control conditions. Although one meta-analysis [92] found that only the combination of exposure and cognitive restructuring produced results that were superior to placebo, the same analysis found no significant difference between the exposure and exposure plus cognitive restructuring conditions, both of which were significantly more effective than waiting list control conditions. Taken together, these results indicate that exposure plus cognitive restructuring and exposure alone are both efficacious treatments for social phobia, and highlight the importance of exposure as the key component in any cognitive-behavioural intervention for social phobia.

Among the exposure-based therapies for social phobia, Heimberg's [95] cognitive-behavioural group treatment (CBGT) is the only one currently listed as an "empirically-supported treatment" by the Society of Clinical Psychology's (Division 12 of the American Psychological Association) Task Force on Promotion and Dissemination of Psychological Procedures. CBGT is a 12-session treatment package that consists of psychoeducation, in-session exposure simulations, cognitive restructuring and homework assignments. Several controlled studies have examined the efficacy of CBGT, and have established its superiority in comparison to waiting list control conditions [96] and credible psychological placebo conditions [97]. In addition, the gains made by patients who receive CBGT have been found to be enduring, even 4–6 years after the end of treatment [98].

Predictors of Treatment Outcome

To our knowledge, little systematic research has been conducted on the role of therapist variables in CBT outcomes in social phobia. However, there has been some research examining the impact of certain patient variables on social phobia treatment outcome. Several researchers have investigated whether treatment for social phobia is moderated by the presence of a generalized subtype of social phobia or an additional diagnosis of avoidant personality disorder (APD). While some studies have suggested that the presence of these two variables in patients with social phobia do lead to poorer CBT outcomes [99,100], other studies have refuted these claims [101–103]. At the present time, the literature suggests that while the overall functioning of individuals with generalized social phobia or individuals with social phobia and other comorbid disorders is lower than individuals with social phobia that is non-generalized or those without comorbid disorders, all individuals with a primary diagnosis of social phobia tend, on average, to improve equally over the course of treatment [104,105].

Chambless et al. [99] studied the effects of disorder severity, treatment expectancy, personality traits, frequency of negative thoughts during social interaction, and symptoms of depression on treatment outcome in 62 patients with social phobia who received Heimberg's CBGT. Patients were assessed at pre- and post-treatment, and at 6-month follow-up on a number of measures, including self-report questionnaires and behavioural tests. The findings indicated that none of the variables predicted treatment outcome across every domain of measurement, and subsequent studies have corroborated these results [106,107]. However, of all the variables examined in the study, pre-treatment depression symptom severity emerged as the most powerful predictor of treatment outcome. A recent study [108] compared CBGT response in three groups of socially phobic patients: individuals with a primary diagnosis of social phobia and no comorbid diagnoses, individuals with a primary diagnosis of social phobia and an additional anxiety disorder diagnosis, and individuals with a primary diagnosis of social phobia and an additional mood disorder diagnosis. Their results indicated that socially phobic patients with comorbid mood disorders, but not comorbid anxiety disorders, were more severely impaired than those with no comorbid diagnosis both before and after 12 weeks of CBGT. However, type of comorbid diagnosis did not predict differential rates of treatment improvement between the different groups. Future research is required to replicate these results and determine the relative efficacy of CBGT and other CBT packages for socially phobic patients who are depressed.

CBT versus Pharmacotherapy

Few controlled studies have directly compared the efficacy of established cognitive-behavioural and pharmacological interventions for social phobia. Gelernter et al. [109] compared treatment outcome among four randomly assigned patient groups: CBGT, alprazolam plus self-directed exposure, phenelzine plus self-directed exposure, and placebo plus self-directed exposure. Results indicated that the active treatment conditions all led to significant but equal improvements in social phobia symptoms after 12 weeks. Similar results were obtained in a study by Otto et al. [107] that compared treatment with clonazepam plus instructions for self-exposure with CBGT. In this study, although a greater number of clonazepam patients dropped out of treatment, those who completed the full 12-week programme were likely to report greater benefits than patients completing CBGT. However, no follow-up data were reported.

Turner et al. [110] followed 72 socially phobic patients for 3 months after randomly assigning them to receive behaviour therapy (flooding), atenolol or a pill placebo. They found that patients who underwent flooding demonstrated significantly greater improvements across a number of outcome measures in comparison to patients who received atenolol or placebo. These findings are consistent with those of similar studies, which have failed to support the efficacy of beta blockers in the treatment of social phobia (for a review, see [83]).

One large, well-controlled study [111] compared the relative efficacy of CBGT, phenelzine, educational-supportive group therapy (psychological placebo) and pill placebo in 133 patients with social phobia who were randomly assigned to one of the four conditions. After the 12-week acute treatment phase, patients who received either CBGT or phenelzine showed substantial but equal reductions in social phobia symptom severity. Both active treatment conditions produced significantly greater improvement rates than either of the placebo conditions. Patients who were classified as treatment responders in the acute phase were eligible to enter a 6-month "maintenance phase", during which CBGT patients received monthly CBGT group sessions and phenelzine patients were maintained on their medication. After the maintenance phase, there were still no differences between the two groups in symptom severity, dropout or relapse. Finally, of those patients who successfully completed the maintenance phase, a number were followed in a 6-month "treatment-free" phase. After the treatment-free phase, 91% of CBGT patients remained well compared with 50% of phenelzine patients. This difference was not statistically significant, due, perhaps, to the low statistical power in this comparison.

Clark et al. [106] recently completed a study comparing the short- and long-term relative benefits of cognitive therapy, fluoxetine plus instructions for self-exposure, and pill placebo plus self-exposure on 60 patients with generalized social phobia, each of whom was randomly assigned to one of the three treatment conditions. The cognitive therapy condition consisted of a variety of cognitive and behavioural procedures designed to modify information-processing biases, which are believed to play an important role in the development and maintenance of social phobia [82]. Assignment to fluoxetine or placebo was double blind. Results suggested a marked advantage of cognitive therapy over fluoxetine plus self-exposure at mid-treatment (8 weeks), post-treatment (16 weeks) and 12-month follow-up on a composite measure of social phobia symptom severity that included both patient self-report and clinician-administered ratings. Patients in the medication and placebo conditions showed small but equal improvements on the composite measure of social phobia at the mid- and end-point assessments. At post-treatment, effect sizes for the social phobia composite were 2.14, 0.92 and 0.56 for cognitive therapy, fluoxetine plus self-exposure and placebo plus self-exposure, respectively. At 12-month follow-up, the gains made by patients who received cognitive therapy relative to those who received fluoxetine plus self-exposure remained significant. The difference in effect size was striking, with cognitive therapy showing an effect size of 2.53, and fluoxetine plus self-exposure an effect size of 1.36.

Summary and Future Directions

Based on the empirical research, it can be concluded that short-term CBTs for social phobia are at least as efficacious as short-term pharmacological treatments. Although the best strategy for treating patients with social phobia in the long term remains to be established, clinicians faced with this difficult question should consider the growing number of studies indicating good long-term maintenance of gains in CBT. Whether the combination of CBT and medications is a more viable and efficacious treatment for social phobia than either type of therapy alone is an issue that has not yet been subjected to close empirical scrutiny.

Future research must also begin to tackle the question "What works for whom and when?" and attempt to determine whether certain subtypes of socially phobic patients respond best to certain types of treatments under particular conditions. A related issue for future research concerns the *effectiveness* of these treatments. It is imperative to begin testing the generalizability and viability of specific treatments beyond academic clinical settings. Little research has been conducted in this area, although preliminary findings have suggested that exposure therapy may be a viable and effective option for treating social phobia in general medical practices [112].

SPECIFIC PHOBIA

Although specific phobia is one of the most common psychological disorders, it is also one of the most treatable disorders, with up to 90% of patients achieving long-term treatment gains in as little as one session of *in vivo* exposure therapy [113–116]. Indeed, exposure-based therapy has emerged as the treatment of choice for specific phobia among experts in the field [113]. Exposure treatment for specific phobia had its origins in systematic desensitization [117,118], a treatment in which the patient imagines the feared stimulus while simultaneously engaging in relaxation exercises. However, early studies revealed that *in vivo* exposure is superior to systematic desensitization in the treatment of phobias [119], and relaxation training alone has not been found to improve treatment outcome [120].

Procedures for conducting *in vivo* exposure for specific phobia are very similar to those described above for agoraphobia and social phobia. The therapist conducts a functional analysis of the patient's phobia, and a fear and avoidance hierarchy is generated. The patient is then exposed to the feared stimulus in a systematic and controlled manner, often facilitated by coping strategies learned in session.

Efficacy of *In Vivo* Exposure

Since the 1970s, researchers have examined the efficacy of *in vivo* exposure for a wide variety of specific phobias, with most studies showing robust treatment effects. Exposure-based treatments have been found to be effective for phobias of spiders [121,122], snakes [123,124], rats [125], thunder and lightning [126], water [127], heights [128], air travel [116,129], enclosed places [130], choking [131,132], dental procedures [114] and blood [133]. These studies have led to the development of detailed treatment manuals for specific phobia, including one developed at our centre [134].

Additional procedures have been added to situational exposure for the blood–injection–injury (BII) subtype of specific phobia. BII phobias are associated with a fainting response upon encountering the feared stimuli, mainly because individuals with BII phobias are more likely than others to experience a reaction known as a *vasovagal syncope*. A vasovagal syncope occurs when an individual experiences a sudden increase in heart rate and blood pressure at the sight of the feared stimulus, followed by an immediate decrease in heart rate and blood pressure, which induces fainting [135]. Kozak and colleagues [136,137] first studied muscle tension as a method of preventing fainting at the sight of blood and injury. Since then, Öst and others have conducted a number of controlled trials of *applied tension*, a procedure that sustains the patient's blood pressure and heart rate at an increased level upon exposure to the feared stimulus. Applied tension involves completely tensing all of the large muscle groups of the body for fifteen seconds, followed by relaxing the muscles for fifteen seconds. The patient tenses and then relaxes the muscles at least five times before encountering the stimulus, and then continues the technique throughout the exposure [138]. Applied tension has been found to be more effective than *in vivo* exposure alone for the treatment of BII phobias [133]. In addition, research indicates that one session of applied tension and continued self-exposure is as effective as five sessions of the same treatment [139].

In Vivo Exposure versus Cognitive Therapy

A few studies have compared the efficacy of *in vivo* exposure with that of cognitive therapy for specific phobia. In one study, cognitive restructuring and applied relaxation (*in vivo* exposure combined with muscle relaxation) were found to be equally efficacious for treating individuals with phobias of dental procedures over nine group sessions [140], with results replicated in a later study [141]. In another study [142], which included a control group, patients with claustrophobia received *in vivo* exposure, interoceptive exposure or cognitive restructuring. Patients in the *in vivo* exposure group showed superior treatment outcome, although the cognitive restructuring group fared better than the control group. These studies and others [143] suggest that cognitive therapy does not significantly add to the efficacy of *in vivo* exposure for specific phobia (see [143] for further review).

Combined *In Vivo* Exposure and Pharmacotherapy

A few studies have examined the benefit of adding medication to exposure-based treatments for specific phobia. Zoellner *et al.* [144] studied the addition of alprazolam to exposure for spider phobics and found that the medication did not lead to better treatment outcome over exposure alone. Two studies found that benzodiazepines reduced fear during initial exposure sessions [145,146]. However, these studies also found that, after discontinuation, benzodiazepines led to greater fear during later exposures for flying phobics when compared to pill placebo [145] and higher relapse rates for dental phobics when compared to cognitive restructuring [146].

A few recent studies of selective serotonin reuptake inhibitors (SSRIs) suggest that fluoxetine and paroxetine may be promising in reducing fear in individuals with specific phobia [147,148]. Further controlled studies in this area are necessary to draw definitive conclusions regarding the efficacy of SSRIs in treating specific phobia, both alone and in combination with exposure-based treatments.

Methods of *In Vivo* Exposure Delivery

As with agoraphobia (reviewed above), research suggests that massed exposures, or exposure sessions conducted within a short amount of time, lead to greater treatment benefits for specific phobia than spaced exposures [8]. A study by Foa *et al.* [42] revealed that ten daily exposure sessions were more effective than ten weekly sessions in reducing fear and avoidance in individuals with specific phobia. As stated above, expanding-spaced schedules of exposure treatment for specific phobia have also shown promise [43], with Rowe and Craske [149] finding that expanding-spaced exposures lead to a decrease in fear of spiders. However, this study also found that massed exposure sessions are more effective than expanding-spaced in reducing relapse rates.

Regardless of treatment intensity, recent research indicates that varying the context of exposure treatment can reduce the risk of relapse for individuals with a phobia of spiders [150,151]. In one study, patients who were repeatedly exposed to a spider in a single context experienced a greater return of fear when later shown a spider in another context [152]. These findings provide initial evidence that *in vivo* exposures should be conducted across a variety of locations and situations.

Research comparing self-guided to therapist-assisted exposures for specific phobia suggests that therapist-assisted treatment leads to significantly greater improvement. For instance, patients with snake phobias who received predominately therapist-assisted treatment experienced greater fear reduction than patients who received less therapist involvement [153]. Similar findings emerged from a study comparing therapist-assisted exposure to a self-help manual for spider phobics [154]. However, a follow-up study [155] revealed that the method of self-help delivery may influence the treatment's efficacy. Patients with a phobia of spiders received one of five treatments: (a) a single session of therapist-assisted exposure, (b) a spider phobia-specific self-help manual used at home, (c) a spider phobia-specific self-help manual used at the clinic, (d) a non-specific self-help manual used at home, and (e) a non-specific manual used at the clinic. The percentages of patients showing significant improvement were 80%, 10%, 63%, 9% and 10%, respectively. These results indicate that, regardless of its specificity, self-help manuals used at home are not effective for the treatment of people with spider phobia. However, phobia-specific self-help manuals can be effective if used in a clinic setting, perhaps because there are fewer distractions in a clinic setting, allowing patients to focus fully on the treatment.

Technological advances in the treatment of specific phobia have also been the subject of recent research. Videotapes are commonly used in exposures to feared stimuli, and computer-administered treatments have been developed for spider phobias [156,157] and dental phobias [158]. Exposure treatments using virtual reality equipment are also available for a number of phobias, including heights, flying and spiders. There have been two published controlled studies of the efficacy of virtual reality treatment. First, Rothbaum *et al.* [159] compared 12 individuals with heights phobia, who received eight sessions of virtual reality exposure, to eight individuals who were placed on a waiting list. Results indicated that those who received the treatment were significantly improved relative to the waiting list group. Second, a larger study [160] examined 45 patients with flying phobia placed in one of three conditions: anxiety management plus virtual reality exposure to a plane, anxiety management plus real exposure to a plane, and waiting list. At post-treatment, both of the treatments were equally effective and better than the waiting list. However, these results may be limited by the fact that both of the treatment groups included a cognitive therapy component. Furthermore, the virtual reality treatment group was exposed to a virtual flight, while the *in vivo* group was only exposed to a stationary plane. Thus, further controlled studies of virtual reality exposure treatment for specific phobia will be important to determine its efficacy and applicability.

Predictors of Treatment Outcome

Because most patients significantly improve after receiving exposure-based treatments for specific phobia, there are few variables that can be identified as predictors of treatment response and relapse [123]. For instance, Hellström and Öst [161] examined a number of variables, including age of onset and duration and severity of the phobia, and no predictors of treatment outcome emerged. However, some variables have been associated with risk of relapse after completion of exposure-based treatment: distraction during exposure [162], depression [163], higher initial heart rate during exposure [164], and both a relatively quick reduction in fear during exposure [162] and a relatively slow reduction in fear [165,166].

Summary and Future Directions

Specific phobia is a remarkably treatable disorder. Exposure-based treatments have proven to be efficacious for all five subtypes of specific phobia in as little as one session of treatment. Recent research has examined different methods of delivering *in vivo* exposure to patients, with results suggesting that intensive, massed exposures are especially effective for the treatment of specific phobia. Exposures conducted via virtual reality equipment are also promising.

However, further research is necessary to better understand the differences between the specific phobia subtypes and how these differences may affect treatment. For example, as more information about BII phobias emerged, *applied tension* was incorporated into treatment, which increased the efficacy of exposure-based therapy for that particular subtype. Exposure may also be tailored for other subtypes, such as situational phobias. Situational phobias have been found to overlap considerably with panic disorder and agoraphobia because individuals with situational phobias appear to be particularly sensitive to the physical sensations of anxiety. Thus, techniques such as interoceptive exposure may increase the effectiveness of *in vivo* exposure for treating situational phobias.

Similarly, more work is necessary to determine which of the specific phobia subtypes can be treated with one-session exposures and massed exposure treatments, a research issue that is particularly important given the increased emphasis on developing cost-effective treatments. It appears that animal and BII phobias respond to such intensive treatments [115,139].

However, other subtypes, such as natural environment and situational phobias, have yet to be examined. Indeed, Öst [115] speculates that claustrophobia would *not* respond well to one-session treatment because this phobia typically encompasses a number of different situations. The answers to this and similar questions await further empirical research.

GENERAL SUMMARY

Consistent Evidence

Agoraphobia and Panic Disorder

The treatment outcome literature has consistently demonstrated the efficacy of *in vivo* exposure for treating agoraphobia. Research has also shown that PCT and other CBTs are efficacious for treating panic disorder with agoraphobia. Such therapies have been found to be more effective than other psychological treatments or waiting list control conditions. These studies indicate that although simultaneously combining exposure therapy with pharmacotherapy may slightly enhance short-term treatment gains, this advantage disappears in the long term and may result in more substantial relapse after the medication has been discontinued.

Social Phobia

Exposure therapy plus cognitive restructuring and exposure therapy alone are both efficacious treatments for social phobia. Research suggests that short-term CBTs are at least as efficacious as short-term pharmacological treatments for social phobia. The gains made by patients who receive CBGT appear to be enduring and long term.

Specific Phobia

The vast majority of patients who complete as little as one session of *in vivo* exposure therapy for specific phobia show considerable clinical improvement. Adding cognitive therapy or benzodiazepines to situational exposure therapy for specific phobia does not significantly increase the efficacy of such treatment. Applied tension in combination with situational exposure is more efficacious than *in vivo* exposure alone for the treatment of BII phobias.

Incomplete Evidence

Agoraphobia and Panic Disorder

Contradictory findings have been reported on the efficacy of adding cognitive therapy to *in vivo* exposure therapy for agoraphobia. While adding this component to situational exposure can be beneficial to people who have both agoraphobia and panic, there has yet to be conclusive evidence for the use of cognitive therapy plus exposure for treating agoraphobia alone. In addition, one study indicating that breathing retraining and relaxation training may put patients with panic and agoraphobia at risk for relapse is awaiting replication.

While initial results appear promising, additional research is needed to demonstrate the efficacy of alternative treatments for panic and agoraphobia, such as PFPP. Furthermore, more research is required to determine if the treatment blend of PCT and pharmacotherapy, particularly in sequential combinations, leads to outcomes that are clinically superior to either treatment alone. Finally, more comprehensive study of predictors of treatment outcome is required. Although initial findings suggest that comorbid depression does not impact negatively on treatment outcomes for PDA, contradictory findings have emerged in the literature about the effects of comorbid personality disorders and certain demographic and cultural variables, such as race, on response to treatment.

Social Phobia

Dismantling studies are necessary to determine the relative efficacy of social skills training, applied relaxation procedures, and cognitive and behavioural skills in the treatment of social phobia. Currently, the prevailing belief among leading researchers in the field is that social skills and relaxation training techniques are only effective in so far as they contain the cognitive and exposure components that have proven efficacious in treating this disorder. As with agoraphobia, more research is required on the impact of patient variables on treatment outcomes for social phobia. Contradictory findings have been reported on the possible treatment-moderating role of variables such as the generalized subtype of social phobia, APD, comorbid depression, treatment expectancy, disorder severity and homework compliance. Finally, the best long-term treatment strategies for social phobia remain unclear, although the emergent literature suggests that CBT may be a more desirable long-term option than pharmacotherapy.

Specific Phobia

Further research is required to establish the efficacy of SSRIs, such as fluoxetine and paroxetine, in treating certain subtypes of specific phobia such as situational phobias, both alone and in combination with exposure-based treatments. Additional research is also needed to determine the most effective methods of delivering *in vivo* exposure for specific phobia. Specifically, the relative efficacy of massed versus expanding-spaced schedules should be further examined empirically, as should the clinical gains attained when exposure is delivered across a variety of different contexts. Lastly, more empirical evidence is necessary to establish the efficacy of self-help manuals and virtual reality approaches in the treatment of specific phobias.

Areas Still Open to Research

Agoraphobia and Panic Disorder

In our current era of managed health care, it is essential to begin to examine the long-term benefits of the abbreviated and self-directed forms of treatment for agoraphobia and panic, which are both more cost-effective than traditional CBT. In addition, it is imperative that researchers begin to recruit and enrol patients with moderate to severe levels of agoraphobia in treatment outcome studies in order to estimate the efficacy of exposure-based therapies for treating individuals with panic disorder and agoraphobia in the general population. Similarly, *effectiveness* studies must begin to be conducted to evaluate the generalizability of findings from well-controlled treatment outcome studies to community mental health centres and other "real world" clinical settings. Finally, much more research is needed to determine the mechanisms of treatment change and predictors of treatment response so that therapies can begin to be tailored and individualized to suit the specific needs and characteristics of particular patients.

Social Phobia

Research is required on the impact of therapist variables on outcomes for CBTs for social phobia. Additionally, although such studies are currently under way, data have yet to be published on the short- and long-term efficacy and viability of combining medications and CBT in the treatment of social phobia. Moreover, *effectiveness* studies should be conducted to determine the transportability of treatments for social phobia from the laboratory to applied clinical settings. The question of "what works for whom and when?" may be best answered in the context of such naturalistic treatment conditions and settings.

Specific Phobia

Whether there are specific patient or therapist variables that significantly influence treatment outcomes in specific phobia has not yet been determined. In addition, research must establish whether differences exist between specific phobia subtypes and, if so, how these differences may affect treatment. Answering such questions could pave the way toward the development of more individualized and phobia-specific therapeutic procedures, such as applied tension for the treatment of BII. Similarly, more research is required to determine which specific phobia subtypes can be treated effectively with massed exposure and which require more traditional, longer-term weekly exposure treatments. Along these lines, it is essential to begin to establish which types and methods of exposure treatment are most effectively and readily transportable from the laboratory to "real world" clinical settings.

REFERENCES

1. Klerman G.L., Weissman M.M., Ouellette R., Johnson J., Greenwald S. (1991) Panic attacks in the community: social morbidity and health care utilization. *JAMA*, **265**: 742–746.
2. Leon A.C., Portera L., Weissman M.M. (1995) The social costs of anxiety disorders. *Br. J. Psychiatry*, **166** (Suppl. 27): 19–22.
3. Craske M.G., Barlow D.H. (1988) A review of the relationship between panic and avoidance. *Clin. Psychol. Rev.*, **8**: 667–685.
4. Turner S.M., Williams S.L., Beidel D.C., Mezzich J.E. (1986) Panic disorder and agoraphobia with panic attacks: covariation along the dimensions of panic and agoraphobic fear. *J. Abnorm. Psychol.*, **95**: 384–388.
5. Barlow D.H. (2002) *Anxiety and its Disorders: The Nature and Treatment of Anxiety and Panic*, 2nd edn. Guilford Press, New York.
6. Craske M.G., Barlow D.H. (2001) Panic disorder and agoraphobia. In *Clinical Handbook of Psychological Disorders*, 3rd edn. (Ed. D.H. Barlow), pp. 1–59. Guilford Press, New York.
7. Gelder M.G., Marks I.M. (1966) Severe agoraphobia: a controlled prospective trial of behavioral therapy. *Br. J. Psychiatry*, **112**: 309–319.
8. Marks I.M. (1987) *Fears, Phobias and Rituals: Panic, Anxiety, and their Disorders*. Oxford University Press, New York.
9. Agras W.S., Leitenberg H., Barlow D.H. (1968) Social reinforcement in the modification of agoraphobia. *Arch. Gen. Psychiatry*, **19**: 423–427.

10. Holden A.E.O., O'Brien G.T., Barlow D.H., Stetson D., Infantino A. (1983) Self-help manual for agoraphobia: a preliminary report of effectiveness. *Behav. Ther.*, **14**: 545–556.
11. Burns L.E., Thorpe C.L., Cavallaro L.A. (1986) Agoraphobia 8 years after behavioral treatment: a follow-up study with interview, self-report, and behavioral data. *Behav. Ther.*, **17**: 580–591.
12. Cohen S.D., Monteiro W., Marks I.M. (1984) Two-year follow-up of agoraphobics after exposure and imipramine. *Br. J. Psychiatry*, **144**: 276–281.
13. Emmelkamp P.M.G., Kuipers A.C.M. (1979) Agoraphobia: a follow-up study four years after treatment. *Br. J. Psychiatry*, **128**: 86–89.
14. Jansson L., Jerremalm A., Öst L.G. (1986) Follow-up of agoraphobic patients treated with exposure in vivo or applied relaxation. *Br. J. Psychiatry*, **149**: 486–490.
15. Jansson L., Öst L.G. (1982) Behavioral treatments for agoraphobia: an evaluative review. *Clin. Psychol. Rev.*, **2**: 311–336.
16. McPherson F.M., Brougham L., McLaren S. (1980) Maintenance of improvement in agoraphobic patients treated by behavioral methods: four-year follow-up. *Behav. Res. Ther.*, **18**: 150–152.
17. Munby J., Johnston D.W. (1980) Agoraphobia: the long-term follow-up of behavioral treatment. *Br. J. Psychiatry*, **137**: 418–427.
18. Mathews A.M. (1978) Fear-reduction research and clinical phobias. *Psychol. Bull.*, **85**: 390–404.
19. Mavissakalian M.R., Barlow D.H. (1981) *Phobia: Psychological and Pharmacological Treatment*. Guilford Press, New York.
20. O'Brien G.T., Barlow D.H. (1984) Agoraphobia. In *Behavioral Treatment of Anxiety Disorders* (Ed. S.M. Turner), pp. 143–185. Plenum Press, New York.
21. Fava G.A., Zielezny M., Savron G., Grandi S. (1995) Long-term effects of behavioural treatment for panic disorder with agoraphobia. *Br. J. Psychiatry*, **166**: 87–92.
22. Emmelkamp P.M.G., Brilman E., Kuiper H., Mersch P.P. (1986) The treatment of agoraphobia: a comparison of self-instructional training, rational emotive therapy, and exposure in vivo. *Behav. Modif.*, **10**: 37–53.
23. Michelson L., Mavissakalian M., Marchione K. (1988) Cognitive, behavioral, and psychophysiological treatments of agoraphobia: a comparative outcome investigation. *Behav. Ther.*, **19**: 97–120.
24. Öst L.G., Hellstrom K., Westling B.E. (1989) Applied relaxation, exposure in vivo, and cognitive methods in the treatment of agoraphobia. Presented at the Meeting of the Association for the Advancement of Behavioral Therapy, Washington, 2–5 November.
25. Michelson L., Marchione K., Greenwald M. (1989) Cognitive behavioral treatments of agoraphobia. Presented at the Meeting of the Association for the Advancement of Behavioral Therapy, Washington, 2–5 November.
26. Bonn J.A., Readhead C.P.A., Timmons B.H. (1984) Enhanced adaptive behavioral response in agoraphobic patients pretreated with breathing retraining. *Lancet*, **2**: 665–669.
27. de Ruiter C., Rijken H., Garssen B., Kraaimaat F. (1989) Breathing retraining, exposure, and a combination of both in the treatment of panic disorder with agoraphobia. *Behav. Res. Ther.*, **27**: 663–672.
28. Schmidt N.B., Woolaway-Bickel K., Trakowski J., Santiago H., Storey J., Koselka M., Cook, J. (2000) Dismantling cognitive-behavioral treatment for

panic disorder: questioning the validity of breathing retraining. *J. Consult. Clin. Psychol.*, **68**: 417–424.
29. Mavissakalian M.R. (1996) Antidepressant medication for panic disorder. In *Anxiety Disorders: Psychological and Pharmacological Treatments* (Eds M. Mavissakalian, R. Prien), pp. 265–284. American Psychiatric Press, Washington, DC.
30. Mavissakalian M.R., Perel J. (1985) Imipramine in the treatment of agoraphobia: dose–response relationships. *Am. J. Psychiatry*, **142**: 1032–1036.
31. Telch M.J., Agras W.S., Taylor C.B., Roth W.T., Gallen C. (1985) Combined pharmacological and behavioral treatment for agoraphobia. *Behav. Res. Ther.*, **23**: 325–335.
32. Mavissakalian M.R. (1993) Combined behavioral therapy and pharmacotherapy of agoraphobia. *J. Psychiatr. Res.*, **27**: 179–191.
33. Mavissakalian M.R., Michelson L. (1986) Two-year follow-up of exposure and imipramine treatment of agoraphobia. *Am. J. Psychiatry*, **143**: 1106–1112.
34. Telch M.J., Lucas J.A. (1994) Combined pharmacological and psychological treatment for panic disorder: current status and future directions. In *Treatment of Panic Disorder: A Consensus Development Conference* (Eds B.E. Wolfe, J.D. Maser), pp. 177–197. American Psychiatric Press, Washington, DC.
35. Marks I.M., Swinsan R.P., Basaglu M., Kuch K., Nashirvani H., O'Sullivan G., Lelliott P.T., Kirby M., McNamee G., Sengun S. *et al.* (1993) Alprazolam and exposure alone and combined in panic disorder with agoraphobia: a controlled study in London and Toronto. *Br. J. Psychiatry*, **162**: 776–787.
36. de Beurs E., van Balkom A.J.L.M., Lange A., Koele P., van Dyck R. (1995) Treatment of panic disorder with agoraphobia: comparison of fluvoxamine, placebo, and psychological panic management combined with exposure and of exposure in vivo alone. *Am. J. Psychiatry*, **152**: 683–691.
37. de Beurs E., van Dyck R., Lange A., van Balkom A.J. (1999) Long-term outcome of pharmacological and psychological treatment for panic disorder with agoraphobia: a two-year naturalistic follow-up. *Acta Psychiatr. Scand.*, **99**: 59–67.
38. Emmelkamp P.M.G., Ultee K.A. (1974) A comparison of ''successive approximation'' and ''self-observation'' in the treatment of agoraphobia. *Behav. Ther.*, **5**: 606–613.
39. Emmelkamp P.M.G., Wessels H. (1975) Flooding in imagination vs. flooding in vivo: a comparison with agoraphobics. *Behav. Res. Ther.*, **13**: 7–15.
40. Hafner R.J. (1976) Fresh symptom emergence after intensive behavior therapy. *Br. J. Psychiatry*, **129**: 378–383.
41. Chambless D.L. (1990) Spacing of exposure sessions in treatment of agoraphobia and simple phobia. *Behav. Ther.*, **21**: 217–229.
42. Foa E.B., Jameson J.S., Turner R.M., Payne L.L. (1980) Massed vs. spaced exposure sessions in the treatment of agoraphobia. *Behav. Res. Ther.*, **18**: 333–338.
43. Lang A.J., Craske M.G. (2000) Manipulations of exposure-based therapy to reduce return of fear: a replication. *Behav. Res. Ther.*, **38**: 1–12.
44. Tsao J.C.I., Craske M.G. (2000) Timing of treatment and return of fear: effects of massed-, uniform-, and expanding-spaced exposure schedules. *Behav. Ther.*, **31**: 479–497.
45. Lang A.J., Craske M.G., Bjork R.A. (1999) Implications of a new theory of disuse for the treatment of emotional disorders. *Clin. Psychol.: Sci. Pract.*, **6**: 80–94.
46. Feigenbaum W. (1988) Long-term efficacy of ungraded versus graded massed exposure in agoraphobics. In *Panic and Phobias: Treatments and Variables*

Affecting Course and Outcome (Eds I. Hand, H. Wittchen), pp. 83–88. Springer-Verlag, Berlin.
47. Ehlers A., Feigenbaum W., Florin I., Margraf J. (1995) Efficacy of exposure in vivo in panic disorder with agoraphobia in a clinical setting. Presented at the World Conference of Behavioural and Cognitive Therapies, Copenhagen, 11–15 July.
48. Heinrichs N., Spiegel D.A., Hofmann S.G. (2002) Panic disorder with agoraphobia. In *Handbook of Brief Cognitive Behavior Therapy* (Eds F. Bond, W. Dryden), pp. 55–76. John Wiley & Sons, Chichester.
49. Spiegel D.A., Barlow D.H. (2000) Intensive treatment for panic disorder and agoraphobia. Presented at the 34th Annual Convention of the Association for the Advancement of Behavior Therapy, New Orleans, 16–19 November.
50. Ghosh R.A., Marks I.M. (1987) Self-treatment of agoraphobia by exposure. *Behav. Ther.*, **18**: 2–16.
51. Swinson R.P., Fergus K.D., Cox B.J., Wickwire K. (1995) Efficacy of telephone-administered behavioral therapy for panic disorder with agoraphobia. *Behav. Res. Ther.*, **33**: 465–469.
52. Barlow D.H., Craske M.G. (2000) *Mastery of Your Anxiety and Panic: Patient Workbook for Anxiety and Panic*. Graywind Psychological Corporation, San Antonio, TX.
53. Barlow D.H., Craske M.G., Cerny J.A., Klosko J.S. (1989) Behavioral treatment of panic disorder. *Behav. Ther.*, **20**: 1–26.
54. Craske M.G., Brown T.A., Barlow D.H. (1991) Behavioral treatment of panic disorder: a two-year follow-up. *Behav. Ther.*, **22**: 289–304.
55. Klosko J.S., Barlow D.H., Tassinari R., Cerny J.A. (1990) A comparison of alprazolam and behavior therapy in treatment of panic disorder. *J. Consult. Clin. Psychol.*, **58**: 77–84.
56. Barlow D.H., Gorman J.M., Shear M.K., Woods S.W. (2000) Cognitive-behavioral therapy, imipramine, or their combination for panic disorder: a randomized control trial. *JAMA*, **283**: 2529–2536.
57. Clark D.M. (1989) Anxiety states: panic and generalized anxiety. In *Cognitive Behavior Therapy for Psychiatric Problems: A Practical Guide* (Eds K. Hawton, P. Salkavakis, J. Kirk, D.M. Clark), pp. 52–96, Oxford University Press, Oxford.
58. Clark D.M., Salkovskis P.M., Hackmann A., Middleton H., Anastasiades P., Gelder M. (1994) A comparison of cognitive therapy, applied relaxation, and imipramine in the treatment of panic disorder. *Br. J. Psychiatry*, **164**, 759–769.
59. Gould R.A., Otto M.W., Pollack M.H. (1995) A meta-analysis of treatment outcome for panic disorder. *Clin. Psychol. Rev.*, **15**: 819–844.
60. Lidren D.M., Watkins P.L., Gould R.A., Clum G.A., Asterino M., Tullach H.L. (1994) A comparison of bibliotherapy and group therapy in the treatment of panic disorder. *J. Consult. Clin. Psychol.*, **62**: 865–869.
61. Carlbring P., Westling B.E., Ljungstrand P., Ekselius L., Andersson G. (2001). Treatment of panic disorder via the Internet: a randomized trial of a self-help program. *Behav. Ther.*, **32**: 751–764.
62. Côté C., Gauthier J.G., Laberge B., Cormier H.J., Plamondon J. (1994) Reduced therapist contact in the cognitive behavioral treatment of panic disorder. *Behav. Ther.*, **25**: 123–145.
63. Shear M.K., Pilkonis P.A., Cloitre M., Leon A.C. (1994) Cognitive behavioral treatment compared to non-prescriptive treatment of panic disorder. *Arch. Gen. Psychiatry*, **51**: 395–401.

64. Shear M.K., Houck P., Greeno C., Masters S. (2001) Emotion-focused psychotherapy for patients with panic disorder. *Am. J. Psychiatry*, **158**: 1993–1998.
65. Milrod B., Busch F., Leon A.C., Aronson A., Roiphe J., Rudden M., Singer M., Shapiro T., Goldman H., Richter D. et al. (2001) A pilot open trial of brief psychodynamic psychotherapy for panic disorder. *J. Psychother. Pract. Res.*, **10**: 239–245.
66. Hoffart A., Martinsen E.W. (1993) The effect of personality disorders and anxious-depressive comorbidity on outcome in patients with unipolar depression and with panic disorder and agoraphobia. *J. Personal. Disord.*, **7**: 304–311.
67. Rathus J.H., Sanderson W.C., Miller A.L., Wetzler S. (1995) Impact of personality functioning on cognitive behavioral treatment of panic disorder: a preliminary report. *J. Personal. Disord.*, **9**: 160–168.
68. Marchand A., Goyer L.R., Dupuis G., Mainguy N. (1998) Personality disorders and the outcome of cognitive-behavioral treatment of panic disorder with agoraphobia. *Can. J. Behav. Sci.*, **30**: 14–23.
69. Dreessen L., Arntz A., Luttels C., Sallaerts S. (1994) Personality disorders do not influence the results of cognitive behavior therapies for anxiety disorders. *Compr. Psychiatry*, **35**: 265–274.
70. Hofmann S.G., Shear M.K., Barlow D.H., Gorman J.M., Hershberger D., Patterson M., Woods S.W. (1998) Effects of panic disorder treatments on personality disorder characteristics. *Depress. Anxiety*, **8**: 14–20.
71. Brown T.A., Antony M.M., Barlow D.H. (1995) Diagnostic comorbidity in panic disorder: effect on treatment outcome and course of comorbid diagnoses following treatment. *J. Consult. Clin. Psychol.*, **63**: 408–418.
72. Laberge B., Gauthier J.G., Côté G., Plamondon J., Cormier H.J. (1993) Cognitive-behavioral therapy of panic disorder with secondary major depression: a preliminary investigation. *J. Consult. Clin. Psychol.*, **61**: 1028–1037.
73. McLean P.D., Woody S., Taylor A., Koch W.J. (1998) Comorbid panic disorder and major depression: implications for cognitive-behavioral therapy. *J. Consult. Clin. Psychol.*, **66**: 240–247.
74. Murphy M.T., Michelson L.K., Marchione K., Marchione N., Testa S. (1998) The role of self-directed in vivo exposure in combination with cognitive therapy, relaxation training, or therapist-assisted exposure in the treatment of panic disorder with agoraphobia. *Behav. Res. Ther.*, **12**: 117–138.
75. Grilo C.M., Money R., Barlow D.H., Goddard A.W., Gorman J.M., Hofmann S.G., Papp L.A., Shear M.K., Woods S.W. (1998) Pre-treatment patient factors predicting attrition from a multicenter randomized controlled treatment study for panic disorder. *Compr. Psychiatry*, **39**: 323–332.
76. Friedman S., Paradis C. (1991) African-American patients with panic disorder and agoraphobia. *J. Anxiety Disord.*, **5**: 35–41.
77. Williams K.E., Chambless D.L. (1994) The results of exposure-based treatment in agoraphobia. In *Anxiety Disorders in African Americans* (Ed. S. Friedman), pp. 111–116. Springer-Verlag, New York.
78. Friedman S., Paradis C.M., Hatch M. (1994) Characteristics of African-American and white patients with panic disorder and agoraphobia. *Hosp. Commun. Psychiatry*, **45**: 798–803.
79. Wade W.A., Treat T.A., Stuart G.L. (1998) Transporting an empirically supported treatment for panic disorder to a service clinic setting: a benchmarking strategy. *J. Consult. Clin. Psychol.*, **66**: 231–239.

80. Stuart G.L., Treat T.A., Wade W.A. (2000) Effectiveness of an empirically based treatment for panic disorder delivered in a service clinic setting: 1-year followup. *J. Consult. Clin. Psychol.*, **68**: 506–512.
81. Rapee R.M., Lim L. (1992) Discrepancy between self- and observer ratings of performance in social phobics. *J. Abnorm. Psychol.*, **101**: 728–731.
82. Clark D.M., Wells A. (1995) A cognitive model of social phobia. In *Social Phobia: Diagnosis, Assessment, and Treatment* (Eds R.G. Heimberg, M.R. Liebowitz, D.A. Hope, F.R. Schneier), pp. 69–93. Guilford Press, New York.
83. Heimberg R.G., Juster H.R. (1995) Cognitive-behavioral treatments: literature review. In *Social Phobia: Diagnosis, Assessment and Treatment* (Eds R.C. Heimberg, M.R. Liebowitz, D.A. Hope, F.R. Schneier), pp. 261–309. Guilford Press, New York.
84. Marzillier J.S., Lambert C., Kelley J. (1976) A controlled evaluation of systematic desensitization and social skills training for socially inadequate psychiatric patients. *Behav. Res. Ther.*, **14**: 225–238.
85. Turner S.M., Beidel D.C., Cooley M.R., Woody S.R., Messer S.C. (1994) A multicomponent behavioral treatment for social phobia: Social Effectiveness Therapy. *Behav. Res. Ther.*, **32**: 381–390.
86. Heimberg R.G. (2001) Current status of psychotherapeutic interventions for social phobia. *J. Clin. Psychiatry*, **62**: 36–42.
87. Al-Kubaisy T., Marks I.M., Lagsdail S., Marks M.P., Lovell K., Sungur M., Araya R. (1992) Role of exposure homework in phobia reduction: a controlled study. *Behav. Ther.*, **23**: 599–621.
88. Alstroem J.E., Nordlund C.L., Persson G., Harding M., Ljungqvist C. (1984) Effects of four treatment methods on social phobic patients not suitable for insight-oriented psychotherapy. *Acta Psychiatr. Scand.*, **70**: 97–110.
89. Öst L.-G. (1987) Applied relaxation: description of a coping technique and review of controlled studies. *Behav. Res. Ther.*, **25**: 397–409.
90. Hofmann S.G., Barlow D.H. (2002) Social phobia (social anxiety disorder). In *Anxiety and its Disorders: The Nature and Treatment of Anxiety and Panic*, 2nd edn. (Ed. D. Barlow), pp. 454–476. Guilford Press, New York.
91. Feske U., Chambless D.L. (1995) Cognitive behavioral versus exposure only treatment for social phobia: a meta-analysis. *Behav. Ther.*, **26**: 695–720.
92. Taylor S. (1996) Meta-analysis of cognitive-behavioral treatments for social phobia. *J. Behav. Ther. Exp. Psychiatry*, **27**: 1–9.
93. Gould R.A., Buckminster S., Pollack M.H., Otto M.W., Yap L. (1997) Cognitive-behavioral and pharmacological treatment for social phobia: a meta-analysis. *Clin. Psychol. Sci. Pract.*, **4**: 291–306.
94. Federoff I.C., Taylor S. (2001) Psychological and pharmacological treatments of social phobia: a meta-analysis. *J. Clin. Psychopharmacol.*, **21**: 311–324.
95. Heimberg R.G. (1991) Cognitive behavioral treatment of social phobia in a group setting: a treatment manual. Unpublished.
96. Hope D.A., Heimberg R.G., Bruch M.A. (1995) Dismantling cognitive-behavioral group therapy for social phobia. *Behav. Res. Ther.*, **33**: 637–650.
97. Heimberg R.G., Dodge C.S., Hope D.A., Kennedy C.R., Zallo L., Becker R.E. (1990) Cognitive-behavioral group treatment for social phobia: comparison to a credible placebo control. *Cogn. Ther. Res.*, **14**: 1–23.
98. Heimberg R.G., Salzman D.G., Holt C.S., Blendell K.A. (1993) Cognitive-behavioral group treatment for social phobia: effectiveness at five-year followup. *Cogn. Ther. Res.*, **17**: 325–339.

99. Chambless D.L., Tran G.Q., Glass C.R. (1997) Predictors of response to cognitive behavioral group therapy for social phobia. *J. Anxiety Disord.*, **11**: 221–240.
100. Feske U., Perry K.J., Chambless D.L., Renneberg B., Goldstein A.J. (1996) Avoidant personality disorder as a predictor for severity and treatment outcome among generalized social phobics. *J. Personal. Disord.*, **10**: 174–184.
101. Hofmann S.G., Newman M.G., Becker E., Taylor C.B., Roth W.T. (1995) Social phobia with and without avoidant personality disorder: preliminary behavior therapy outcome findings. *J. Anxiety Disord.*, **9**: 427–438.
102. Hope D.A., Herbert J.D., White C. (1995) Diagnostic subtype, avoidant personality disorder, and efficacy of cognitive behavioral group therapy or social phobia. *Cogn. Ther. Res.*, **19**: 399–417.
103. Turner S.M., Beidel D.C., Townsley R.M. (1992) Social phobia: a comparison of specific and generalized subtype and avoidant personality disorder. *J. Abnorm. Psychol.*, **101**: 326–331.
104. van Velzen C.M.J., Emmelkamp P.M.G., Scholing A. (1997) The impact of personality disorders on behavioural treatment outcome for social phobia. *Behav. Res. Ther.*, **35**: 889–900.
105. Turner S.M., Beidel D.C., Wolff P.L., Spaulding S., Jacob R.G. (1996) Clinical features affecting treatment outcome in social phobia. *Behav. Res. Ther.*, **34**: 795–804.
106. Clark D.M., Ehlers A., McManus F., Hackmann A., Fennell M., Campbell H., Flower T., Davenport C., Louis B. (submitted) Cognitive therapy vs. fluoxetine plus self-exposure in the treatment of generalized social phobia (social anxiety disorder): a randomized placebo controlled study.
107. Otto M.W., Pollack M.H., Gould R.A., Worthington J.J., McArdle E.T., Rosenbaum J.F., Heimberg R.G. (2000) A comparison of the efficacy of clonazepam and cognitive-behavioral group therapy for the treatment of social phobia. *J. Anxiety Disord.*, **14**: 345–358.
108. Erwin B.A., Heimberg R.G., Juster H., Mindlin M. (2002) Comorbid anxiety and mood disorders among persons with social anxiety disorder. *Behav. Res. Ther.*, **40**: 19–35.
109. Gelernter C.S., Uhde T.W., Cimbolic P., Arnkoff C.B., Vittone B.J., Tancer M.E., Bartko J.J. (1991) Cognitive-behavioral and pharmacological treatments for social phobia: a controlled study. *Arch. Gen. Psychiatry*, **48**: 938–945.
110. Turner S.M., Beidel D.C., Jacob R.G. (1994) Social phobia: a comparison of behavior therapy and atenolol. *J. Consult. Clin. Psychol.*, **62**: 350–358.
111. Heimberg R.G., Liebowitz M.R., Hope D.A., Schneier F.R., Holt C.S., Welkowitz L.A., Juster H.R., Campeas R., Bruch M.A., Cloitre M. *et al.* (1998) Cognitive-behavioral group therapy versus phenelzine therapy for social phobia: 12-week outcome. *Arch. Gen. Psychiatry*, **55**: 1133–1141.
112. Haug T.T., Hellstrøm K., Blomhoff S., Humble M., Madsbu H.-P., Wold J.E. (2000) The treatment of social phobia in general practice: is exposure therapy feasible? *Family Practice*, **17**: 114–118.
113. Antony M.M., Barlow D.H. (2002) Specific phobias. In *Anxiety and its Disorders: The Nature and Treatment of Anxiety and Panic*, 2nd edn. (Ed. D. Barlow), pp. 380–417. Guilford Press, New York.
114. Gitin N.M., Herbert J.D., Schmidt C. (1996) One-session in vivo exposure for odontophobia. Presented at the 30th Annual Meeting of the Association for the Advancement of Behavior Therapy, New York, 21–24 November.

115. Öst L.G. (1989). One-session treatment for specific phobias. *Behav. Res. Ther.*, **21**: 1–7.
116. Öst L.G., Brandberg M., Alm T. (1997) One versus five sessions of exposure in the treatment of flying phobia. *Behav. Res. Ther.*, **35**: 987–996.
117. Wolpe J. (1958) *Psychotherapy by Reciprocal Inhibition*. Stanford University Press, Stanford, CA.
118. Wolpe J. (1973) *The Practice of Behavior Therapy*, 2nd edn. Pergamon Press, New York.
119. Emmelkamp P.M.G., Wessels H. (1975) Flooding in imagination vs. flooding in vivo: a comparison with agoraphobics. *Behav. Res. Ther.*, **13**: 7–15.
120. Öst L.G., Lindahl I.L., Sterner U., Jerremalm A. (1984) Exposure in vivo vs. applied relaxation in the treatment of blood phobia. *Behav. Res. Ther.*, **22**: 205–216.
121. Muris P., Mayer B., Merckelbach H. (1998) Trait anxiety as a predictor of behavior therapy outcome in spider phobia. *Behav. Cogn. Psychother.*, **26**: 87–91.
122. Öst L.G., Ferebee I., Furmark T. (1997) One session group therapy of spider phobia: direct versus indirect treatments. *Behav. Res. Ther.*, **35**: 721–732.
123. Gauthier J., Marshall W.L. (1977) The determination of optimal exposure to phobic stimuli in flooding therapy. *Behav. Res. Ther.*, **15**: 403–410.
124. Hepner A., Cauthen N.R. (1975) Effect of subject control and graduated exposure on snake phobias. *J. Consult. Clin. Psychol.*, **43**: 297–304.
125. Foa E.B., Blau J.S., Prout M., Latimer P. (1977) Is horror a necessary component of flooding (implosion)? *Behav. Res. Ther.*, **15**: 397–402.
126. Öst L.G. (1978) Behavioral treatment of thunder and lightning phobias. *Behav. Res. Ther.*, **16**: 197–207.
127. Menzies R.G., Clark J.C. (1993) A comparison of in vivo and vicarious exposure in the treatment of childhood water phobia. *Behav. Res. Ther.*, **31**: 9–15.
128. Bourque P., Ladouceur R. (1980) An investigation of various performance-based treatments with acrophobics. *Behav. Res. Ther.*, **18**: 161–170.
129. Beckham J.C., Vrana S.R., May J.G., Gustafson D.J., Smith G.R. (1990) Emotional processing and fear measurement synchrony as indicators of treatment outcome in fear of flying. *J. Behav. Ther. Exp. Psychiatry*, **21**: 153–162.
130. Craske M.G., Mohlman J., Yi J., Glover D., Valeri S. (1995) Treatment of claustrophobia and snake/spider phobias: fear of arousal and fear of context. *Behav. Res. Ther.*, **33**: 197–203.
131. McNally R.J. (1986) Behavioral treatment of choking phobia. *J. Behav. Ther. Exp. Psychiatry*, **17**: 185–188.
132. McNally R.J. (1994) Choking phobia: a review of the literature. *Compr. Psychiatry*, **35**: 83–89.
133. Öst L.G., Fellenius J., Sterner U. (1991) Applied tension, exposure *in vivo*, and tension-only in the treatment of blood phobia. *Behav. Res. Ther.*, **29**: 561–574.
134. Antony M.M., Craske M.G., Barlow D.H. (1995) *Mastery of Your Specific Phobia*. Graywind Psychological Corporation, San Antonio, TX.
135. Page A.C. (1994) Blood-injury phobia. *Clin. Psychol. Rev.*, **14**: 443–461.
136. Kozac M.J., Montgomery G.K. (1981) Multimodal behavioral treatment of recurrent injury-scene elicited fainting (vasodepressor syncope). *Behav. Psychother.*, **9**: 316–321.

137. Kozac M.J., Miller G.A. (1985) The psychophysiological process of therapy in a case of injury-scene-elicited fainting. *J. Behav. Ther. Exp. Psychiatry*, **16**: 139–145.
138. Öst L.G., Sterner U. (1987) Applied tension: a specific behavioral method for treatment of blood phobia. *Behav. Res. Ther.*, **25**: 25–29.
139. Hellström K., Fellenius J., Öst L.G. (1996) One versus five sessions of applied tension in the treatment of blood phobia. *Behav. Res. Ther.*, **34**: 101–112.
140. Jerremalm A., Jansson L., Öst L.G. (1986) Individual response patterns and the effects of different behavioral methods in the treatment of dental phobia. *Behav. Res. Ther.*, **24**: 587–596.
141. Getka E.J., Glass C.R. (1992) Behavioral and cognitive-behavioral approaches to the reduction of dental anxiety. *Behav. Ther.*, **23**: 433–448.
142. Booth R., Rachman S. (1992) The reduction of claustrophobia: I. *Behav. Res. Ther.*, **30**: 207–221.
143. Craske M.G., Rowe M.K. (1997) A comparison of behavioral and cognitive treatments for phobias. In *Phobias: A Handbook of Theory, Research, and Treatment* (Ed. G.C.L. Davey). John Wiley & Sons, Chichester.
144. Zoellner L.A., Craske M.G., Hussain A., Lewis M., Echeveri A. (1996) Contextual effects of alprazolam during exposure therapy. Presented at the 30th Annual Meeting of the Association for the Advancement of Behavior Therapy, New York, 21–24 November.
145. Wilhelm F.H., Roth W.T. (1996) Acute and delayed effects of alprazolam on flight phobics during exposure. Presented at the 30th Annual Meeting of the Association for the Advancement of Behavior Therapy, New York, 21–24 November.
146. Thom A., Sartory G., Jöhren P. (2000) Comparison between one-session psychological treatment and benzodiazepine in dental phobia. *J. Consult. Clin. Psychol.*, **68**: 378–387.
147. Abene M.V., Hamilton J.D. (1998) Resolution of fear of flying with fluoxetine treatment. *J. Anxiety Disord.*, **12**: 599–603.
148. Benjamin J., Ben-Zion I.Z., Karbofsky E., Dannon P. (2000) Double-blind placebo-controlled pilot study of paroxetine for specific phobia. *Psychopharmacology*, **149**: 194–196.
149. Rowe M.K., Craske M.G. (1998) Effect of an expanding-spaced vs. massed exposure schedule on fear reduction and return of fear. *Behav. Res. Ther.*, **36**: 701–717.
150. Bouton M.E., Mineka S., Barlow D.H. (2001) A modern learning-theory perspective on the etiology of panic disorder. *Psychol. Rev.*, **108**: 4–32.
151. Gunther L.M., Denniston J.C., Miller R.R. (1998) Conducting exposure treatment in multiple contexts can prevent relapse. *Behav. Res. Ther.*, **36**: 75–91.
152. Mineka S., Mystowski J.L., Hladek D., Rodriguez B.I. (1999) The effects of changing contexts on return of fear following exposure therapy for spider fear. *J. Consult. Clin. Psychol.*, **67**: 599–604.
153. O'Brien T.P., Kelley J.E. (1980) A comparison of self-directed and therapist-directed practice for fear reduction. *Behav. Res. Ther.*, **18**: 573–579.
154. Öst L.G., Salkovskis P.M., Hellström K. (1991) One-session therapist directed exposure versus self-exposure in the treatment of spider phobia. *Behav. Ther.*, **22**: 407–422.
155. Hellström K., Öst L.G. (1995) One-session therapist directed exposure vs. two forms of manual directed self-exposure in the treatment of spider phobia. *Behav. Res. Ther.*, **33**: 959–965.

156. Nelissen I., Muris P., Merckelbach H. (1995) Computerized exposure and in vivo exposure treatments of spider fear in children: two case reports. *J. Behav. Ther. Exp. Psychiatry*, **26**: 153–156.
157. Smith K.L., Kirkby K.C., Montgomery I.M., Daniels B.A. (1997) Computer-delivered modeling of exposure for spider phobia: relevant versus irrelevant exposure. *J. Anxiety Disord.*, **11**: 489–497.
158. Coldwell S.E., Getz T., Milgrom P., Prall C.W., Spadafora A., Ramsey D.S. (1998) CARL: a LabVIEW 3 computer program for conducting exposure therapy for the treatment of dental injection fear. *Behav. Res. Ther.*, **36**: 429–441.
159. Rothbaum B.O., Hodges L.F., Kooper R., Opdyke D., Williford J.S., North M. (1995) Effectiveness of computer-generated (virtual reality) graded exposure in the treatment of acrophobia. *Am. J. Psychiatry*, **152**: 626–628.
160. Rothbaum B.O., Hodges L.F., Smith S., Lee J.H., Price L. (2000) A controlled study of virtual reality exposure therapy for the fear of flying. *J. Consult. Clin. Psychol.*, **68**: 1020–1026.
161. Hellström K., Öst L.G. (1996) Prediction of outcome in the treatment of specific phobia: a cross-validation study. *Behav. Res. Ther.*, **34**: 403–411.
162. Rose M.P., McGlynn F.D. (1997) Toward a standard experiment for studying post-treatment return of fear. *J. Anxiety Disord.*, **11**: 263–277.
163. Salkovskis P.M., Mills I. (1994) Induced mood, phobic responding, and the return of fear. *Behav. Res. Ther.*, **32**: 439–445.
164. Craske M.G., Rachman S.J. (1987) Return of fear: perceived skill and heart rate responsivity. *Br. J. Clin. Psychol.*, **26**: 187–199.
165. Rachman S.J., Lopatka C. (1988) Return of fear: underlearning and overlearning. *Behav. Res. Ther.*, **26**: 99–104.
166. Rachman S.J., Whittal M. (1989) The effect of an aversive event on the return of fear. *Behav. Res. Ther.*, **27**: 513–520.

Commentaries

4.1
Phobias: A Suitable Case for Treatment
Anthony D. Roth[1]

Behavioural therapy gained its therapeutic spurs with the treatment of phobias. Learning theory underpinned the development of systematic desensitization and other exposure techniques, and research demonstrated the efficacy of a relatively simple and brief intervention. At the time they emerged, behavioural approaches were revolutionary; psychoanalytic therapies were predominant, relating the etiology of most psychiatric conditions to distal events whose meaning was inchoate in the absence of lengthy therapy. As evidence emerged for the efficacy of behavioural techniques, behaviourists challenged conventional psychotherapists not only on theoretical and empirical grounds but also in relation to clinical utility. In some sense then, the roots of evidence-based practice lie in exposure-based approaches to phobias.

Reviewing treatment techniques for anxiety disorders—and especially for phobic disorders—makes it clear that this is one area where there is a therapeutic hegemony. The opportunity for the dodo-bird to make its presence felt is limited by the fact that beyond behavioural and cognitive-behavioural approaches, there are few well-conducted comparative treatment trials. There are some trials of non-prescriptive or non-directive therapy (e.g. [1,2]), though the evidence for this approach is not compelling [3,4]. A small number of studies explore the benefits of eye-movement desensitization and reprocessing (EMDR) for specific phobia, panic and agoraphobia (e.g. [5–7]), though EMDR could be seen as a variation on exposure, and its benefits for phobias are not clear. Finally, there appears to be one open trial examining the benefit of interpersonal psychotherapy (IPT) for social phobia [8] and two of psychodynamic therapy for panic disorder [9,10]. Intriguingly, these provide some limited evidence for the efficacy of each of these methods, though without replication and methodological improvements their status remains uncertain. Although rarely contrasted to alternative psychological approaches, the efficacy of

[1] Sub-Department of Clinical Health Psychology, University College London, Gower Street, London, WC1E 6BT, UK

cognitive-behavioural therapy (CBT) in relation to a range of medications has been explored. Though some have questioned the methodological adequacy of these studies (e.g. [11]), there is robust evidence for the efficacy of behavioural and cognitive techniques in this field—though questions remain about a range of process issues, and the applicability of some techniques in routine clinical contexts.

Faced with this picture, a naïve observer might expect a comparatively comfortable transition between research and practice; in fact, there is evidence that (even in an era of managed care), most patients with anxiety disorders treated in routine practice receive psychodynamic therapy [12]. This could be seen as perverse, though it has to be recognized that research evidence is only one element in the application of evidence-based practice [13], and under some conditions clinical judgement has an important role, especially where clinical presentations do not mirror those in research trials. People presenting with phobias represent a broad span of complexity, and their aggregation within classificatory systems belies differences in etiology and the likely challenge they pose to treatment. For example, a person with a specific phobia may well have no associated psychopathology, and on that basis be quite likely to respond rapidly to focused treatment. Conversely, the "phobic" element in a person with generalized and severe social phobia may reflect a broader spectrum of anxieties with deeper roots, and the social withdrawal inherent in this presentation acts to reduce the likely resources and resourcefulness of the patient.

Sceptical clinicians tend to point out that this admixture of diagnoses (which often includes mood disorder and is often complicated by poor levels of functioning) makes research findings hard to apply, and perhaps even irrelevant to everyday practice. Certainly some force is given to this argument when meta-analysis of outcome studies suggests a link between larger effect sizes and the proportion of patients excluded from a trial [14]. Equally, however, there is evidence that clinical judgement is not always based on accurate appraisal of what is or is not helpful. Schulte et al. [15] looked at treatment outcomes for specific phobias, contrasting standardized *in vivo* exposure against an individualized treatment where therapists were free to implement any therapeutic approach. The greatest benefit was found with *in vivo* exposure, and those who did well with an individualized approach had been given *in vivo* exposure. This result is salutary: specific phobia is a condition with a straightforward treatment approach of known efficacy, and yet at least some clinicians elected to employ alternative and less effective techniques. This study raises questions about how therapists manage more complex conditions, where more sophisticated treatment decisions are needed (an issue discussed in Wilson's [16] thought-provoking paper). It also emphasizes the efficacy of a technique which is pragmatically (if not theoretically) simple to grasp.

One very evident shift reflected in the 40 years of research covered by Barlow et al.'s review is the development of cognitive therapy, focusing attention on the meaning and interpretation of events (both external and internal to the patient). In relation to phobic disorders this makes much clinical sense, but it is interesting to note that evidence for the benefit of adding cognitive to behavioural techniques is not always consistent. Nonetheless, a striking aspect of this field is the development of cognitive models which propose mechanisms for the maintenance of disorders, and which imply a route of action for their treatment. Panic control therapies are one such example, but a more recent one would be Clark and Wells's [17] model of social phobia. Given that social phobics do not benefit from naturalistic exposure to social events, Clark and Wells hypothesize that their problems are maintained by engaging in a number of counter-productive cognitive and behavioural strategies. This model does not supersede others, since it incorporates techniques known to be of value, such as exposure. Nor is it unique (e.g. [18]). However, it does demonstrate how therapeutic technique can grow out of astute clinical observation, experimental scrutiny (e.g. [19]) and successful clinical test [20], a powerful cycle of activity which links experimental and clinical psychology, to the benefit of patients and clinicians alike.

Contrast of the status of treatments for anxiety disorders with those in other diagnostic areas suggests that this is a somewhat unusual area, partly in terms of the clarity of outcomes achieved, and partly because of evidence of technical innovation linked to explicit modelling of disorders. There are fewer examples of this approach elsewhere, and a current overview of progress in other diagnostic areas [21] suggests that the impact of many interventions (whether psychological or pharmacological) is less than optimal. That this should be so represents a challenge, and whether this situation resolves is a matter for the future. The hope has to be that the progress made in the management of anxiety disorders will at some point be reflected elsewhere in the field.

REFERENCES

1. Shear M.K., Pilkonis P.A., Cloitre M., Leon A.C. (1994) Cognitive behavioral treatment compared with non-prescriptive treatment of panic disorder. *Arch. Gen. Psychiatry*, **51**: 395–401.
2. Teusch L., Bohme H., Gastpar M. (1997) The benefit of an insight-oriented and experiential approach on panic and agoraphobia symptoms. Results of a controlled comparison of client-centered therapy alone and in combination with behavioral exposure. *Psychother. Psychosom.*, **66**: 293–301.

3. Craske M.G., Maidenberg E., Bystritsky A. (1995) Brief cognitive-behavioral versus nondirective therapy for panic disorder. *J. Behav. Ther. Exp. Psychiatry*, **26**: 113–120.
4. Shear M.K., Houk P., Greeno C., Masters S. (2001) Emotion focused psychotherapy for patients with panic disorder. *Am. J. Psychiatry*, **158**: 1993–1998.
5. Muris P., Merckelbach H., van Haaften H., Mayer B. (1997) Eye movement desensitisation and reprocessing versus exposure in vivo: a single session crossover study of spider-phobic children. *Br. J. Psychiatry*, **171**: 82–86.
6. Feske U., Goldstein A.J. (1997) Eye-movement desensitization and reprocessing treatment for panic disorder: a controlled outcome and partial dismantling study. *J. Consult. Clin. Psychol.*, **65**: 1026–1035.
7. Goldstein A.J., de Beurs E., Chambless D.L., Wilson K.A. (2000) EMDR for panic disorder with agoraphobia: comparison with waiting list and credible attention-placebo control conditions. *J. Consult. Clin. Psychol.*, **68**: 947–956.
8. Lipsitz J.D., Markowitz J.C., Cherry S., Fyer A.J. (1999) Open trial of interpersonal psychotherapy for the treatment of social phobia. *Am. J. Psychiatry*, **156**: 1814–1816.
9. Wiborg I.M., Dahl A.A. (1996) Does brief dynamic psychotherapy reduce the relapse rate of panic disorder? *Arch. Gen. Psychiatry*, **53**: 689–694.
10. Milrod B., Busch F., Leon A.C., Aronson A., Roiphe J., Rudden M., Singer M., Shapiro M., Goldman H., Richter D. et al. (2001) A pilot open trial of brief psychodynamic psychotherapy for panic disorder. *J. Psychother. Pract. Res.*, **10**: 239–245.
11. Sharpe D.M., Power K.G. (1997) Treatment-outcome research in panic disorder: dilemmas in reconciling the demands of pharmacological and psychological methodologies. *J. Psychopharmacol.*, **11**: 373–380.
12. Goisman R.M., Warshaw M.G., Keller M. (1999) Psychosocial treatment prescriptions for generalized anxiety disorder, panic disorder, and social phobia, 1991–1996. *Am. J. Psychiatry*, **156**: 1819–1821.
13. Roth A.D., Parry G. (1997) The implications of psychotherapy research for clinical practice and service development: lessons and limitations. *J. Ment. Health*, **6**: 367–380.
14. Westen D., Morrison, K. (2001) A multidimensional meta-analysis of treatments for depression, panic and generalized anxiety disorder: an empirical examination of the status of empirically supported therapies. *J. Consult. Clin. Psychol.*, **69**: 875–899.
15. Schulte D., Kunzel R., Pepping G., Schulte B. (1992) Tailor-made versus standardized therapy of phobic patients. *Adv. Behav. Res. Ther.*, **14**: 67–92.
16. Wilson G. (1996) Manual-based treatments: the clinical application of research findings. *Behav. Res. Ther.*, **34**: 295–314.
17. Clark D.M., Wells A. (1995) A cognitive model of social phobia. In *Social Phobia: Diagnosis, Assessment and Treatment* (Eds R. Heimberg, M. Liebowitz, D.A. Hope, F.R. Schneider), pp. 69–93. Guilford Press, New York.
18. Rapee R.M., Heimberg R.G. (1997) A cognitive behavioural model of anxiety in social phobia. *Behav. Res. Ther.*, **35**: 741–756.
19. Clark D.M., McManus F. (2002) Information processing in social phobia. *Biol. Psychiatry*, **51**: 92–100.
20. Clark D.M., Ehlers A., McManus F., Hackmann A., Fennell M., Campbell H., Flower T., Davenport C., Louis B. (2003) Cognitive therapy vs fluoxetine in generalized social phobia: a randomized placebo controlled trial. *J. Consult. Clin. Psychol.*, **71**: 1058–1067.

4.2
Cognitive-Behavioural Interventions for Phobias: What Works for Whom and When
Richard G. Heimberg and James P. Hambrick[1]

The question of "what works for whom and when" is a major theme of this chapter, encompassing issues such as comorbidity and the relationship of cognitive-behavioural therapy (CBT) and pharmacotherapy. Although this argument can be overstated, controlled studies often exclude patients with comorbid disorders. These patients can be among the most challenging and difficult to treat. For example, a recent review of the literature found that the presence of personality disorders negatively affected the outcome of CBT for panic disorder [1]. Similarly, a recent empirical study found that patients with social phobia and a comorbid mood disorder were more impaired before and after CBT than patients with a comorbid anxiety disorder or no comorbid disorder [2]. In contrast, patients with social phobia with and without comorbid generalized anxiety disorder responded similarly to CBT [3]. More research into the treatment of patients with panic disorder and social phobia and comorbid disorders is clearly indicated.

Although there is considerable evidence from controlled studies for the *efficacy* of CBT in the treatment of panic disorder, social phobia and specific phobias, there is as yet little evidence regarding CBT's *effectiveness* when applied to patients with these disorders in community settings. Wade *et al.*'s [4] bench-marking study of panic disorder and agoraphobia suggested that CBT was about as effective as it was in controlled studies when delivered by therapists in a community mental health centre, and gains were maintained after a 1-year follow-up [5]. However, this is only one study, in one disorder.

As Barlow *et al.*'s review indicates, most research involving CBT and pharmacotherapy has explored how they compare to each other, not how well they work together. However, in a large multicentre trial [6], the combination of CBT and imipramine conferred no additional advantage over CBT plus placebo, and the combination may have resulted in increased chance of relapse. In an earlier study [7], agoraphobic patients who responded well to the combination of alprazolam and exposure were more

---
[1] *Adult Anxiety Clinic of Temple University, 1701 North Thirteenth Street, Philadelphia, PA 19122-6085, USA*

likely to relapse if they attributed their change predominantly to medication rather than their own efforts. In examining the efficacy of combined treatments (or medications alone, for that matter), it will be very important to examine how psychological variables such as attributions for change affect response and relapse.

The results of these studies do not suggest that psychotherapy and pharmacotherapy should not be combined. In fact, preliminary results from our recently completed study of phenelzine and CBT for social phobia suggest superior response among patients in the combined treatment condition [8]. Instead, these studies make the case that the relationship between psychotherapy and medication can be a complicated one and deserves further study. Combined treatments may increase the overall efficacy of individual treatments, reduce it or leave it unchanged [9]. The review's call for novel treatment approaches, such as sequential combination of treatments, exemplifies what Stein calls "cognitively-behaviourally informed pharmacotherapy" [10]. The approach emphasizes integrating resources in the most effective fashion to produce the best overall level of care. To accomplish this goal, community-based research may be critical. Although only controlled studies are capable of answering questions regarding the active ingredients or components of treatment, conducting more disciplined research in community settings may answer broader questions regarding whether different varieties of CBT and particular medications form effective partnerships.

In summary, the evidence in support of the efficacy of CBT for panic disorder, social phobia and specific phobias is impressive, but evaluation of its effectiveness for these disorders in the community is incomplete. If past performance is the best predictor of future behaviour, there is reason to believe that CBT will demonstrate persuasive effectiveness in the treatment of phobias, and we can keep working toward the ideal answer to "what works for whom and when"—all of our patients, all of the time.

REFERENCES

1. Mennin D.S., Heimberg R.G. (2000) The impact of comorbid mood and personality disorders in the cognitive-behavioral treatment of panic disorder. *Clin. Psychol. Rev.*, **20**: 339–357.
2. Erwin B.A., Heimberg R.G., Juster H.R., Mindlin M. (2002) Comorbid anxiety and mood disorders among persons with social anxiety disorder. *Behav. Res. Ther.*, **40**: 19–35.
3. Mennin D.S., Heimberg R.G., Jack M.S. (2000) Comorbid generalized anxiety disorder in primary social phobia: symptom severity, functional impairment, and treatment response. *J. Anxiety Disord.*, **14**: 325–343.

4. Wade W.A., Treat T.A., Stuart G.L. (1998) Transporting an empirically supported treatment for panic disorder to a service clinic setting: a benchmarking strategy. *J. Consult. Clin. Psychol.*, **66**: 231–239.
5. Stuart G.L., Treat T.A., Wade W.A. (2000) Effectiveness of empirically based treatment for panic disorder delivered in a service clinic setting: 1-year follow-up. *J. Consult. Clin. Psychol.*, **68**: 506–512.
6. Barlow D.H., Gorman J.M., Shear M.K., Woods S.W. (2000) Cognitive-behavioral therapy, imipramine, or their combination for panic disorder: a randomized control trial. *JAMA*, **283**: 2529–2536.
7. Basoglu M., Marks I.M., Kilic C., Brewin C.R., Swinson R.P. (1994) Alprazolam and exposure for panic disorder with agoraphobia: attribution of improvement to medication predicts subsequent relapse. *Br. J. Psychiatry*, **164**: 652–659.
8. Heimberg R.G. (2002) The understanding and treatment of social anxiety: what a long strange trip it's been (and will be). Presented at the Annual Meeting of the Association for Advancement of Behavior Therapy, Reno, NV, 16 November.
9. Heimberg R.G. (2002) Cognitive-behavioral therapy for social anxiety disorder: current status and future directions. *Biol. Psychiatry*, **51**: 101–108.
10. Stein M.B. (2002) Is the combination of medication and psychotherapy better than either alone? Presented at the Annual Meeting of the Anxiety Disorders Association of America, Austin, TX, 24 March.

4.3
Practical Comments on Exposure Therapy
Matig R. Mavissakalian[1]

The development of effective behavioural and cognitive behavioural therapies of phobias is one of the major advances in modern psychiatry. The empirical evidence presented by Barlow *et al.* is overwhelming and leaves no doubt that the exposure-based treatments are effective in a variety of phobic disorders. This research effort culminates in the validation of phobic anxiety as a useful model of neurotic anxiety and the emergence of exposure as a robust and generalizable treatment principle that, like serotonergic antidepressants and benzodiazepines, transcends diagnostic boundaries between anxiety disorders. Elsewhere I have proposed a functional integrated approach to the treatment of anxiety disorders with the use of these three specific treatment modalities [1]. Here I present a simple conceptualization of the exposure paradigm for application in everyday psychiatric practice.

Phenomenology and process. From the phenomenological perspective it is essential that the patient have insight into the neurotic nature of phobic

---

[1] *Anxiety Disorders Program, University Hospitals of Cleveland, 11100 Euclid Avenue, Cleveland, OH 44106, USA*

anxiety, i.e. realize and accept that the fear is unrealistic and that the perceived danger is at the very least highly exaggerated and improbable. Most neurotic patients readily differentiate between their fears and real danger and come to see the reinforcing nature of avoidance/escape in the vicious cycle of fear→avoidance/escape behaviours→temporary relief from fear/anxiety that maintains the fear and strengthens the tendency to avoid/escape.

Rationale. This conceptualization that phobic anxiety is maintained despite effective management of fear or anxiety symptoms with avoidance/escape strategies and the established fact that phobic anxiety habituates (decreases and abates) upon repeated or prolonged exposure to the very stimuli that elicit fear form the basis of the exposure paradigm. Practically speaking then, the therapeutic task would consist in having patients identify and block all anxiety management strategies in response to fear, thus delivering exposure systematically without interference with the process of habituation of fear. It is important to underscore that exposure is exposure to fear and not to actual danger and that the experience of discomfort and anxiety/fear expected from exposure is nothing new to the patient. The reasoning is relatively easy to accept when the source of phobic anxiety is internal, such as in obsessive–compulsive disorder when the dreaded event has never occurred. This is also true in panic disorder/ agoraphobia, because the essential fear of panicking has to do with the fear of fainting, having a heart attack or losing one's mind, events that have not occurred even in the midst of their worst panic attacks. It is somewhat more difficult when the source of the perceived danger is external, particularly when tied to real possibilities, no matter how remote (e.g. in specific fears of thunderstorms). Social phobia also presents the same type of difficulty, because the dreaded consequence is also external to the patient in the form of being ridiculed or at the very least of being seen as anxious by others. In these cases a cognitive behavioural therapeutic approach is often needed to ensure that the patient differentiates between his fears and real danger before proceeding with exposure.

Application. The dismantling of escape/avoidance mechanisms need not be complete or start with exposure to the most feared situation at first. The pace of treatment needs to be individualized depending on the readiness and tolerance of the patient for anxiety. It is a good principle to follow a hierarchy of contexts from least distressful to most distressful. Concomitant treatment with antidepressants and even benzodiazepines can be useful as long as benzodiazepines are not taken contingently to decrease anxiety nor given in large doses that could interfere with the ability to experience the process of habituation. Once patients experience this process they become convinced of its therapeutic usefulness and they can and very often do apply the exposure principle at every occasion. A point comes in treatment where they spontaneously take the initiative of abandoning the most tacit of avoidance and escape mechanisms such as mental distractions, applied relaxation or breathing techniques, the anxiolytic they carried in their pockets for many months or years, praying etc. The goal of treatment is to approximate a situation where the patient no longer takes precautionary measures to avoid experiencing anxiety/fear and where the only response elicited by fear, less and less frequent and severe, is to simply acknowledge its neurotic nature. The approach is both therapeutic and prophylactic and may underlie the lasting effects of behavioural treatment.

Research questions. The empirical evidence shows lasting improvement with behavioural treatments. Whether this is due to the enduring effects of acute treatment or to ongoing maintenance treatment warrants investigation. One way of addressing this question would be to monitor the use of anxiety management strategies, in addition to symptom severity, over the follow-up period.

The evidence presented by Barlow *et al.* clearly suggests that the effectiveness of exposure depends on self-exposure regardless of whether instructions are provided by a therapist or not. Questions have also been raised regarding the specific role of cognitive therapy independent of exposure. Given the importance of translating evidence into practical experience, it may be valuable therefore to ascertain the extent to which patients require a fully manualized cognitive behaviour approach above and beyond the simple formulation of therapeutic rationale and instructions for self-directed exposure in everyday clinical practice.

REFERENCE

1. Mavissakalian M. (1993) Combined behavioral and pharmacological treatment of anxiety disorders. In *American Psychiatric Press Annual Review of Psychiatry*, vol. 12 (Eds J.M. Oldham, M.B. Riba, A. Tasman), pp. 565–584. American Psychiatric Press, Washington, DC.

4.4
The Treatment of Phobic Disorders: Is Exposure still the Treatment of Choice?
Paul M.G. Emmelkamp[1]

The review by Barlow et al. provides a fair evaluation of the progress that has been achieved in the treatment of phobias, particularly in the past decade. As noted by these authors, exposure *in vivo* is consistently effective across the various phobic conditions. Exposure therapy is based on the notion that anxiety subsides through a process of habituation after a person has been exposed to a fearful situation for a prolonged period of time, without trying to escape. Several studies [1] have provided supportive evidence for the role of habituation in exposure therapy, with self-reported fear and physiological arousal showing a declining trend across exposures, consistent with habituation.

The success of exposure *in vivo* has also been explained by the acquisition of fresh, disconfirmatory evidence, which weakens the catastrophic cognitions. From this perspective, exposure is viewed as a critical intervention through which catastrophic cognitions may be tested. Results of a study [2] showed that cognitive change (decrease in frequency of negative self-statements) indeed was achieved by exposure *in vivo* therapy. However, cognitive change *per se* was not related to a positive treatment outcome.

A recent development consists of exposure by using virtual reality (VR). VR integrates real-time computer graphics, body tracking devices, visual displays and other sensory inputs to immerse individuals in a computer-generated virtual environment. VR exposure has several advantages over exposure *in vivo*. The treatment can be conducted in the therapist's office rather than the therapist and patient having to go outside to do the exposure exercises in real phobic situations. Hence, treatment may be more cost-effective than therapist-assisted exposure *in vivo*. Further, VR treatment can also be applied on patients who are too anxious to undergo real-life exposure *in vivo*.

In a study at the University of Amsterdam [3], the effectiveness of two sessions of VR versus two sessions of exposure *in vivo* was investigated in a within-group design in individuals suffering from acrophobia. VR exposure was found to be at least as effective as exposure *in vivo* on anxiety and avoidance. The aim of a following study [4] was to compare the effectiveness of exposure *in vivo* versus VR exposure in a between-group design

---

[1] *Department of Clinical Psychology, University of Amsterdam, Roetersstraat 15, 1018 WB Amsterdam, The Netherlands*

with acrophobic patients. In order to enhance the comparability of exposure environments, the locations used in the exposure *in vivo* programme were exactly reproduced in virtual worlds that were used in VR exposure. VR exposure was found to be as effective as exposure *in vivo* on anxiety and avoidance and also reflected in a reduction of actual avoidance behaviour. Recently, we completed a study [5] in which the role of feelings of presence during VR was investigated. High presence (Computer Automatic Virtual Environment, CAVE) and low presence (Head Mounted Display, HMD) were compared. Both VR exposure conditions were more effective than no-treatment, but high presence did not enhance treatment effectiveness. Taken together, the results of these studies show considerable evidence that VR exposure is an effective treatment for patients with specific phobias.

In agoraphobia, exposure *in vivo* not only leads to a reduction of anxiety and avoidance, but also to a reduction of panic attacks [6]. A number of studies with agoraphobics have shown that exposure *in vivo* is superior to cognitive therapy consisting of insight into irrational beliefs and training of incompatible positive self-statements. Current cognitive-behavioural approaches focus more directly on the panic attacks than is the case in rational emotive therapy and self-instructional training, but, in the case of agoraphobia, there is no evidence that cognitive therapy is as effective as exposure *in vivo* [6]. For example, in patients with panic disorder and agoraphobia, cognitive therapy led to a reduction of panic attacks, but this did not automatically lead to an abandonment of the agoraphobic avoidance behaviour. Also other studies did not find that cognitive therapy enhanced the effectiveness of exposure alone in agoraphobic patients [7]. There is now considerable evidence that the degree of agoraphobic disability has a significant bearing on panic treatment effectiveness. When panic treatment research excludes people with severe agoraphobic avoidance, as it has routinely done, an overtly positive estimate of cognitive treatment effectiveness can result.

Although the effectiveness of exposure *in vivo* in social phobia is well established [6], the effectiveness of cognitive therapy is divergent. In one study [7] 70% of patients treated with exposure were rated as clinically improved, in contrast to only 36% of patients treated with cognitive-behavioural group therapy. For patients with a more specific social phobia (e.g. fear of writing, blushing, trembling or sweating), exposure *in vivo* seems indispensable and it is doubtful whether cognitive strategies do have additional value [8].

Social skills training has also been shown to be an effective treatment in a number of studies conducted outside the US [9–11]. It must be noted that the effects of social skills training, when conducted in groups (as is usually the case), can be explained in terms of *in vivo* exposure. Group treatment provides a continuous exposure to a group—for many social phobics one of the most anxiety-provoking situations.

The emphasis in the review is on the effects of psychotherapeutic interventions in adults. However, in recent years the same type of cognitive-behavioural interventions has been applied in phobic children. In 1994 the first controlled study [12] on the effects of cognitive-behavioural therapy (CBT) in children with an anxiety disorder was published. CBT was rather effective, approximately 70% of children no longer meeting criteria for an anxiety disorder after treatment. Since then, a number of studies from different research centres have been reported [13], yielding approximately the same positive results. Although the results of CBT in children with anxiety disorders are positive, it should be noted that most of the findings are reported from university centres, rather than mental health centres.

Since parents play an important role in both the etiology and maintenance of their children's anxiety, dealing with inadequate parental rearing style and addressing parental cognitions may strengthen the effects of behavioural interventions. In a study by our research group [14], 79 phobic children in mental health clinics were randomly assigned to a CBT condition or a waiting list control condition. Half of the families received an additional cognitive parent training programme. Phobic children showed more treatment gains from CBT than from a waiting list control condition. At three-months follow-up, 68% of the children no longer met the criteria for any anxiety disorder. No significant outcome differences were found between families with or without additional parent training. Thus, phobic children as well as adults may profit from CBT.

In conclusion, the effects of exposure *in vivo* are now well established for agoraphobia, simple phobia and social phobia, not only in adults, but also in children. Although recent years have witnessed a number of alternative approaches for the treatment of phobias (e.g. cognitive interventions, medications, applied relaxation), there is neither evidence that these treatments are more effective than exposure *in vivo*, nor that these treatments enhance the effects of exposure *in vivo*. If anything, stopping taking medications is the most robust variable predicting relapse. Exposure *in vivo* is still the treatment of choice for specific phobia, social phobia, agoraphobia and childhood phobias.

REFERENCES

1. van Hout W.J.P.J., Emmelkamp P.M.G. (2002) Exposure in vivo. In *The Encyclopedia of Psychotherapy* (Eds M. Hersen, W. Sledge), pp. 693–697. Academic Press, New York.

2. van Hout W.J.P.J., Emmelkamp P.M.G., Scholing A. (1994) The role of negative self-statements in agoraphobic situations: a process study of eight panic disorder patients with agoraphobia. *Behav. Modif.*, **18**: 389–410.
3. Emmelkamp P.M.G., Bruynzeel M., Drost L., van der Mast C.A.P.G. (2001) Virtual reality exposure in acrophobia: a comparison with exposure in vivo. *CyberPsychol. Behav.*, **4**: 335–339.
4. Emmelkamp P.M.G., Krijn M., Hulsbosch L., de Vries S., Schuemie M.J., van der Mast C.A.P.G. (2002) Virtual reality treatment versus exposure in vivo: a comparative evaluation in acrophobia. *Behav. Res. Ther.*, **40**: 509–516.
5. Krijn M., Emmelkamp P.M.G., Biemond R., de Wilde de Ligny, Schuemie M.J., van der Mast C.A.P.G. (submitted) Treatment of acrophobia in virtual reality: the role of immersion and presence. *Behav. Res. Ther.*
6. Emmelkamp P.M.G. (2003) Behavior therapy with adults. In *Bergin and Garfield's Handbook of Psychotherapy and Behavior Change*, 4th edn (Ed. M. Lambert). John Wiley & Sons, New York.
7. Hope D.A., Heimberg R.G., Bruch M.A. (1995) Dismantling cognitive-behavioral group therapy for social phobia. *Behav. Res. Ther.*, **33**: 637–650.
8. Scholing A., Emmelkamp P.M.G. (1993) Cognitive and behavioral treatments of fear of blushing, sweating or trembling. *Behav. Res. Ther.*, **31**: 155–170.
9. Mersch P.P.A., Emmelkamp P.M.G., Lips C. (1991) Social phobia: individual response patterns and the long-term effects of behavioral and cognitive interventions: a follow-up study. *Behav. Res. Ther.*, **29**: 357–362.
10. Mersch P.P., Jansen M., Arntz A. (1995) Social phobia and personality disorder: severity of complaints and treatment effectiveness. *J. Personal. Disord.*, **9**: 143–159.
11. Öst L.G., Jerremalm A., Johansson J. (1981) Individual response patterns and the effect of different behavioral methods in the treatment of social phobia. *Behav. Res. Ther.*, **19**: 1–16.
12. Kendall P.C. (1994) Treating anxiety disorders in children: results of a randomized clinical trial. *J. Consult. Clin. Psychol.*, **62**: 100–110.
13. Nauta M.H., Scholing A., Emmelkamp P.M.G., Minderaa R.B. (2001) Cognitive-behavioural therapy for anxiety disordered children in a clinical setting: does additional cognitive parent training enhance treatment effectiveness? *Clin. Psychol. Psychother.*, **8**: 330–340.
14. Nauta M.H., Scholing A., Emmelkamp P.M.G., Minderaa R.B. (2003) Cognitive-behavioural therapy for anxiety disordered children in a clinical setting: no additional effect of a cognitive parent training. *J. Am. Acad. Child Adolesc. Psychiatry*, **42**: 1270–1278.

4.5
"Behavioural Experimentation" and the Treatment of Phobias

Yiannis G. Papakostas, Vasilios G. Masdrakis and George N. Christodoulou[1]

Barlow *et al.*'s critical and comprehensive review of an extensive body of research demonstrates the efficacy of current psychological treatments in

---

[1] *Department of Psychiatry, Athens University Medical School, 74 Vasilissis Sophias Avenue, Athens, GR 115 28, Greece*

the management of phobias. Among these treatments, *in vivo* exposure, alone or in combination with cognitive therapy (for panic disorder and social phobia) and applied tension (for blood phobia), stands predominantly as a key therapeutic strategy for these disorders. In clinical practice, this intervention refers to a systematic exposure to the feared stimulus (rapid, slow, continuous, intermittent), aiming at fear reduction which is called "habituation" or, if the fear response had initially been conditioned, "extinction" [1].

Naturally, such concepts as "exposure" and "extinction" do not fit comfortably into the cognitive school of thought. In this approach the elicitation of cognitions and their subsequent treatment as "hypotheses" to be tested represent the dual task of the therapist. Both tasks are achieved verbally—merely through a Socratic type of questioning—and by conducting so-called "behavioural experiments", the latter being considered as the cognitive counterpart of exposure. Thus defined, behavioural experimentation differs, in principle, from the concept of exposure in at least two main aspects [2]. First, the former is presented to the patient as a method of identifying and testing (confirming or disconfirming) cognitions–hypotheses, whereas in the latter the therapist tries to convince the patient of the therapeutic merits of systematically approaching the fearful situations. Second, behavioural experimentation is characterized by a greater variety of procedures than merely the "exposure" paradigm.

After conducting a brief survey on more than 60 studies cited in Barlow *et al.*'s review, we found that the majority of them (around 75%) employ the "exposure" protocol. Most of these studies have been conducted under the label of "cognitive behaviour therapy" where behavioural experimentation was diminished to and/or replaced by exposure. Only in a few studies (i.e. around 20%) was the behavioural experimentation paradigm faithfully followed, mainly in the ones deriving from the leading proponents of the cognitive approach, such as Beck and Clark.

These observations, of course, do not dispute or negate the overwhelming experimental evidence on the outcome efficacy of psychological therapies, and "exposure" in particular, in the treatment of phobias, so amply presented in Barlow *et al.*'s review. If anything they make exposure's contribution to this outcome clearer. On the other hand, it seems equally clear that behavioural experimentation, as opposed or compared to exposure, has not been systematically applied and tested. Partly, this is due to the considerable, mainly clinical, overlap between exposure and behavioural experimentation, a major obstacle in conducting meaningful comparative studies. The typical, yet questionable, research manoeuvre to reduce the overlap with the exposure treatment is to keep the number of the behavioural experiments low (if any) in the cognitive approach, the latter being restricted to a merely verbal task of cognition identification and disputation. Nevertheless, the findings from a recent study [3] that adopted this strategy while comparing cognitive therapy (CT) to interoceptive exposure (IE) in the treatment of panic disorder without agoraphobia are interesting and may be relevant to our discussion. While both treatments were equally effective, "the IE seemed, at least when applied in isolated format, somewhat less acceptable for patients than CT. Some patients found IE exercises strange, shameful, and aversive. Some patients also complained about the IE rationale, which they found not very convincing. The higher drop out rate may be related to this issue" [3]. Thus, the possibility that the rationale given to patients might have an impact on the attrition rate, as this study implies, an issue stressed by other investigators as well [4], needs to be systematically addressed in future studies.

At least theoretically, behavioural experimentation, as a "hypothesis to be empirically tested" strategy, may be more suitable whenever advanced cognitive formulations about a clinical condition exist. Regarding phobias, this might be the case with panic disorder and social phobia. However, in specific phobias—perhaps because of their circumscribed nature, their possible relationship to conditioned fear [5] and the paucity of empirically tested cognitive models—the application of behavioural experimentation seems less guaranteed. Things seem more complicated in agoraphobia, whose conceptualization still poses a dilemma for clinicians. Whereas early behaviourists targeted agoraphobia and ignored panic or considered it as a secondary phenomenon, nowadays cognitive-behavioural therapists view agoraphobia as secondary to panic. Therefore, as long as the cognitive approach runs short of theories about agoraphobia as an entity on its own— a notable exception is the, as yet untested, theory of Guidano and Liotti [6]—the merits of behavioural experimentation employed in this condition are questionable.

In conclusion, while the efficacy of evidence-based psychotherapy in the treatment of phobias is well established, future studies are indicated to investigate the relative effectiveness of the cognitive-theory-driven key concept of behavioural experimentation.

REFERENCES

1. Marks I., Dar R. (2000) Fear reduction by psychotherapies: recent findings, future directions. *Br. J. Psychiatry*, **176**: 507–511.
2. Clark D.M. (1999) Anxiety disorders: why they persist and how to treat them. *Behav. Res. Ther.*, **37** (Suppl.): S5–S27.
3. Arntz A. (2002) Cognitive therapy versus interoceptive exposure as treatment of panic disorder without agoraphobia. *Behav. Res. Ther.*, **40**: 325–341.
4. Snaith P. (2000) Invited commentary on: fear reduction by psychotherapies. *Br. J. Psychiatry*, **176**: 512–513.

5. Fyer A.J. (1998) Current approaches to etiology and pathophysiology of specific phobia. *Biol. Psychiatry*, **44**: 1295–1304.
6. Guidano V.F., Liotti G. (1983) *Cognitive Processes and Emotional Disorders*. Guilford Press, New York.

4.6
Evaluating the Durability of Cognitive-Behavioural Therapy
Eberhard H. Uhlenhuth, Deepa Nadiga and Paula Hensley[1]

Barlow *et al.*, like so many others, espouse the view that relatively brief cognitive-behavioural interventions in agoraphobia and panic disorder bring about "durable" improvement; that is, improvement lasts well beyond the termination of therapy. If this is a fact, it is of far-reaching importance, as no other treatment short of psychoanalysis makes that claim.

The evidence to support this view derives from numerous studies of cognitive-behavioural therapy with post-treatment follow-up. These studies commonly are "naturalistic": a group of patients who have responded well to an acute treatment phase receives cross-sectional re-evaluations periodically after the conclusion of active therapy. The usual, though not universal, finding is that a gratifying majority of patients "maintained their gains". While this type of information is useful to clinicians, it does not establish a scientific basis for concluding that the *long-term outcome* of cognitive-behavioural therapies is superior to that of other treatments. In a recent review of follow-up studies limited to individual cognitive-behavioural therapy in panic disorder, we found only three that met scientific requirements [1]. This being said, the design and execution of valid long-term studies clearly present the clinical investigator with daunting challenges.

First, one should consider the standard of "durability". In many studies "durability" refers to effects lasting three or six months beyond the termination of active therapy. Effects of such short duration, even if clearly demonstrated, have little practical significance in the context of chronic fluctuating illnesses like anxiety disorders that often span the better part of a lifetime. Furthermore, it seems likely that improvement induced by other acute treatments, including medications, can be sustained over similar time periods using attenuated maintenance regimens that demand little effort and expense. Although the choice of any time period to define "durability" is necessarily arbitrary, it seems reasonable to suggest at least one to two years beyond the termination of acute therapy.

---

[1] *Department of Psychiatry, University of New Mexico, Albuquerque, NM 87131-0001, USA*

Second, to evaluate long-term treatment effects, a credible comparison group is necessary, as with short-term treatment effects. A group receiving an acute treatment with no claim to durability, e.g. medication, is one possibility. Another is a group receiving a dummy treatment. Without other design modifications, a medication comparator may be too lenient, since patients suddenly withdrawn from medication are at risk of early relapse. A dummy comparator may be too stringent, as patients who survive 12–16 weeks of inactive treatment are likely to maintain gains without additional intervention. Barlow et al. [2] furnish an excellent example: only 3 of 24 patients assigned to pill placebo completed the acute treatment and maintenance phases, and all 3 went on do well at the subsequent six-month follow-up, yielding 100% durability!

Third, purely cross-sectional evaluations provide data only at follow-up visits. Relapse and additional treatment to avoid relapse between evaluations may go undetected without specific inquiry, and analyses refer to the condition of the group at each evaluation rather than to the course of the individual patient. This issue becomes increasingly important as intervals between follow-up visits increase. With chronic fluctuating disorders, data covering the individual patient's entire course is needed. The Longitudinal Interval Follow-up Evaluation (LIFE) [3] is one instrument designed to obtain such information. The duration of treatment effects should be measured by the time to the first relapse (clearly defined by protocol) or the institution of additional treatment.

Fourth, patients who fail to respond to acute treatment should be included in the follow-up. Such patients may improve later, because the full effect of a short-term therapy may take more time to develop, because of spontaneous fluctuations in the illness etc. The effect of this design element on the study's outcome, of course, depends on the distribution of non-responders among treatment groups.

Fifth, dropouts should be taken into account in the main analyses of the study. In short-term pharmacotherapy studies, patients usually drop out because of adverse events (in the experimental treatment group) or because the treatment is ineffective (in the comparison group), regardless of the reasons they supply when questioned. Subtler issues may be more prominent in psychotherapy studies, including dissatisfaction with the patient–therapist relationship. In any event, it seems reasonable to consider patients who drop from the acute phase as treatment failures. The reasons for dropping from follow-up may be more varied and complex, including sustained improvement and changes in life circumstances. The problem increases in complexity and magnitude as the length of follow-up increases. It may be justifiable to rely on the last available evaluation in long-term studies, particularly if survival analysis is appropriate. The only fully satisfactory solution, however, is to expend major resources on securing full participation in follow-up.

Considering all of these issues, long-term treatment effects ideally would be evaluated in one continuous study designed for the purpose from the start, rather than as an after-thought to an acute study. From this perspective, it would be possible to take account of all patients who originally were assigned to treatment and to use appropriate measures and analyses, including intent-to-treat analyses, consistently throughout the course of treatment and follow-up. These procedures would provide a more level playing field for comparing the long-term outcomes of different treatments. The recent study by Barlow et al. [2] offers a provisional template for the conduct of such studies, incorporating several of the features suggested above.

REFERENCES

1. Nadiga D.N., Hensley P.L., Uhlenhuth E.H. (2003) A review of the long-term effectiveness of cognitive behavioral therapy compared to medication in panic disorder. Depress. Anxiety, 17: 58–64.
2. Barlow D.H., Gorman J.M., Shear M.K., Woods S.W. (2000) Cognitive-behavioral therapy, imipramine, or their combination for panic disorder. JAMA, 283: 2529–2536.
3. Keller M.B., Lavori P.W., Friedman B., Nielsen E., Endicott J., McDonald-Scott P., Andreason N.C. (1987) The Longitudinal Interval Follow-up Evaluation: a comprehensive method for assessing outcome in prospective longitudinal studies. Arch. Gen. Psychiatry, 44: 540–548.

4.7
Some Comments on Psychological Treatment of Phobias
Lars-Göran Öst[1]

Barlow et al. have produced an excellent and up-to-date review of the state of the art regarding psychological treatment of phobias. I provide here some comments concerning treatment of the various types of phobia.

Agoraphobia. The authors conclude that breathing retraining and relaxation training may put patients with panic and agoraphobia at risk of relapse, because they teach patients to minimize physical anxiety reactions. However, there is only one study, by Schmidt et al. [1], on breathing retraining to support this notion. In my own research on panic disorder with [2,3] or without [4,5] agoraphobia, I have evaluated applied relaxation (AR) [6]. In the first agoraphobia study [2], the proportion of patients

---

[1] Department of Psychology, University of Stockholm, Sweden

clinically significantly improved after AR was 58% at post-treatment and 83% at the 15-month follow-up, while the corresponding figures in the second study [3] were 65% and 70%. In the first panic disorder study [4], 100% of the AR-treated patients were panic-free both at post-treatment and at the 19-month follow-up, whereas in the second study [5] the figures were 65% and 82%, respectively. Thus, it seems that the AR coping technique does not lead to relapse at follow-up: the effects are maintained or a further improvement takes place.

Barlow et al. refer to the intriguing ungraded exposure treatment developed by Fiegenbaum [7] in Germany. However, there is no information in the original publication about the proportion of patients who, during the contemplation phase after having had the treatment described to them, decided to drop out of the study. An effectiveness study on this treatment from three outpatient clinics in Germany [8] showed that 13% decided not to start the treatment and another 8.5% dropped out during the treatment. The former figure is probably higher than is common for in vivo exposure, whereas the latter is lower. In a meta-analysis of cognitive-behavioural therapy (CBT) for anxiety disorders [9], I found a dropout rate of 15.2% across 73 studies published between 1966 and 2002.

Barlow et al. also describe the necessity of doing effectiveness studies on panic disorder treatments and mention the study by Wade et al. [10]. However, there are also three effectiveness studies from European countries: Norway [11], Germany [7] and Spain [12]. The general conclusion that can be drawn from these is that the effect sizes obtained by these studies are approximately of the same magnitude as those obtained in efficacy studies.

Social phobia. When it comes to AR for social phobia [13,14], the authors say that it is likely that the treatment effects are due to the patient's exposure to feared situations. This might be true, but it should be kept in mind that only 20% of the therapy sessions consist of application training, during which the patients are briefly exposed to phobic situations in order to experience the anxiety increase, use the relaxation skills, and notice the drop in anxiety that follows. Thus, the exposure is much briefer than is usual in exposure *in vivo* and for only two sessions followed by homework. A dismantling study is necessary to find out if it is the use of the relaxation skills or the exposure that is responsible for the effects of applied relaxation.

Heimberg's cognitive-behavioural group therapy (CBGT) is described as an empirically supported treatment. However, it should be noticed that a meta-analysis [9] found that the effect sizes in Heimberg's three studies were gradually deteriorating; from 0.75 in the 1990 to 0.12 in the 1998 study (calculated for the most important self-report measure). Heimberg has also developed an individual version of his group treatment and the pilot data [15] indicated clearly higher effect sizes than ordinarily obtained in the group treatment. Furthermore, the individual CBT developed by Clark yielded effect sizes of 2.14 at post-treatment and 2.53 at the 1-year follow-up. This means that we need to reconsider before deciding that CBGT is the treatment of choice for social phobia. Perhaps the advantage of doing the treatment in a group is outweighed by the disadvantage of not being able to deal with each individual patient's catastrophic beliefs in a detailed and individualized way.

There is also a lack of effectiveness studies for social phobia. The only one I am familiar with was done in Italy by Fava *et al.* [16]. Patients were given only eight 30-min sessions of exposure (biweekly) and at post-treatment 83% were considered recovered. At follow-up 2–12 years later (median 6 years) the relapse rate was only 13%.

Specific phobia. The authors describe technical advances in the treatment of specific phobias. The most advanced of these are virtual reality treatments, but so far no study has compared it with state-of-the-art exposure *in vivo* treatment, which means that it can only be regarded as a promising treatment. However, it usually takes longer than the one-session treatment that I have developed, and requires expensive computer hardware and software. Furthermore, a computer-aided exposure was found significantly inferior to exposure *in vivo* for children with spider phobia in Australia [17].

When it comes to blood phobia, the applied tension treatment is described. However, it is necessary to mention that in one study we found that tension-only without any exposure to blood stimuli was as effective as applied tension when given for five sessions [18] and, in a subsequent study, one session of tension-only was as effective as one session of applied tension when both were given for two hours [19].

The issue of which subtypes of specific phobias can be treated successfully with one-session treatment is interesting. We have done studies on animals [20–23], blood–injury–injection [19,24], and situational type (flying phobia and claustrophobia) [25,26]. Clinically, patients with natural environment type (heights, slopes) and other type (vomiting, choking and, in children, avoidance of loud sounds and costumed characters) have been successfully treated with one-session exposure treatment. The results of our randomized controlled trials have been replicated by researchers in Norway, the UK, Holland, Germany, Canada and the USA. Thus, I think that it is possible to conclude that one-session treatment can be used for any type of specific phobia, even though it would be difficult when it comes to thunder and lightning phobia, since the therapist has to be on call during the thunder storm season.

In addition to the point that the authors raise under the headings of "Incomplete evidence" and "Areas still open to research", I would like to add that more basic research concerning the psychopathology (primarily maintenance factors) for the different phobias is needed. I believe that we need to learn more about these issues before we can improve our treatment methods. While our best treatments yield 80–90% clinically significantly improved patients with specific phobias, the figures are 65–75% for social phobia and agoraphobia. Thus, there is still room for improvement.

REFERENCES

1. Schmidt N.B., Woolaway-Bickel K., Trakowski J., Santiago H., Storey J., Koselka M., Cook J. (2000) Dismantling cognitive-behavioral treatment for panic disorder: questioning the validity of breathing retraining. *J. Consult. Clin. Psychol.*, **68**: 417–424.
2. Öst L.-G., Jerremalm A., Jansson L. (1984) Individual response patterns and the effects of different behavioral methods in the treatment of agoraphobia. *Behav. Res. Ther.*, **22**: 697–707.
3. Öst L.-G., Westling B., Hellström K. (1993) Applied relaxation, exposure in-vivo, and cognitive methods in the treatment of panic disorder with agoraphobia. *Behav. Res. Ther.*, **31**: 383–394.
4. Öst L.-G. (1988) Applied relaxation vs. progressive relaxation in the treatment of panic disorder. *Behav. Res. Ther.*, **26**: 13–22.
5. Öst L.-G., Westling B.E. (1995) Applied relaxation vs. cognitive therapy in the treatment of panic disorder. *Behav. Res. Ther.*, **33**: 145–158.
6. Öst L.-G. (2002) Applied relaxation. In *Encyclopedia of Psychotherapy*, vol. 1 (Eds M. Hersen, W. Sledge), pp. 95–102. Academic Press, New York.
7. Fiegenbaum W. (1988) Long-term efficacy of ungraded versus graded massed exposure in agoraphobics. In *Panic and Phobias: Treatments and Variables Affecting Course and Outcome* (Eds I. Hand, H. Wittchen), pp. 83–88. Springer-Verlag, Berlin.
8. Hahlweg K., Fiegenbaum W., Frank M., Schroeder B., von Witzleben I. (2001) Short- and long-term effectiveness of an empirically supported treatment for agoraphobia. *J. Consult. Clin. Psychol.*, **69**: 375–382.
9. Öst L.-G. (2002) CBT for anxiety disorders. What progress have we made after 35 years of randomized clinical trials? Presented at the British Association for Behavioural and Cognitive Psychotherapy Annual Convention, Warwick, 19 July.
10. Wade W.A., Treat T.A., Stuart G.L. (1998) Transporting an empirically supported treatment for panic disorder to a service clinic setting: a benchmarking strategy. *J. Consult. Clin. Psychol.*, **66**: 231–239.
11. Martinsen E.W., Olsen T., Tonset E., Nyland K.E., Aarre T.F. (1998) Cognitive behavioral group therapy for panic disorder in the general clinical setting: a naturalistic study with 1-year follow-up. *J. Clin. Psychiatry*, **59**: 437–442.
12. Garcia-Palacios A., Botella C., Robert C., Banos R., Perpina C., Quero S., Ballester R. (2002) Clinical utility of cognitive-behavioural treatment for panic disorder. *Clin. Psychol. Psychother.*, **9**: 373–383.
13. Öst L.-G., Jerremalm A., Johansson J. (1981) Individual response patterns and the effects of different behavioral methods in the treatment of social phobia. *Behav. Res. Ther.*, **19**: 1–16.
14. Jerremalm A., Jansson L., Öst L.-G. (1986) Cognitive and physiological reactivity and the effects of different behavioral methods in the treatment of social phobia. *Behav. Res. Ther.*, **24**: 171–180.

15. Heimberg R.G. (2002) The understanding and treatment of social anxiety. Presented at the Association for the Advancement of Behavior Therapy Annual Convention, Reno, NV, 16 November.
16. Fava G.A., Grandi S., Rafanelli C., Ruini C, Conti S., Belluardo P. (2001) Long-term outcome of social phobia treated by exposure. *Psychol. Med.*, **31**: 899–905.
17. Dewis L.M., Kirkby K.C., Martin F., Daniels B.A., Gilroy L.J., Menzies R.G. (2001) Computer-aided vicarious exposure versus live graded exposure for spider phobia in children. *J. Behav. Ther. Exp. Psychiatry*, **32**: 17–27.
18. Öst L.-G., Fellenius J., Sterner U. (1991) Applied tension, exposure *in vivo*, and tension-only in the treatment of blood phobia. *Behav. Res. Ther.*, **29**: 561–574.
19. Hellström K., Fellenius J., Öst L.-G. (1996) One versus five sessions of applied tension in the treatment of blood phobia. *Behav. Res. Ther.*, **34**: 101–112.
20. Öst L.-G., Salkovskis P.M., Hellström K. (1991) One-session therapist directed exposure versus self-exposure in the treatment of spider phobia. *Behav. Ther.*, **22**: 407–422.
21. Hellström K., Öst L.-G. (1995) One-session therapist directed exposure vs. two forms of manual directed self-exposure in the treatment of spider phobia. *Behav. Res. Ther.*, **33**: 959–965.
22. Öst L.-G. (1996) One-session group treatment of spider phobia. *Behav. Res. Ther.*, **34**: 707–715.
23. Öst L.-G., Ferebee I., Furmark T. (1997) One session group therapy of spider phobia: direct versus indirect treatments. *Behav. Res. Ther.*, **35**: 721–732.
24. Öst L.-G., Hellström K., Kåver A. (1992) One vs. five sessions of exposure in the treatment of injection phobia. *Behav. Ther.*, **23**: 263–282.
25. Öst L.-G., Brandberg M., Alm T. (1997) One versus five sessions of exposure in the treatment of flying phobia. *Behav. Res. Ther.*, **35**: 987–996.
26. Öst L.-G., Alm T., Brandberg M., Breitholtz E. (2001) One vs. five sessions of exposure and five sessions of cognitive therapy in the treatment of claustrophobia. *Behav. Res. Ther.*, **39**: 167–183.

4.8
Pushing the Envelope on Treatments for Phobia
Michael J. Telch[1]

Barlow *et al.* provide a thoughtful review of the evidence on empirically supported treatments and factors that predict treatment response in patients with phobias. Not surprisingly, exposure to fear-eliciting cues appears as a common therapeutic strategy across phobia types. In this commentary, I raise the following question: "What does our science tell us about how to conduct therapeutic exposure more effectively?". Although Barlow *et al.* cite selected studies investigating several exposure parameters

---

[1] *Laboratory for the Study of Anxiety Disorders, University of Texas at Austin, 108 Dean Keaton, Austin, TX 78712, USA*

(i.e. spacing and intensity), recent studies [1,2] that have experimentally manipulated other exposure parameters provide additional guidance on the procedural dos and don'ts for enhancing the effects of exposure therapy.

Manipulation of cognitive parameters. Two recent investigations with claustrophobics have shown that, after controlling for total duration of exposure, patients who are instructed to focus on their identified core threats during exposure and provided brief guidance in threat re-evaluation between exposure trials fare significantly better than those who receive exposure without threat focus and re-evaluation [3,4]. In contrast, recent data suggest that having phobics engage in a demanding cognitive load task during exposure significantly weakens therapeutic efficacy [3–5]. Moreover, treatment process analyses showed that the cognitive load task exerted its disruptive effects by interfering with between-trial habituation as opposed to fear activation or within-trial habituation. These data help to resolve the mixed findings that have been reported on the effects of distraction during exposure [6], namely it is not distraction *per se* but the extent to which the distracter task makes attentional resources less available for cognitive processing during exposure.

Feedback manipulations during exposure. Recent evidence suggests that providing relevant feedback during exposure may facilitate its therapeutic efficacy. In one study, claustrophobics who were provided audio heart-rate feedback during exposure fared significantly better than those who received either no feedback or audio feedback unrelated to heart rate [7]. In a study just completed, social phobics who received video feedback of their performance following each of 15 three-minute public speaking exposure trials displayed significantly greater fear reduction than those receiving exposure with no feedback [8].

Manipulation of safety behaviours during exposure. Ironically, the safety strategies that patients engage in during exposure therapy may inadvertently impede their recovery. Barlow *et al.* note the importance of fading safety behaviours during exposure. There is now compelling evidence from well-controlled experiments attesting to: (a) the disruptive effects of safety behaviours on fear reduction during exposure [4,9,10], (b) the beneficial effects of fading safety behaviours during exposure [11–14], and (c) the potential mechanisms through which safety behaviours undermine therapeutic exposure [10].

Clinical implications. One common therapeutic principle may help explain the above-mentioned findings and offers a heuristic for clinicians in working with phobic patients. The principle could be crudely stated as: exposure interventions will be maximally effective when they include procedural elements that maximize the salience of threat disconfirmation. Carrying out this strategic principle requires that the clinician identify the specific core phobic threat(s) of the individual patient and creatively design exposure interventions that are likely to provide potent disconfirmation of those threats.

REFERENCES

1. Tsao J.C.I., Craske M.G. (2000) Timing of treatment and return of fear: effects of massed-, uniform-, and expanding-spaced exposure schedules. *Behav. Ther.*, **31**: 479–497.
2. Lang A.J., Craske M.G., Bjork R.A. (1999) Implications of a new theory of disuse for the treatment of emotional disorders. *Clin. Psychol. Sci. Pract.*, **6**: 80–94.
3. Kamphuis J., Telch M.J. (2000) Effects of distraction and guided threat reappraisal on fear reduction during exposure-based treatments for specific fears. *Behav. Res. Ther.*, **38**: 1163–1181.
4. Sloan T., Telch M.J. (2002) The effects of safety-seeking behavior and guided threat reappraisal on fear reduction during exposure: an experimental investigation. *Behav. Res. Ther.*, **40**: 235–251.
5. Telch M.J., Valentiner D.P., Ilai D., Young P.R., Powers M.B., Smits J.A.J. (submitted) Fear activation and distraction during the emotional processing of claustrophobic fear. *J. Behav. Ther. Exp. Res.*
6. Rodriguez B.I., Craske M.G. (1993) The effects of distraction during exposure to phobic stimuli. *Behav. Res. Ther.*, **31**: 549–558.
7. Telch M.J., Valentiner D.P., Ilai D., Petruzzi D., Hehmsoth M. (2000) The facilitative effects of heart-rate feedback in the emotional processing of claustrophobic fear. *Behav. Res. Ther.*, **38**: 373–387.
8. Smits J.A.J., Powers M.B., Cho Y., Wimmer M., Roddy S.K., Telch M.J. (2003) Facilitating public speaking fear reduction by increasing the salience of disconfirmatory evidence: work in progress. Presented at the Annual Meeting of the Anxiety Disorders Association of America, Toronto, 29 March.
9. Rentz T., Powers M., Smits J., Cougle J., Telch M. (2003) Active-imaginal exposure: examination of a new behavioral treatment for cynophobia (dog phobia). *Behav. Res. Ther.*, **41**: 1337–1353.
10. Powers M.B., Smits J.A.J, Telch M.J. (in press) Disentangling the effects of safety behavior utilization and availability during exposure-based treatment: a placebo-controlled study. *J. Consult. Clin. Psychol.*
11. Williams S.L., Dooseman G., Kleifield E. (1984) Comparative effectiveness of guided mastery and exposure treatments for intractable phobias. *J. Consult. Clin. Psychol.*, **52**: 505–518.
12. Salkovskis P.M., Clark D.M., Hackman A., Wells A., Gelder M.G. (1999) An experimental investigation of the role of safety-seeking behaviours in the maintenance of panic disorder with agoraphobia. *Behav. Res. Ther.*, **37**: 559–574.
13. Wells A., Clark D.M., Salkovskis P.M., Ludgate J., Hackmann A., Gelder M. (1995) Social phobia: the role of in-situation safety behaviors in maintaining anxiety and negative beliefs. *Behav. Ther.*, **26**: 153–161.
14. Telch M.J., Sloan T., Smits J. (2000) Safety-behavior fading as a maintenance treatment for panic disorder. Presented at the Annual Meeting of the Association for Advancement for Behavior Therapy, New Orleans, 18 November.

4.9
Treatment of Phobic Disorders from a Public Health Perspective
Ronald M. Rapee[1]

The review by Barlow et al. provides a clear and succinct overview of the state of our current knowledge of the treatment of phobic disorders. The review describes this literature from a primarily clinical perspective; that is, a perspective that places traditional treatment with a clinician at the centre of the treatment process. Our knowledge at present suggests that this style of treatment delivery is extremely efficacious in the reduction of phobic behaviour. As cogently argued by the authors, an area that requires considerable future research is the issue of effectiveness of treatment and its generalization to the community situation. Another important issue raised by the authors lies in alternative methods of treatment delivery that may have greater cost-effectiveness, including bibliotherapy and computer-assisted delivery.

A public health perspective on phobic disorders sees these problems as ones that produce major life interference and societal costs. In the context of restricted health budgets, any changes to services need to be achieved within existing budgets. Phobic disorders do indeed produce a major burden on Western society. As an example, it has been estimated that social phobia is the 24th greatest source of disability adjusted life years (DALYs) for females (and 37th for males) of any disease [1]. Panic disorder is ranked number 50 and is responsible for a greater burden than diseases such as colon and rectal cancers, leukaemia, breast cancer, and hepatitis B and C [2]. Others have expressed this burden in economic terms. Greenberg et al. [3] estimated the cost of anxiety disorders to the US economy in 1990 to be $42.3 billion, while Rice and Miller [4] used a different methodology to estimate the burden at $44.6 billion. This marked burden is largely due to the relatively high prevalence of these disorders, with phobic disorders representing some of the most common mental health problems [5]. Yet, despite their high prevalence, phobic disorders represent a small fraction of the load typically presenting to mental health professionals. Data from the Australian National Mental Health Survey has indicated that less than 30% of individuals with phobic disorders used any mental health services in the preceding year, with only around 20% seeing a general practitioner and 5% seeing a psychiatrist or psychologist [5]. It is clear from these figures that for treatments to reach those in the population who need them, alternative modes of delivery need to be identified.

---

[1] Department of Psychology, Macquarie University, Sydney, NSW, Australia

One such alternative which we have tested through our centre involves a stepped care approach to the management of panic attacks. Our justification was based on the reasoning that panic attacks represent a trigger for the seeking of help and a marker for the existence of mental health difficulties [6]. The stepped care approach is based on the principle that the minimal extent of intervention should be used with increasing treatment intensity accompanying unsuccessful intervention. Specifically, upon initial experience of a panic attack, individuals were given a brief information booklet. Six weeks later, only if panic attacks continued, individuals were given a five-week self-help manual. The final step involved standard group cognitive-behavioural therapy conducted by a therapist in those cases where self-help was not successful. The data indicated that 29.4% of individuals did not need to proceed to the self-help stage and only 51.0% needed to proceed to the group treatment stage. Compared with treatment as usual, the stepped care approach represented a saving of $647 in November 2000 Australian dollars (about $323 US dollars) for each client (Baillee and Rapee, unpublished work).

Another potential cost-saving approach to treatment delivery is self-help. The review by Barlow et al. describes some data demonstrating the value of self-help and minimal therapist assistance approaches to the treatment of panic disorder and specific phobias. However, to date there has been virtually no similar research into the management of social phobia. Social phobia is a highly debilitating problem but, because of its personality-like features, has perhaps been seen as a less likely target for self-help. At our centre we have recently been trialling a self-help programme for the management of social phobia [7]. In order to maximize generalizability, we specifically selected individuals with severe levels of social phobia coexisting with high levels of avoidant personality disorder. Individuals in the self-help condition were given a book [8] which describes treatment strategies based on a recent theoretical conceptualization of social phobia [9]. Another group received standard therapist-led treatment that involved the same treatment components in a 10-session group format. Finally, another group received five sessions of therapist-assisted treatment that involved using the self-help book and having five problem-solving sessions with a therapist. Thus this condition represented half the cost of the standard group treatment. Results indicated that those individuals receiving the book alone showed a significantly greater improvement than individuals on the waiting list. In particular, individuals who stated reading and using the majority of the book showed especially large gains. Perhaps of greatest interest, however, was the fact that those in the therapist-assisted condition did just as well as those in the standard group treatment, but at half the cost. Thus, these results show that a debilitating personality style like severe social phobia can be helped by delivery of treatment strategies through a self-help book and that the use of such materials can halve the burden placed on limited therapeutic resources.

REFERENCES

1. Mathers C., Vos T., Stevenson C. (1999) *The Burden of Disease and Injury in Australia*. Australian Institute of Health and Welfare, Canberra.
2. Murray C.J.L., Lopez A.D. (1996) *The Global Burden of Disease: A Comprehensive Assessment of Mortality and Disability from Diseases, Injuries, and Risk Factors in 1990 and Projected to 2020*. Harvard University Press, Cambridge, MA.
3. Greenberg P.E., Sisitsky T., Kessler R.C., Finkelstein S.N., Berndt E.R., Davidson J.R.T., Ballenger J.C., Fyer A.J. (1999) The economic burden of anxiety disorders in the 1990s. *J. Clin. Psychiatry*, 60: 427–435.
4. Rice D.P., Miller L.S. (1998) Health economics and cost implications of anxiety and other mental disorders in the United States. *Br. J. Psychiatry*, 173 (Suppl. 34): 4–9.
5. Andrews G., Hall W., Teesson M., Henderson S. (1999) *The Mental Health of Australians*. Mental Health Branch, Commonwealth Department of Health and Aged Care, Canberra.
6. Baillie A.J., Rapee R.M. (submitted) Panic attacks as risk markers for mental disorders.
7. Rapee R.M., Abbott M., Gaston J. (2000) Self help for social phobia: preliminary results from a controlled trial of bibliotherapy vs therapist treatment. Presented at the World Congress of Behavioral and Cognitive Therapies, Vancouver, 17–21 July.
8. Rapee R.M. (2001) *Overcoming Shyness and Social Phobia: A Step by Step Guide*, 2nd edn. Lifestyle Press, Sydney.
9. Rapee R.M., Heimberg R.G. (1997) A cognitive-behavioral model of anxiety in social phobia. *Behav. Res. Ther.*, 35: 741–756.

4.10
Psychotherapeutic Interventions for Phobia: A Psychoanalytic-Attachment Perspective

Jeremy Holmes[1]

Immediately following the singles finals at Wimbledon, the UK's annual Grand Slam tennis tournament, the participants are interviewed on TV, starting with the dejected losers, who typically concede that their opponent was the best player "on the day". Asking a psychodynamic psychotherapist to comment on Barlow *et al.*'s triumphant survey of the benefits of behavioural and cognitive approaches in the treatment of phobias provides

---

[1] Psychoanalysis Unit, University College, London, UK

some insight into how losers feel—except that we analytic sophomores would probably not even have reached the final, which, according to Barlow et al., is mainly a struggle between cognitive-behavioural therapy (CBT) and pharmacotherapy, with the former, with its "sleeper effects", which mean that benefits continue after therapy has ceased, a narrow winner.

By contrast, psychodynamic approaches to phobic disorders, with one or two honourable exceptions [1,2], are nowadays conspicuous by their absence from the literature. To date there have been few if any controlled trials of psychodynamic therapy for anxiety disorders, although a retrospective note-based study from the Anna Freud Centre showed that children with anxiety disorders responded well to psychoanalytic play therapy. Nevertheless, my aim in this brief commentary, while lauding the rigour and comprehensiveness of Barlow et al.'s work, is to adopt a psychodynamic perspective, expressing firstly a number of reservations about a purely cognitive therapy approach, and secondly drawing some integrative lessons from their review.

Diagnostic issues. The authors stick firmly to DSM categories for the different, if overlapping, categories of anxiety disorders. This gives an appearance of precision to their article that bears but tenuous relationship to clinical reality. In practice the different types of anxiety disorders often coexist, as Barlow et al. acknowledge in the case of agoraphobia and panic disorder. The drive further to create ever more specific sub-categories of psychiatric illness is to an extent driven by a global pharmaceutical industry which profits from a conceptual universe in which each spuriously specific disorder can be targeted by a particular new drug [3]. This "drug metaphor" has in turn influenced a comparable proliferation of variants of psychotherapy, each of which claims distinctive features which make it unlike competitors. This process is strikingly at variance with the "common factors" literature, which suggests that different therapies on the whole produce similar outcomes [4].

Anxiety as a manifestation of depressive illness is probably its commonest mode of presentation and is associated with greater severity of anxiety than autonomous anxiety syndromes [5]. Shorter and Tyrer [6] have recently suggested that the diagnostic "firewall" between anxiety and depression is an artefact and should be lifted. This undermines the idea that there are necessarily specific treatments—whether psychological or pharmaceutical—for specific anxiety disorders. There may be general psychotherapeutic mechanisms producing change, and we have yet to determine what, if any, is the "added value" of particular psychotherapeutic modalities. Nevertheless, the literature review does suggest that *exposure* and *cognitive restructuring* are crucial components of therapies that led to improvement in anxiety-based symptoms. Marks and Dar [7] point out that the CBT literature is strong on efficacy, but relatively weak on mechanism-of-action studies. Cognitive restructuring and exposure might better be seen as general psychotherapeutic tools, of value in a range of different conditions, component parts of several different therapeutic modalities.

Effectiveness. At more than one point in their review the authors call for a move from efficacy studies to those looking at effectiveness. There is an urgent need to see how the approaches they advocate stand up in the "real world" of office or community mental health centre practice, targeted at "real" (i.e. difficult, multifaceted, comorbid and complex) cases, as opposed to volunteers and highly selected patients to be found in university research settings. Here the issue of comorbidity becomes crucial. Again, the use of the term lends a pseudo-scientific aura to what essentially is a reification of the complexity of psychiatric presentation. Does a patient "have" two separate "disorders"—generalized anxiety disorder, say, and borderline personality disorder—or is the anxiety a manifestation of untoward developmental experiences which have inscribed themselves on the psyche? If so, will treating the anxiety by itself leave untouched the "underlying" (there is an inescapable spatial onion-skin type metaphor here) personality disorder? The authors suggest, correctly in my view, that specific treatment for the anxiety components of a personality disorder, while lessening the chances of good outcomes for anxiety generally, is a worthwhile enterprise in its own right. Nevertheless, treatments that focus exclusively on the "illness" and fail to take account of the sufferer are as likely to be unsatisfactory in psychiatry as they are in general medicine. And we psycho-professionals, it might be said, should know better than that.

Meaning and etiology. Once one moves from a purely symptomatic approach, which I take to be the preferred position of Barlow *et al.*, then the question of the *meaning* of the anxiety in the life of the patient, its precipitants and possible developmental origins begin to come into focus. Panic-focused psychodynamic psychotherapy (PFPP) is one of the two specifically psychodynamic approaches to an anxiety disorder mentioned, although its conceptual basis and clinical ambience are not. Milrod and his co-workers [8] identify a number of psychodynamic factors relevant to anxiety disorders. There is usually a *precipitant* for the onset of anxiety which has personal salience, with both *proximate* and *developmental implications*. Thus, to take a fictional example, imagine the onset of panic disorder in a middle-aged man whose wife, on whom he is highly dependent, has just recovered from a serious but non-fatal bout of asthma for which she has had to be hospitalized. As a child his relationship with his mother was characterized by "affectionless control". Now his secure base has been compromised: his wife can no longer be seen as the rock to which he can always turn; at the same time his repressed hostility towards a controlling care-giver in childhood and to an extent reproduced in his spousal relationship, is activated. He is anxious precisely because of unexpressed but hostile feelings towards the wife on whom he also depends. He dared not bite the hand that feeds, yet fate seems to have done so on his behalf. The patient is caught in a vicious circle in which the more he senses abandonment, the more angry he becomes, yet the more angry he becomes, the more his dependency on the object needs to be strengthened. His anxiety can be seen as a manifestation both of this external threat and this inner conflict. In this formulation anxiety is both a by-product of internal conflict (between dependency and aggression) and also a "signal" of threatened separation, thereby aligning itself with both the early and late Freudian models of anxiety [9]. Often there are specific links between anxiety-based symptoms and traumatic experiences. Bush et al. [10] illustrate this with a case in which a woman suffering from panic attacks could trace her escalating anxiety about the possibility of not being able to breathe with the experience as a child of witnessing her dying mother's dyspnea.

Anxiety and the therapeutic relationship. A simple psychodynamic model of anxiety derives from attachment theory [11]. Separation, or threat of separation, from a "secure base" leads to the negative affect of anxiety, which provokes strenuous efforts to become reunited, thereby assuaging the unpleasant feeling. Insecurely attached individuals are compromised in their ability to tolerate separation and tend either to cling to their secure base (care-giver in the case of children, partner or spouse for most adults) or to hover anxiously nearby, denying fear while remaining enslaved to it. The agoraphobic can be thought of as "clinging" to his or her familiar environment, and resisting what by him or her is perceived as the threat implicit in being away from home. Psychotherapy can be construed in part as an attempt to create through the therapeutic relationship a secure base for patients whose prior experience has been that of inconsistency or partial rejection. Psychotherapy research has consistently shown that a good therapeutic alliance is the best predictor of outcome for psychological treatments. Forming an alliance is a precondition of successful therapy of whatever modality. The establishment of such an alliance is anxiolytic in itself. This suggests a relational perspective on anxiety, viewing anxiety syndromes as the consequence of disturbed interpersonal relationships with significant others, usually characterized by the developmental precursors of insecure attachment—inconsistency or aggressive care-giving. The therapeutic implications are that the therapist must provide a secure base for the client, comprising (a) personal predictability and integrity, (b) a stable therapeutic setting and (c) a clear (and therefore secure-making) theoretical framework. Currently, CBT provides all three, while psychodynamic psychotherapies often lack a good specific theoretical rationale for their approach to anxiety.

A dynamic context for "exposure". An exception is "emotion-focused psychotherapy" as developed by Shear and others [1]. The hypothesis underlying this treatment is that avoidance of experienced emotion underlies panic disorder. Rather than feeling specific negative affects such as anger, fear, disappointment, lack of control and sadness, the sufferer is prey to sudden eruptions of anxiety. At the same time such individuals fail to make links between provoking events such as interpersonal friction and their experienced emotion. The aim of treatment is to help the patients see how their panics "represent" interpersonal dynamics, and to find more appropriate ways of handling these situations and the negative affects they arouse. For example, a patient who develops "inexplicable" panic attacks during the evening is helped see that these occur when her husband is back late from the office, to explore and verbalize her fantasies about possible car crashes or infidelity, and to find ways to tell him about her fears so that his returns can be more predictable, or he can ring her when necessary. This approach links *meaning* with "exposure" in a psychodynamic context. In the context of a secure therapeutic relationship the patient can begin to expose him or herself to negative affect, and to tolerate fear and anxiety without pathologizing either. "Transference" in this context can be seen as a variety of "exposure" in that the patient is exposed to the vicissitudes of the therapeutic relationship—mis-attunements by the therapist, holiday breaks, minor frame irregularities—and will have an opportunity to examine his or her reactions to these in a safe setting.

Freud famously described the aim of psychoanalysis as exchanging neurotic misery for ordinary human unhappiness. A psychodynamic approach to anxiety aims to transform overwhelming fear into useful negative affect that can act as a guide to action and interpersonal satisfaction. There is always a second chance for "losers", whether at Wimbledon, in psychotherapy, or in "real life".

REFERENCES

1. Shear M.K., Weiner K. (1997) Psychotherapy for panic disorder. *J. Clin. Psychiatry*, **58**: 38–43.
2. Gabbard G. (1992) Psychodynamic approaches to anxiety disorders. *Bull. Menninger Clin.*, **56**: A3–13.
3. Healy D. (2000) Some continuities and discontinuities in the pharmacotherapy of nervous conditions before and after chlorpromazine and imipramine. *Hist. Psychiatry*, **11**: 393–412.
4. Shapiro D. (1995) Finding out how psychotherapies help people change. *Psychother. Res.*, **5**: 1–21.

5. Coryell W., Endicott J., Winokur G. (1992) Anxiety syndromes as epiphenomena of primary major depression: outcome and familial psychopathology. *Am. J. Psychiatry*, **149**: 100–107.
6. Shorter E., Tyrer P. (2003) Separation of anxiety and depressive disorders: blind alleys in classification of disease. *Br. Med. J.*, **327**: 158–160.
7. Marks I., Dar R. (2000) Fear reduction by psychotherapies. *Br. J. Psychiatry*, **176**: 507–511.
8. Milrod B., Busch F., Leon A.C., Aronson A., Roiphe J., Rudden M., Singer M., Shapiro T., Goldman H., Richter D. *et al.* (2001) A pilot of brief psychodynamic psychotherapy for panic disorder. *J. Psychother. Pract. Res.*, **10**: 239–245.
9. Bateman A., Holmes J. (1995) *Introduction to Pyschoanalysis: Models and Methods*. Routledge, London.
10. Bush F., Cooper A., Klerman G. (1997) Neurophysiological, cognitive-behavioural and psychoanalytic approaches to panic disorder. *Psychoanal. Inquiry*, **11**: 316–332.
11. Holmes J. (1992) *John Bowlby and Attachment Theory*. Routledge, London.

4.11
Psychotherapy in the Treatment of Phobias: A Perspective from Latin America

Flávio Kapczinski[1]

The treatment of fear/avoidance states has been managed with either psychotherapy or drug treatments. Some types of psychotherapy, but not all of them, have been shown to be highly effective in the treatment of anxiety/avoidance symptoms. Some authors argue that psychotherapies may be, in some anxiety disorders, a better choice, as they are not associated with side effects. This may be the case for a variety of situations, but it is certainly not the case for all anxiety disorders and all psychosocial interventions. A very good example of that is the harm associated with certain techniques of psychological debriefing after acute exposure to trauma. A recent meta-analysis has shown that psychological debriefing may increase the odds of the development of post-traumatic stress disorder (PTSD) after a one-year follow up [1].

A large body of evidence drawn from randomized controlled trials supports the efficacy of cognitive-behavioural techniques in the treatment of panic disorder and phobias. There is a variety of technical differences in how the therapy should be delivered in such patients. A good example is provided by the need for the development of new social skills in patients with social phobia. This means that, before hoping that patients with social

---

[1] *Department of Psychiatry, UFRGS, Rua Tobias da Silva 99/502, Porto Alegre RS, 90570-020, Brazil*

phobia will have a real-life exposure, they should be trained in how to deal with social situations in the first place. This specific characteristic of these patients has prompted the development of specific group treatments which are as effective as the standard pharmacological treatments for this condition [2]. In the case of patients with social phobia, using a group treatment setting brings some additional advantages. For instance, social skills are developed naturally during the therapy and exposure to social interactions is carried out in each session [3].

In the case of panic disorder, it is interesting to notice that naturalistic studies indicate that, despite the availability of effective treatments, many patients in the community setting are left untreated. The Harvard/Brown Anxiety Research Program assessed 323 patients with panic disorder with agoraphobia and 73 without agoraphobia who were treated naturalistically. Twenty-two months after the index episode, only 43% patients without agoraphobia and 18% of patients with agoraphobia had recovered [4]. Among recovered patients, a follow-up of 18 months showed that 40% of those without agoraphobia and 60% of those with agoraphobia had relapsed. Part of these high rates of relapse may be related to the fact that many of these patients did not receive empirically validated psychosocial treatments for their conditions [5–7]. One of the reasons may be the lack of availability, especially in primary care settings, of clinicians who are trained in the effective techniques available [8].

In the case of social phobia, the cognitive-behavioural approaches have been the best studied both individually and in group settings. Concerning other types of psychotherapy in social phobia, we have carried out in Brazil a randomized single-blind clinical trial using psychodynamic group therapy in 40 patients [9]. In this trial we have compared the efficacy of 12 sessions of psychodynamic group therapy and 12 sessions of a credible placebo procedure, as described by Heimberg *et al.* [3]. We have found that the effect of psychodynamic group treatment was equivalent to that of credible plabebo on the primary outcome measures. Our findings should be interpreted within the limits of a small sample study and short-term therapy design. However, we found that the effect size of the active and control groups were almost the same, which indicates that the results would not be substantially changed if we increased the sample size.

REFERENCES

1. Rose S., Bisson J., Wessely S. (2002) Psychological debriefing for preventing post traumatic stress disorder (PTSD) (Cochrane Review). In *The Cochrane Library*, Issue 4. John Wiley & Sons, Chichester.

2. Heimberg R.G., Liebowitz M.R., Hope D.A., Schneier F.R., Holt C.S., Welkowitz L.A., Juster H.R., Campeas R., Bruch M.A., Cloitre M. et al. (1998) Cognitive behavioral group therapy versus phenelzine in social phobia: 12 week outcome. *Arch. Gen. Psychiatry*, **55**: 1133–1141.
3. Heimberg R.G., Dodge C.S., Hope D.A., Kennedy C.R., Zallo L., Becker R.E. (1990) Cognitive-behavioral group treatment for social phobia: comparison to a credible placebo control. *Cogn. Ther. Res.*, **14**: 1–23.
4. Keller M.B., Yonkers K.A., Warshaw M.G., Pratt L.A., Gollan J.K., Massion A.O., White K., Swartz A.R., Reich J, Lavori P.W. (1994) Remission and relapse in subjects with panic disorder and agoraphobia. *J. Nerv. Ment. Dis.*, **182**: 290–296.
5. Breier A., Charney D.S., Heninger G.R. (1986) Agoraphobia with panic attacks: development, diagnostic stability, and course of illness. *Arch. Gen. Psychiatry*, **43**: 1029–1036.
6. Goisman R.M., Warshaw M.G., Peterson L.G. (1993) Utilization of behavioral methods in a multi center anxiety disorders study. *J. Clin. Psychiatry*, **54**: 213–218.
7. Taylor C.B., King R., Margraf J., Ehlers A., Telch M., Roth W.T., Agras W.S. (1989) Use of medication and in vivo exposure in volunteers for panic disorder research. *Am. J. Psychiatry*, **146**: 1423–1426.
8. Barlow D.H., Hoffmann S.G. (1997) Efficacy and dissemination of psychosocial treatment expertise. In *Science and Practice of Cognitive Behaviour Therapy* (Eds D.F. Clark, C.G. Fairburn), pp. 95–117. Oxford University Press, Oxford.
9. Knijnik D.Z., Kapczinski F., Chachamovich E., Margis R., Eizirik C.L. (submitted) Psychodynamic group therapy in social phobia.

CHAPTER

5

Phobias in Children and Adolescents: A Review

Thomas H. Ollendick
Department of Psychology, Child Study Center, Virginia Polytechnic Institute and State University, 3110 Prices Fork Road, Blacksburg, VA 24061, USA

Neville J. King
Faculty of Education, Monash University, Melbourne, Victoria, Australia

Peter Muris
Department of Medical, Clinical, and Experimental Psychology, Maastricht University, Maastricht, The Netherlands

INTRODUCTION

Fear is a normal part of life. Whether we learn to fear or come "prepared" to develop certain fears, the result is the same. It is common for children sitting around a campfire to become entranced by ghost stories, for teenagers at movies to recoil in their seats from horror films, and for adults to enthusiastically read mystery books with fear-producing outcomes. As evident in these everyday examples, we do not always avoid becoming scared or frightened. At times we seem to actually invite it. Of course, we are usually able to shake these everyday fears off by pulling the covers tight, checking under the bed or around the corner, and making sure to turn the locks on our doors. We tell ourselves the feared event is unlikely to happen and we muster up enough courage to go on with whatever we are doing. Not so with a phobia.

A phobia can be a particularly crippling disorder, at least in part because it is poorly understood. A phobia, like so many psychological disorders, is characterized by affective, behavioural, cognitive and physiological responses whose intensity is sufficient to cause distress and interference in our lives. Adults, at least, have some measure of insight into their phobia

Phobias. Edited by Mario Maj, Hagop S. Akiskal, Juan José López-Ibor and Ahmed Okasha.
©2004 John Wiley & Sons Ltd: ISBN 0-470-85833-8

and recognize it as excessive or unreasonable, even though the fear may be so intense that it leads to active avoidance or extreme anxiety if it cannot actually be avoided. Adults seem to know that the level of their fear is unwarranted. Children, by contrast, frequently do not have this awareness. All a child may know is that he or she is scared of a dog, getting a shot at the doctor's office, or speaking in front of his or her school mates and wants to get away and to avoid the event or situation at all costs, and as soon as possible [1–3].

CLINICAL PICTURE AND DIFFERENTIAL DIAGNOSIS

According to Marks [4], "fear is a normal response to active or imagined threat in higher animals, and comprises an outer behavioural expression, an inner feeling, and accompanying physiological changes". As we have noted elsewhere [2,5–7], nearly all children experience some degree of fear during their development. Furthermore, although such fears vary in frequency, intensity and duration, they tend to be mild, age-specific and transitory. Typically, children evince fear reactions to everyday stimuli such as strangers, separation, new situations, loud noises, darkness, water, imaginary creatures, and small animals such as snakes and spiders, as well as other circumscribed or specific events or objects. For the most part, these fears appear to result from day-to-day experiences of growing children and to reflect the children's emerging cognitive and representational abilities. Moreover, most of these fears do not involve intense or persistent reactions, are short-lived, are adaptive and enhance the child's quality of life.

In contrast to normal fears, according to Marks [4], phobias (a) are out of proportion to the demands of the situation, (b) cannot be explained or reasoned away, (c) are beyond voluntary control and (d) lead to avoidance of the feared situation. In an early paper, we [8] expanded upon Marks' definition of a phobia, as it pertains to children, and suggested that phobias in childhood also (e) persist over an extended period of time, (f) are not developmentally adaptive or appropriate, (g) are not age- or stage-specific and (h) lead to considerable distress.

In recent years, the two most widely accepted diagnostic classification systems for psychiatric disorders have incorporated these criteria into their definitions of a phobia [9,10]. For example, the DSM-IV provides the following criteria for specific phobia: (a) marked and persistent fear that is excessive or unreasonable, cued by the presence or anticipation of a specific object or situation (e.g. flying, heights, animals, receiving an injection, seeing blood); (b) exposure to the phobic stimulus provokes an immediate anxiety response, which may take the form of a situationally-bound or situationally-predisposed panic attack; (c) the individual recognizes that the fear is excessive or unreasonable; (d) the phobic situation(s) is avoided, or else endured with intense anxiety or distress; (e) the avoidance, anxious anticipation or distress in the feared situation(s) interfere significantly with the person's normal routine, occupational (or academic) functioning, or social activities or relationships, or there is marked distress about having the phobia; and (f) in individuals under 18 years, the duration is at least 6 months.

Of importance to the study of phobias in children, the framers of DSM-IV recognized that children may not view their fears as excessive or unreasonable; furthermore, the DSM-IV allowed that children's fears may be expressed in "childhood" ways such as crying, tantrums, freezing or clinging. These are important acknowledgements, since these criteria accommodate the developmental nature of children and the developmental course of their fears [11–13]. In addition, DSM-IV has provided specific criteria for the duration of phobias in children (i.e. 6 months). In previous editions of the DSM, duration was not specified. Such a criterion ensures that the phobia is not a transitory nor developmentally idiosyncratic one and that the fear causes significant distress to the child (and frequently his or her parents) over an extended period of time.

Social phobia and agoraphobia also occur in childhood [2,3], albeit less commonly than the specific phobias. Although social phobia tends to emerge out of a childhood history of social inhibition and shyness, it is less evident in childhood and is known to have its primary onset in mid-teens. Very similar criteria and developmental considerations to those offered for specific phobia are put forth for social phobia in the DSM-IV. Social phobia (also referred to as social anxiety disorder) is defined as a marked and persistent fear of one or more social or performance situations in which the person is subject to possible scrutiny by others, especially strangers. Basically, the person fears that he or she will act in a way that will be embarrassing or humiliating to her or him. Of importance, DSM-IV also specifies that, in children, "there must be evidence of the capacity for age-appropriate social relationships with familiar people and the anxiety must occur in peer settings, not just in interactions with adults". The duration is also specified to be 6 months. Emerging research suggests that the assessment and treatment of social phobia, especially in adolescence, closely parallel the practices and findings obtained with adults. The same applies to agoraphobia (including fears such as being outside the home alone, being in a crowd, travelling in a bus, train or automobile). Therefore, the remainder of this review will not focus on these conditions.

EPIDEMIOLOGY

In recent years, several epidemiological studies have estimated that the prevalence of anxiety disorders (including phobias) in non-selected community samples of children and adolescents ranges from 5.7% to 17.7% [14]. In general, anxiety disorders tend to be more prevalent in girls than boys and in older than younger subjects. For phobias, several studies report relatively low prevalence rates: Anderson *et al.* [15] reported a 2.4% rate for 11-year-old children from New Zealand, whereas McGee *et al.* [16] reported a rate of 3.6% for 15-year-old adolescents in that same birth cohort of New Zealand children; Bird *et al.* [17] reported an overall rate of 2.6% in children and adolescents between 4 and 16 years of age from Puerto Rico; Steinhausen *et al.* [18] reported a 2.6% rate in children and adolescents between 7 and 16 years of age in Switzerland; Costello *et al.* [19] reported a 3.6% rate in 12–18-year-olds from the United States; Essau *et al.* [20] indicated a 3.5% rate in 12–17-year-old adolescents in Germany; Verhulst *et al.* [21] indicated a 4.5% rate in Dutch adolescents between 13 and 18 years of age; finally, Wittchen *et al.* [22] reported a 2.3% rate in a sample of 14–24-year-old community respondents. Slight differences in prevalence rates appear to be due to differences in ascertainment practices, criterion definitions of diagnosis, and functional impairment associated with the phobias. These differences notwithstanding, it is evident that phobias range in prevalence from 2.6% to 4.5% of children and adolescents, and they average about 3.5% across studies. Thus, although phobias are not highly prevalent in children and adolescents, they do occur with considerable frequency and result in considerable distress for them [23].

Two additional epidemiological findings are of considerable interest. First, although the findings are not conclusive, it appears that comorbidity within the anxiety disorders is less frequent for phobic disorders than it is for other anxiety disorders in community samples of children and adolescents [14]. That is, phobic disorders tend to be relatively "pure" in community samples, whereas other anxiety disorders tend to overlap and coexist with one another. Furthermore, these other anxiety disorders tend to co-occur with other internalizing (e.g. especially depression) and externalizing (e.g. conduct disorder, attention-deficit/hyperactivity disorder) disorders, whereas phobic disorders in community samples do not. Second, there appears to be a modest level of continuity (between 20% and 40%) for the anxiety disorders in general, as well as the phobias in particular, across intervals varying from 2 to 5 years. That is, about 30% of children with a phobic disorder at one point in time had such a disorder at an earlier point in time. This conclusion is based on studies conducted in New Zealand, Germany, Canada and the United States. These findings indicate that childhood phobias are moderately stable and relatively "pure" in community samples.

However, different conclusions can be drawn from clinical samples. In an early review of comorbidity in clinical samples, Brady and Kendall [24] reported that comorbidity between anxiety disorders and other internalizing and externalizing disorders was as high as 61.9%. This very high rate was found in a group of children and adolescents referred to an outpatient clinic for school-refusing children, followed by rates of 55.2% in a sample of psychiatric inpatient children (mixed diagnoses), 36.4% in a sample of children with primary affective disorders, and 31.5% in a sample of 8–13-year-old mental health outpatients (mixed diagnoses). Unfortunately, the studies reviewed by Brady and Kendall [24] did not isolate comorbidity associated with phobias *per se*. Fortunately, one early study [25] and one recently published study [23] have done so. Last *et al.* [25], in a sample of children and adolescents between the ages of 5 and 18 referred to an anxiety disorder outpatient clinic, found that 15% of the children met criteria for a primary diagnosis of simple (i.e. specific) phobia. Furthermore, they reported that 64% of children and adolescents with a primary diagnosis of simple (i.e. specific) phobia presented with one or more additional diagnoses, including overanxious disorder, social phobia, obsessive–compulsive disorder, panic disorder, major depressive disorder, dysthymia and oppositional defiant disorder. Similar results were obtained by Silverman *et al.* [23]. In their study of 104 children and adolescents between 6 and 16 years of age referred to a phobia outpatient treatment programme, the majority (72%) of the children were found to have at least one comorbid diagnosis: 19% had an additional specific phobia, 16% had separation anxiety disorder, 14% had overanxious disorder, and 6% were diagnosed with attention-deficit/ hyperactivity disorder. The remaining 17% of the 72% who had a comorbid diagnosis were distributed over eight additional diagnostic categories. We have obtained very similar findings in our ongoing study on the treatment of phobias in children and adolescents: 75% of our sample have been found to have at least one other psychiatric disorder (most commonly another phobic or anxiety disorder, but also major depressive disorder, attention deficit disorder and oppositional defiant disorder), and a substantial minority (nearly 40%) to have a third psychiatric disorder.

Collectively, these findings indicate that clinically significant phobias are present in about 3.5% of children and adolescents in community samples and in about 15% of outpatient, clinic-referred samples. Furthermore, these findings indicate that clinic-referred children and adolescents who present with phobias are more likely to have other comorbid disorders than are community samples. These findings undoubtedly have important implications for the assessment and treatment of these phobic youths [24,26,27].

ETIOLOGY

The etiology of childhood phobias is not fully understood at this time [2,3,6]. Although childhood phobias may result from terrifying or frightening experiences, they may also be due to less direct influences such as observing a fearful reaction in another child or reading about or hearing about fears and phobias in others. Still, other childhood phobias apparently have no obvious environmental cause, direct or indirect, and reportedly "have always been present" in the child. In this latter instance, the child, according to parental report, has always been afraid of the phobic object, apparently in the absence of direct or indirect conditioning experiences. For example, an intense fear and avoidance of snakes or spiders may develop in a child who has never been traumatized directly or indirectly. Yet the child is terrified of snakes or spiders and actively avoids going on excursions into the countryside due to fear of some frightening event occurring. To the parent's knowledge and the child's recollection, no terrifying events that might have served to "condition" the child have ever occurred.

Menzies and Clarke [28] have illustrated this etiological conundrum in a study of 50 water-phobic children (mean age 5½ years). Parents of these children were administered a questionnaire that consisted of a list of commonly reported origins of phobias, including all three of Rachman's [29,30] now classic pathways to fear acquisition (i.e. direct classical conditioning, vicarious conditioning and information/instruction). In addition, parents were allowed to indicate that they did not know how the phobia developed or that their child had always been afraid of the water (i.e. "fearful upon their very first contact with water"). Although 2% of parents attributed their child's phobia to a direct conditioning episode and another 26% reported vicarious conditioning episodes, the majority of the parents (56%) believed that their child's fear had been present from their child's very first contact with water. The remaining 16% of the parents were not able to offer any explanation of onset, recalling no traumatic experience but reporting nonetheless that their child had not always displayed a fear of water. These findings from parents of water-phobic children are similar to those reported by McNally and Steketee [31] for 22 adults who evidenced severe animal phobias (e.g. snake, cat, bird, dog and spider). In their study, a structured interview was conducted to obtain information regarding the mode of onset, course of development and frequency of natural exposure to the phobic stimulus. Information was also obtained regarding the feared consequences that the phobic adults expected to occur following unavoidable encounters with the feared animal, as well as the specific stimulus characteristics of the feared animal that they found particularly upsetting. As with Menzies and Clark [28], a majority of the adults (68%) could not recall the onset of their phobia, reporting that they had had the fear "as long as they could remember". Of the remaining adults, 23% attributed their fear to a frightening encounter with the animal and thus were classified as conditioning cases. The remaining 9% of phobic adults were classified as vicarious and instructional cases. In one instance, the patient reportedly acquired a bird phobia after her father teasingly told her that a bird "might swoop down and get her" (instructional onset), whereas in another instance a patient attributed her snake phobia to watching frightening movies that depicted snakes as dangerous (vicarious conditioning). Interestingly, of those who could recall the origin of their phobia, all indicated that it began before the age of 10 and that the intensity of the phobia remained constant over the years (on average for 24 years).

Collectively, findings by Menzies and Clarke [28] for young children and McNally and Steketee [31] for adults stand in sharp contrast to those obtained by Öst and colleagues for adult phobic patients [32,33]. In a study of 110 patients undergoing behavioural treatment of phobias—41 with small animal phobias (snakes, spiders, rats), 34 with social phobias and 35 with claustrophobia—Öst and Hugdahl [32] reported that only 15.1% could *not* recall experiences of any kind regarding the onset of their phobias. In contrast, more than half (57.5%) ascribed their phobias to direct conditioning experiences, with 17% attributing their phobias to vicarious conditioning experiences and 10.4% to informational or instructional experiences. Thus, in this sample, very few patients could not recall the origins of their phobias and twice as many patients recalled acquiring their phobias through direct conditioning experiences as through indirect experiences (vicarious or instructional). As in the McNally and Steketee study [31], duration of the phobias was extended (average of 24 years), with most patients reporting childhood onset and unrelenting intensity over the intervening years. Inconsistencies in origins of phobias in these studies are difficult to reconcile, but may be due, at least in part, to differences in questionnaires used, operational definitions of conditioning events and severity of the phobias [2,34].

From a methodological standpoint, it is important to note that these studies did not include a comparison group of non-fearful participants. In order to establish the etiological significance of conditioning events or negative expected consequences in the development of phobias, such a contrast group is imperative. If painful or frightening experiences with the stimulus are equally prevalent among non-fearful controls, or if expectations of panic or harm are equally high among controls, then such experiences or expectations alone cannot be a sufficient explanation for development of the phobia. Fortunately, at least two adult studies and one child study have included non-fearful groups and have made such comparisons. In the first study, DiNardo *et al.* [35] examined these issues in 16 dog-phobic young adults and 21 non-fearful matched controls. Similar to the Öst and Hugdahl [32] findings, 56% of these phobic adults reported direct conditioning events associated with the origin of their phobia; unexpectedly, however, 66% of the non-fearful subjects also reported direct conditioning events. Obviously, reliable differences between the two groups were not observed. In fact, direct conditioning experiences were reported by more of the non-fearful controls than the phobic group! Furthermore, the majority of encounters for both phobic and non-fearful adults were similar and consisted of painful events involving bites or scratches. Although the two groups had similar experiences with dogs, they had very different *expectations* about the consequences of an encounter with a dog. Not surprisingly, and consistent with the findings of McNally and Steketee [31], 100% of phobic subjects expected to experience fear and harm upon an encounter with a dog, whereas only a small minority (14%) of non-fearful subjects expected similar outcomes. DiNardo et al. [35] concluded that high expectancies of fear and harm served to maintain phobic avoidance in the phobic group. In a second study with adults, Menzies and Clarke [36] reported similar findings in 50 height phobic young adults and 50 non-fearful matched controls: there were no differences between the phobic and non-fearful groups in acquisition pathways. However, the groups did differ on expected consequences upon encounter with heights, as they did in the DiNardo *et al.* [35] study on fear of dogs: a majority of the height-phobic young adults reported extreme fear and panic associated with heights.

Interestingly, even though many specific phobias are acquired in childhood and adolescence [32,33,37], efforts to explore pathways of acquisition have relied largely on retrospective reports of adults, frequently 20 or more years after the onset of their phobias. As noted above, many adults report that they are simply unable to recall the onset of their phobias with sufficient specificity or, due to time and associated life experiences, recall events that help them make "sense" of their fears or phobias. To date, only one study has specifically addressed these issues in a child and adolescent sample. In this study, Ollendick and King [38] explored Rachman's [30] three pathways of fear acquisition in 1092 Australian and American children between 9 and 14 years of age. In response to ten commonly reported fears in children, the youth were asked to indicate their own level of fear and then whether (a) they remembered having a bad or frightening experience with the feared object (direct conditioning experience), (b) their parents, friends or other acquaintances showed fear or avoidance of the feared object (vicarious conditioning) and (c) they had been told, or heard stories about, frightening things regarding the feared object (instruction or information pathway). Responses to acquisition routes varied and were dependent on specific fear stimuli. For example, 36% of the sample indicated a bad or frightening experience with snakes, whereas 70% indicated a similarly frightening experience with "not being able to breathe" (i.e. choking, gasping, not able to catch breath). Moreover, 65% indicated that someone they knew showed extreme fear of snakes, whereas 46% indicated that someone they knew showed extreme fear of "not being able to breathe". Finally, 89% of the youth indicated they had heard or been told frightening stories about snakes, whereas 76% indicated similar instruction/information about "not being able to breathe". (Percentages do not add up to 100% since youth could endorse more than one pathway.) These findings suggest that pathways may be phobia-specific and that the causes may be multiply determined, if not over-determined [8].

Of course, it should be noted that these findings and those of others are based on retrospective reports and are therefore subject to limitations attendant to self-report studies. Although the children and adolescents in our study were "closer" in time to the onset of their fears than adults whose fears had a childhood onset and prolonged course, they still had to rely on their recollections to identify the likely sources of onset. As such, these findings really speak to the causal attributions of children and adolescents to account for the onset of their fears. These attributions may or may not reflect actual causes and, accordingly, may or may not reflect the "real" sources of acquisition. In future research, these self-reports should be supplemented with intensive structured interviews, behavioural observations and use of other informants (e.g. parents, teachers) to determine their validity.

Overall, these findings suggest that not all phobias are acquired through individual-specific learning histories and other causal factors need to be considered. Among these other factors are those related to the heritability of phobias, biological-constitutional factors of the child and parenting influences on the growing child. Early on, Darwin (see [37]) asked: "May we not suspect that . . . fears of children, which are quite independent of experience, are the inherited effects of real dangers . . . during savage times?". Basically, Darwin was suggesting that aversive experiences with certain stimuli were not necessary for the acquisition of fear; rather, some fears were "independent of experience" and were largely innate. Advancing this notion, Seligman [39] hypothesized that associations between certain stimuli and fear responses were more likely to be formed than others (i.e. "prepared" and constituting non-cognitive forms of associative learning). The status of this notion of "inherited phobia proneness" is certainly controversial and well beyond the scope of this review (see [34,37,40–42] for discussion of issues related to these theories).

Nonetheless, the pursuit of heritability estimates has continued to fuel this controversy. Although no known studies of heritability exist for children with phobias, studies with adults suggest that phobias may be largely due to non-genetic factors [43,44]. In discussing the role of genetics in specific phobias, social phobia and agoraphobia, Kendler *et al.* [44] proposed that these subtypes of phobias can be placed along an etiologic continuum: at the one end of the continuum lies agoraphobia, which has the latest age of onset, the highest heritability estimate and the least specific environmental influences. At the other end of the continuum lie the specific phobias, which have the earliest age of onset, the lowest heritability estimates and the highest specific environmental influences. They conclude: "The estimated heritability of liability of phobias . . . indicates that genetic factors play a significant but by no means overwhelming role in the etiology of phobias. Individual-specific environment appears to account for approximately twice as much variance in liability to phobias as do genetic factors." Overall, genetic factors appear to be associated with a general state or propensity toward "fearfulness" (although Stevenson *et al.* [45] question this conclusion with high fearful—albeit not phobic—children), whereas the environment plays a stronger role in making an individual afraid of, say, snakes rather than heights or enclosed places. Specificity is afforded by the environment [2].

Along with genetic factors, constitutional (i.e. temperament) characteristics of the child may play a role in the onset and maintenance of phobias in children. Temperament refers to stable response dispositions that are evident early in life, observable in a variety of settings and relatively persistent across time [46,47]. Two of the most important temperamental categories are based on responses or initial reactions to unfamiliar people and novel situations, frequently referred to as "shyness versus sociability", "introversion versus extroversion", or "withdrawal versus approach". In unfamiliar situations or upon meeting new people, "shy" or "inhibited" children typically withhold responding or interrupt ongoing behaviour, show vocal restraint and withdraw. In contrast, "sociable" and "uninhibited" children typically seek out novelty, engage in conversation, smile and explore the environment around them. Data from Chess and Thomas' New York Longitudinal Study [46] show that these tendencies to approach or withdraw are relatively enduring dimensions of behaviour.

In recent years, Kagan and colleagues [48–50] have demonstrated that approximately 10% to 15% of American Caucasian children are predisposed to be fussy and irritable as infants, shy and fearful as toddlers, and cautious, quiet and introverted when they reach school age; in contrast, about 15% of the population show the opposite profile, with the remainder of the population intermediate on these dimensions. Kagan and his colleagues hypothesize that inhibited children, compared with uninhibited children, have a low threshold for arousal in the amygdala and hypothalamic circuits, especially to unfamiliar events, and that they react under such conditions with sympathetic arousal [51]. In general, sympathetic activation is indicated by high heart rate, low heart-rate variability, and acceleration of heart rate under stressful conditions. Indeed, inhibited children have been shown to have higher and more stable heart rates and to show greater heart-rate acceleration under stressful and novel conditions than uninhibited children. Furthermore, inhibited children have been shown to have a greater increase in diastolic blood pressure when changing their posture from a sitting to a standing position than uninhibited children, suggesting increased noradrenergic tone [52]. Collectively, these findings indicate a more reactive sympathetic influence on cardiovascular functioning in inhibited children. The behavioural response of withdrawal and avoidance shown by children with behavioural inhibition, along with the considerable evidence of increased arousal in the limbic-sympathetic axes, fits well with current hypotheses of the neurobiological underpinnings of anxiety disorders (see [53–55] for discussions).

The sample of inhibited and uninhibited children studied by Kagan and colleagues has been described in detail elsewhere [49,50]. Briefly, children were identified at 21 months of age for a study on the preservation of temperamental differences in normal children. The children were selected from a larger group of 305 Caucasian children whose mothers described them as displaying inhibited or uninhibited behaviour across different situations. On the basis of the interviews, 117 children were invited to the Harvard Infant Study Laboratory and were studied more extensively. Initially, 28 children were identified as the most extremely inhibited and 30 as the most extremely uninhibited. Subsequent to identification, 22 inhibited and 19 uninhibited children were available for follow-up at 4, 5 and 7 years of age. Biederman *et al.* [56] reasoned that the inhibited children identified by Kagan and his colleagues would be at risk for the development of anxiety disorders. Their hypothesis was based on earlier work they had conducted with the offspring of parents with panic disorder and agoraphobia (PDAG). In that study, they reported a high prevalence of behavioural inhibition in children born to adults with PDAG compared with control children of parents without anxiety disorder [57]. They then examined the Kagan *et al.* longitudinal sample of "normal" children when the children were 7 to 8 years of age. Mothers of the 22 inhibited and 19 uninhibited children were systematically interviewed using a structured diagnostic interview. Findings revealed that the rates of all anxiety disorders were higher in inhibited than uninhibited children: overanxious disorder (13.6% versus 10.5%), separation anxiety disorder (9.1% versus 5.3%), avoidant disorder (9.1% versus 0%) and phobic disorders (31.8% versus 5.3%, including both specific phobia and social phobia). Only the difference for phobic disorders was statistically significant. Clearly, the inhibited group was found to be at risk for anxiety disorders, particularly phobic disorders. It should be recalled that designation of group status as inhibited versus uninhibited occurred at 21 months of age and that assessment for psychopathology in the present study occurred when the children were approximately 7 years of age.

In a subsequent study, Hirshfeld *et al.* [58] re-examined these findings by contrasting children who remained inhibited or uninhibited throughout childhood with those who were less stable across the four assessment periods (21 months, 4 years, 5 years and 7 years). Four groups of children were formed: stable inhibited ($n = 12$), unstable inhibited ($n = 10$), stable uninhibited ($n = 9$) and unstable uninhibited ($n = 10$). As is evident, 54.5% of the inhibited children and 47.4% of the uninhibited children maintained stable group status across the assessment periods. The researchers showed the following rates of phobic disorders (both specific and social phobia) at age 7 years: stable inhibited 50%, unstable inhibited 10%, stable uninhibited 11.1% and unstable uninhibited 0%. (Rates for the other anxiety disorders were also higher for the stable inhibited group compared to the other groups.) Thus, children who remained consistently inhibited from 21 months through 4, 5 and 7 years of age accounted for the high rates of phobic disorders found to be associated with behavioural inhibition in the earlier study [56]. In this stability study, Hirshfeld et al. also obtained diagnostic interviews on the parents themselves. Comparison between parents of the stable inhibited group and the other three groups indicated that the parents of the stable inhibited group themselves were also characterized by a greater prevalence of phobic disorders and related anxiety disorders. Again, it should be noted that the children and parents in the Kagan et al. [50,51] longitudinal cohort were selected for a study on the preservation of temperamental differences in normal children. They were not selected because they were thought to be at risk or because they presented with anxious symptomatology.

The increased rates of anxiety disorders and phobic disorders in parents of stable inhibited children (as well as heightened levels of behavioural inhibition in children born from anxiety disorder parents) raise the possibility that the association between stable behavioural inhibition and anxiety disorder is familial, perhaps genetic. If genetic, it is probable that the link is one that predisposes the child to a heightened level of general fearfulness or anxiety sensitivity, as suggested by Kendler et al. [44]. As noted by Hirshfeld et al. [58], "whether behavioural inhibition is under genetic influence remains unresolved and can be elucidated ultimately only by carefully controlled twin or adoption studies and by genetic linkage studies".

Alternatively, stable behavioural inhibition in the child might be related to having a parent with an anxiety disorder. Continued exposure to a parent's anxious symptomatology might lead a child to remain cautious, uncertain and fearful in novel or unfamiliar situations. Furthermore, phobic parents might model phobic avoidance on a regular basis and have difficulty encouraging their youngsters to explore their surroundings and take risks [58]. Parents of anxious children have long been described as "overprotective" and shielding their children from potential misfortunes. Recent studies using direct behavioural observations of parent–child interactions in ambiguous and stressful situations confirm such "protective" and "insulating" patterns [59–62]. Finally, it is interesting to note that Kagan suggested early on that children who did not remain inhibited seemed to come from families in which children were encouraged to be more sociable and outgoing [51]. In the absence of such encouragement and the direct modelling of avoidance, behavioural inhibition might be expected to persist and be resistant to change. In all probability, stability of behavioural inhibition may be related to a combination of genetic influences, parental psychopathology and environmental factors that transact in a reciprocal manner.

In the final analysis, a host of factors converge to occasion the onset and maintenance of phobias in children. Genetic influences and temperamental tendencies may predispose the child to general fearfulness, behavioural inhibition and phobic disorder; however, particular forms of parental psychopathology and specific conditioning histories are seemingly necessary to set the stage for the development of any one phobia such as fear of heights or fear of dogs.

PRINCIPLES OF TREATMENT

Prior to illustrating some of the procedures that have been found to work with phobias, it is important for us to state the underlying premises that guided our selection of effective treatments. For us, treatment programmes should rest on a sound, theoretical rationale that addresses both the determinants of the disorder and the purported mechanisms for bringing about the desired changes in the disorder. The treatments we next review possess these characteristics.

Acute Treatment: Psychosocial Interventions

In earlier reviews of the psychosocial treatment of phobic disorders in childhood and adolescence [51], we have reported that behavioural and cognitive-behavioural procedures demonstrate considerable promise. Much of this early promise, however, was based on single-case and uncontrolled group outcome studies. Moreover, little or no support was found for the use of other psychosocial treatment procedures, including those based on psychodynamic, non-directive and family systems perspectives. However, it should be noted that in recent years, Fonagy and Target [63] have suggested, based on retrospective chart reviews of 196 children meeting "anxiety disorder diagnoses" at the Anna Freud Centre in London, that child psychoanalysis may be effective (but then only for younger children who receive treatment four or five times weekly for an average of two years). Strong empirical support for these other procedures is notably lacking. Such a conclusion is consistent with Weisz *et al.*'s meta-analysis of 108 treatment studies conducted between 1970 and 1985 [64], and their more recent meta-analytic review of an additional 150 studies published between 1967 and 1993 [65]. They concluded that behavioural treatments proved more effective than non-behavioural treatments regardless of client age, therapist experience or treated problem. As a result, the current review will be restricted to behavioural and cognitive-behavioural procedures that have been used to treat phobic disorders of childhood and adolescence and that have empirical support for their use. Consistent with recent developments in the classification of effective psychotherapy procedures [66], we will classify procedures as well established when they have been shown to be more effective than some credible placebo control or alternate treatment condition in at least two controlled trials, as probably efficacious if they have been shown to be more effective than only a waiting list or no-treatment condition in at least two controlled trials (or superior to a credible control condition in at least one study and to waiting list or no-treatment controls in other studies), and as experimental if they have been shown to be more effective than either a credible placebo control or waiting list condition but only in one study. In all instances the studies must have been randomized controlled clinical trials.

Our review will address the following behavioural and cognitive-behavioural procedures: systematic desensitization (both imaginal and *in vivo*), emotive imagery, modelling, reinforced practice, verbal self-instruction, and integrated cognitive-behavioural interventions.

Systematic Desensitization and its Variants

Wolpe [67] first formulated the systematic desensitization procedure. In this paradigm, fears and phobias were viewed as classically conditioned responses that could be unlearned through specific counter-conditioning procedures. In counter-conditioning, fear-producing stimuli are presented imaginally or *in vivo* (real-life) in the presence of other stimuli that elicit responses incompatible with fear. In this manner, fear is counter-conditioned and inhibited by the incompatible response. In its most basic form, systematic desensitization consists of three components: (a) induction of an incompatible response (e.g. relaxation), (b) development of a fear-producing hierarchy and (c) the systematic and graduated pairing of items in the hierarchy with the incompatible response. Generally, fear-producing stimuli are presented imaginally (in order of least to most fear-producing) while the child is engaged in an incompatible behaviour (e.g. relaxation).

This aspect of treatment is the desensitization proper and is thought to lead to direct inhibition of the fear response. Although studies have questioned the active mechanisms and the necessary ingredients of systematic desensitization [8], there is little doubt that it and its variants are frequently used procedures with children.

How effective is systematic desensitization and its variants in the treatment of childhood and adolescence fears and phobias? Four controlled group outcome studies support the likely effectiveness of systematic desensitization. In the first examination of standard (i.e. imaginal) systematic desensitization with children, Kondas [68] randomly assigned 23 "stage-fright" boys and girls (ages ranged from 11 to 15 years of age) to one of four conditions: (a) relaxation training, (b) imaginal systematic desensitization, (c) presentation of hierarchy items without relaxation training and (d) no-treatment control. Systematic desensitization was found to be superior to the two other active treatments and to the no-treatment control group.

In the second study, Mann and Rosenthal [69] randomly assigned 50 high test-anxious 12- and 13-year-old children to one of five treatment conditions: (a) individual desensitization, (b) vicarious individual desensitization (these children observed a child in the former condition receive individual desensitization), (c) group desensitization, (d) vicarious group desensitization (groups of students observed the group treatment of other children) and (e) vicarious group desensitization (groups of children observed desensitization of a single peer model). A further 21 test-anxious children served as no-treatment controls. Although findings were somewhat mixed, the five treatment conditions proved superior to the no-treatment condition with no significant differences among the treatment groups. Thus, in comparison to a no-treatment control condition, support was found for both individual and group imaginal systematic desensitization and individual and group "live" modelling (see below).

In still another early study, Barabasz [70] randomly assigned 47 high test-anxious children (fifth and sixth grades) to imaginal systematic desensitization or no-treatment control group conditions. Results indicated that children in the imaginal systematic desensitization group exhibited lower autonomic indices of test anxiety and showed significant improvement on a criterion performance measure.

In the last controlled study, Miller *et al.* [71] randomly assigned 67 phobic children aged 6–15 to three treatments: standard systematic desensitization, psychotherapy (verbal or play, dependent upon the age of the child), and a waiting list control condition. All children were clinic-referred. Unfortunately, although the two treatments differed substantially in terms of in-session activities with the children, work with the parents and those outside the family (e.g. teachers) was "essentially the same" across both active treatments. Parents of both groups of children were exposed to standard behavioural treatment involving contingency management and parent training to help manage the children's behaviour at home and in school. Given this confound, perhaps the equivalence of the groups on parental reports of target fears and general fear behaviours following treatment should not have been unexpected. Essentially, Miller et al. [71] found that the two treatments were equally effective in reducing phobic behaviours (per parental report, and only for 6- to 10-year-old children and not 11- to 15-year-old children) and that both treatments were more effective than the waiting list condition. Thus, limited support for the effectiveness of imaginal systematic desensitization was garnered: it was more effective than a waiting list control condition (at least as reported by parents) but not more effective than a standard psychotherapy intervention (plus behavioural parent management).

In sum, imaginal systematic desensitization has been found to be more effective than no treatment in four randomized control trials [68–71]. Furthermore, it has been found to be more effective than some alternative treatments (e.g. relaxation training) but not others (e.g. live modelling). On the basis of these studies, imaginal systematic desensitization can be said to be a probably efficacious treatment [72,73].

In one later study, however, the effectiveness of imaginal systematic desensitization was questioned. In this study, Ultee et al. [74] randomly assigned 24 water-phobic children between the ages of 5 and 10 years to two treatment groups and a no-treatment control group. One of the groups was treated with four sessions of imaginal systematic desensitization, followed by four sessions of *in vivo* desensitization (graduated real-life exposure to fear-producing stimuli plus relaxation). The second treatment group received eight sessions of *in vivo* desensitization. The control group participated only in the assessments that occurred prior to the beginning of treatment, after four sessions, and at the end of the course of treatment. Results favoured *in vivo* systematic desensitization over both imaginal systematic desensitization and the control condition. In fact, no differences were found between the latter two groups. Overall, findings indicated that real-life exposure to the feared stimuli was superior to exposure in imagination for reduction of water phobias. As noted by Ultee et al. [74], an important aspect of the avoidance behaviour treated was the lack of skill and familiarity with the aquatic environment. If the children were deficient in the very skills that lead to fear reduction, real-life desensitization would be expected to be more effective because it incorporates skill training (i.e. actual practice) in its application. Thus, *in vivo* desensitization is thought to include a critical component in the treatment package in addition to the graduated pairing of the fear-producing stimuli and the incompatible response that characterizes imaginal desensitization. Findings in this study support the superiority of *in vivo* desensitization over imaginal desensitization.

The effectiveness of *in vivo* desensitization has also been supported in another randomized control trial. Kuroda [75] treated two groups of Japanese children: one fearful of frogs, the other fearful of cats. Children between 3 and 5 years of age were assigned randomly to *in vivo* desensitization or no-treatment control groups. In the first study, 35 children fearful of frogs were treated. Treatment was implemented in "brief" sessions using a game-like format (e.g. children sang songs or told stories about frogs and dramatized the movements of frogs via dance). Hence, Kuroda [75] used fun and games, rather than relaxation, as the competing response. The modified *in vivo* procedure was found to be highly effective. In the second study, Kuroda treated 23 children fearful of cats using a similarly modified *in vivo* desensitization procedure. Once again, the procedure was demonstrated to be more effective than no treatment.

Thus, in both the Ultee *et al.* [74] and Kuroda [75] studies, *in vivo* desensitization was found to be superior to no-treatment control conditions. Furthermore, in the Ultee *et al.* study, it was found to be superior to imaginal systematic desensitization. On the basis of these findings, *in vivo* procedures also can be viewed as probably efficacious.

Yet another variant of systematic desensitization that has been used with children is emotive imagery [76]. As in imaginal and *in vivo* desensitization, emotive imagery involves development of a fear hierarchy. However, rather than using muscular relaxation as the anxiety inhibitor, the child is instructed to imagine an exciting story involving his or her favourite hero. Items from the fear hierarchy are interwoven at various stages of the story. Feelings of "positive affect" created by the story serve to counter or inhibit feelings of anxiety that might be elicited by the fear-related stimuli.

Unfortunately, the effectiveness of this procedure has been examined in only one randomized controlled trial [77]. In this study, Cornwall *et al.* examined the effectiveness of emotive imagery in the treatment of darkness phobia in 24 7–10-year-old children. Children were assigned randomly to the emotive imagery treatment group or to a waiting list control condition. Results indicated the superiority of emotive imagery over the waiting list control condition on multiple outcome measures, including general fearfulness and trait anxiety, child ratings on a fear thermometer, behaviour during a darkness tolerance test, and their parents' ratings of fear of darkness.

Although the utility of this procedure has also been demonstrated in a single case controlled design study [78], it must be viewed as an "experimental" procedure at this time. It must be demonstrated to be more effective than a waiting list control group in at least one more study before it can be designated as probably efficacious [72].

In sum, imaginal desensitization and *in vivo* desensitization enjoy probably efficacious status; however, emotive imagery must be viewed as an "experimental" treatment at this time. Inasmuch as systematic desensitization and its variants are frequently used and often viewed as effective treatments for childhood phobias [79], our conclusion does not support clinical lore. Quite obviously, empirical support for these procedures is not extensive at this time. Most studies examining the efficacy of these procedures are also quite old at this time and systematic replication with carefully diagnosed and characterized children is called for before their efficacies can be viewed as well established.

Modelling and its Variants

Drawing on vicarious conditioning principles, modelling capitalizes on the power of observational learning to overcome children's fears and phobias [80]. Theoretically, the extinction of avoidance responses is thought to occur through observation of modelled approach behaviour directed toward a feared stimulus without adverse consequences accruing to the model. In its most basic procedural form, it entails demonstrating non-fearful behaviour in the anxiety-provoking situation and showing the child a more adaptive and appropriate response for handling or dealing with the feared object or event. Modelling can be symbolic (filmed) or live; furthermore, the phobic child can be assisted in approaching the feared stimulus (participant modelling) or prompted to display the modelled behaviour without such assistance. In all of these procedural variations, anxiety is thought to be reduced and a new skill to be acquired [81].

Several randomized control trials, in addition to the one reported by Mann and Rosenthal [69] and reviewed earlier, support the effectiveness of modelling and its variants. In the first systematic evaluation of this procedure, Bandura *et al.* [82] randomly assigned children who displayed excessive fearful and avoidant behaviour to dogs to one of the following treatment conditions: (a) modelling sessions in which they observed, within a highly positive context (party), a fearless peer exhibit progressively stronger approach responses to the dog, (b) sessions in which they observed the graduated modelling stimuli, but in the absence of a positive context (neutral context), (c) sessions in which the children observed the dog in the positive context but in the absence of modelling and (d) sessions in which the children simply participated in the party but were not exposed either to the dog or the modelled display. A group of 48 children, ranging in age from 3 to 5 years, participated. Results indicated that children in the modelling positive-context condition displayed significantly more approach behaviour than children in either the exposure alone or positive-context alone groups. Similarly, children who had observed the model within the neutral context exceeded both the exposure-alone and positive-context-alone groups in approach behaviour. No significant differences were obtained between the two modelling groups. Thus, contrary to expectation, the positive-context condition, which was designed to induce anxiety-competing responses, did not enhance extinction effects produced through modelling in the neutral context (children in this condition simply observed the same sequence of approach responses performed by the same peer model except that the parties were omitted).

In a related study, Bandura and Menlove [83] examined the effectiveness of filmed (symbolic) modelling by randomly assigning 32 children, 3 to 5 years of age, who were markedly fearful of dogs, to one of three conditions in which: (a) children observed a graduated series of films in which a peer model displayed progressively more intimate interactions with a dog, (b) children were exposed to a similar set of graduated films depicting a variety of models interacting non-anxiously with numerous dogs varying in size and fearfulness and (c) children were shown movies containing no animals. Results indicated that children who received the multiple-modelling and single-modelling treatments achieved greater increases in approach behaviour than did the controls. The two modelling conditions did not differ from one another on this measure. Of importance, however, when the terminal approach response was examined (i.e. remaining with the dog in the playpen for a brief period of time), the two groups did differ, suggesting the superiority of the multiple-model condition.

A third randomized control trial [84] also explored the utility of filmed modelling. In this study, 18 "preschool" boys who were fearful of dogs were randomly assigned to groups. Children in the filmed modelling group watched a filmed sequence depicting a series of interactions between a large dog and a child of their age and sex. The children in the control group, matched for initial avoidance of dogs, were not exposed to the film. Findings supported the effectiveness of the film on post-treatment performance.

In a fourth study, Lewis [85] explored the relative effectiveness of three modelling-based techniques in the reduction of avoidance behaviour towards water activities in 40 black, male children between 5 and 12 years of age. Specifically, Lewis compared the following conditions: (a) modelling, in which the children were shown a film of three peers engaged in progressively more interactive activities in the swimming pool, (b) participation, in which the therapist prompted and assisted the children to engage in various swimming activities on a progressive basis, but did not actually model the requisite behaviours, (c) combined modelling and participation (participant modelling), in which the children were shown the film and then assisted in engaging in the various water activities and (d) control, in which the children participated in various non-water fun activities. Children were randomly assigned to the conditions. Results indicated that the conditions that included assisted participation showed greater change in avoidance behaviour than filmed modelling alone and control conditions, which did not differ from one another. Furthermore, a combination of modelling and participation was the most effective intervention, surpassing both the modelling-alone and participation-alone conditions, as well as the control condition. This study suggests that assisted participation may be superior to modelling alone.

In yet another early study, Ritter [86] examined the effectiveness of live modelling and participant modelling in 44 boys and girls (5 to 11 years of age) who evinced snake-avoidant behaviour. Children in the live modelling condition observed the adult therapist and five peer models engage in gradually bolder interactions with a tame 4-foot Gopher snake. In the participant modelling condition, the children not only observed the therapist and peers perform as in the modelling alone condition, but also had opportunities for physical contact with the model-therapists (adult and peers) and the phobic object. For example, initially the children were asked to put on gloves and to place their hands on the therapist's hand while the therapist stroked the snake; subsequently, the children were eased into stroking the snake with their gloved hand unaided. This was then repeated with bare hands. Children were randomly assigned to one of these conditions or to a control condition. Results indicated that both treatments produced greater decrements in avoidance than the control condition and that the participant modelling condition produced greater effects than the modelling alone condition. Thus, although support for the efficacy of both procedures was garnered in this study (when compared to a no-treatment control group), the superiority of participant modelling was shown.

The superiority of participant modelling was also demonstrated in another study [87]. In this study, snake-phobic individuals (determined by self-report and behavioural avoidance measures) who varied in age from 13 to 59 years were randomly assigned to one of four conditions: (a) standard (i.e. imaginal) systematic desensitization, (b) symbolic (i.e. filmed) modelling, (c) live modelling combined with guided participation and (d) no-treatment control. All three treatment approaches produced generalized and enduring reductions in fear arousal and behavioural avoidance. However, of the three methods, modelling with guided participation proved most powerful, achieving virtually complete elimination of phobic behaviour in all participants. In related studies, Blanchard [88] demonstrated that the participant component of the guided participation approach was critical to its outcome, whereas Murphy and Bootzin [89] showed that the participation could be child-initiated (active) or therapist-initiated (passive). In the latter study, both active and passive guided participation were equally effective with snake-phobic young children (enrolled in the early grades of elementary school). In both studies, participant modelling was found to be superior to no-treatment conditions.

Thus, on the basis of these nine studies, it can be concluded that filmed modelling and live modelling are probably efficacious procedures. Both have been shown to be superior to no-treatment conditions with a variety of excessive fears and phobias. Participant modelling, on the other hand, enjoys well-established status. It is not only more effective than filmed and live modelling, but it is also more effective than standard (imaginal) systematic desensitization.

Contingency Management

In contrast to systematic desensitization, modelling and their variants, which make the assumption that fear must be reduced or eliminated before approach behaviour will occur, contingency management procedures make no such assumption. Derived from principles of operant conditioning, contingency management procedures attempt to alter phobic behaviour by manipulating its consequences [90]. Operant-based procedures assert that acquisition of approach responses to the fear-producing situation is sufficient and that anxiety reduction, *per se*, is not necessary. Shaping, positive reinforcement and extinction are the most frequently used contingency management procedures to reduce phobic behaviour.

In the first systematic application of these principles to the reduction of phobic avoidance, Obler and Terwilliger [91] randomly assigned 30 "emotionally disturbed, neurologically impaired" children (7 to 12 years old) to a reinforced practice condition or to a no-treatment control condition. The children all presented clinically with severe monophobic disorders of either riding on a public bus or the sight of a live dog. In the reinforced practice condition, children obtained graduated and repeated practice in approaching the actual feared stimulus and were reinforced for doing so. Modelling was not used, nor was a specific counter-conditioning agent employed. Results indicated that treated children were less phobic and avoidant, and they were able to perform approach tasks (i.e. ride the bus, pet a dog) that they were unable to do prior to treatment. Control children did not evince such changes.

In a second examination of this procedure, Leitenberg and Callahan [92] randomly assigned 14 nursery and kindergarten children who showed extreme fear and avoidance of the dark to a reinforced practice condition or to a no-treatment control condition. As in the Obler and Terwilliger [91] study, significant changes in dark tolerance were evinced for the reinforced practice group only; changes were not evident in the control group.

Sheslow et al. [93] provided yet another demonstration of the effectiveness of reinforced practice. This study compared reinforced practice (labelled graduated exposure by the authors), verbal coping skills and their combination in treating fear of the dark in 32 young children (4 to 5 years old). The children were randomly assigned to one of the three treatment conditions or to a control group condition. Reinforced practice consisted of graduated exposure to dark stimuli accompanied by reinforcement. Verbal coping skills consisted of teaching children a set of self-instructions that would assist them in coping with, and handling, their fears while in the dark. Graduated exposure was not used in this condition. In the combined group, verbal coping skills were practised while graduated exposure occurred. Results indicated that the reinforced practice group and the combined verbal self-instruction plus reinforced practice group demonstrated significant changes on the behavioural avoidance task; such changes were not evinced for the verbal-coping-only group or the control group.

Similarly, positive support for the effectiveness of reinforced practice was found in a study conducted by Menzies and Clarke [28]. They examined the relative effectiveness of reinforced practice and modelling in reducing children's phobic anxiety and avoidance of water. Forty-eight water-phobic children between the ages of 3 and 8 years were randomly assigned to one of four groups: (a) reinforced practice, (b) live (therapist) modelling, (c) reinforced practice plus live modelling and (d) assessment-only control. At the conclusion of treatment, the reinforced practice condition had produced statistically and clinically significant gains that had generalized to other water-related activities. In contrast, the live modelling condition did not lead to greater treatment benefits than those observed in the control children. Moreover, modelling did not appear to enhance the effects of reinforced practice, as was anticipated. This combined condition was no more effective than the reinforced-practice-alone condition.

Thus, on the basis of these four randomized control studies, it can be concluded that reinforced practice has also earned well-established status: it has been shown to be more effective than no-treatment control conditions in two studies [91,92] and to be superior to two other treatment modalities, verbal coping skills [93] and live (adult) modelling [28,36], both of which have been shown to be more effective than no treatment.

Cognitive-Behavioural Procedures

Cognitive-behavioural procedures include a variety of strategies designed to alter perceptions, thoughts, images and beliefs of phobic children by manipulating and restructuring their distorted, maladaptive cognitions.

Because these maladaptive cognitions are assumed to lead to maladaptive behaviour (e.g. phobic avoidance), it is asserted that cognitive changes will produce behaviour changes. In support of this underlying hypothesis, a limited amount of research has confirmed the presence of maladaptive thoughts and beliefs in phobic and anxious children. During testing situations, for example, test-phobic children frequently report having more off-task thoughts, more negative self-evaluations and fewer positive self-evaluations [94,95]. Verbal self-instruction procedures are used to teach phobic children how to generate positive self-statements using cognitive modelling, rehearsal and social reinforcement. Positive self-statements typically include instructions to aid the child in developing a plan to deal with the feared situation, coping with the anxiety experienced by using relaxation or other problem-solving strategies, and evaluating ongoing performance.

Support for the "probably efficacious" status for cognitive-behavioural procedures (as defined above) is available. Kanfer *et al.* [96] first demonstrated the potential utility of this approach. They randomly assigned 45 children, 5 to 6 years of age, who demonstrated "strong fear of the dark" to one of three experimental groups which varied in the verbal self-instructions used during treatment: (a) competence group, in which the children were taught to say such phrases as "I am a brave boy (girl). I can take care of myself in the dark", (b) stimulus control group, in which the children were instructed to say such words as "The dark is a fun place to be. There are many good things in the dark", and (c) neutral group, in which the children simply rehearsed nursery rhymes. Results revealed that the "competence" group was superior to the "stimulus" and "neutral" groups on fear of dark measures.

In a clinical outcome trial, Graziano and Mooney [97] randomly assigned 33 children, 6 to 13 years of age, with severe night-time fears of long duration (over 2 years) and their families to a verbal self-instruction group or a waiting list control group. In the self-instruction group, children were taught a series of exercises to use on a nightly basis and parents were instructed in how to supervise, monitor and reward their children with praise and "bravery" tokens. Nightly exercises included muscle relaxation, imagining a pleasant scene and reciting "brave" statements. After training, the self-instruction group had significantly less night-time fear than did the control group. Following the clinical trial, the waiting list group was also provided treatment. At 6- and 12-month follow-up, the treated children revealed maintenance of and steady improvement in night-time fearless behaviour. Subsequent to this report, Graziano and Mooney [98] conducted a 2.5- to 3-year follow-up of these children. Gains persisted over this extended period of time, and no new problems were reported.

In a recent study, Silverman *et al.* [23] examined the benefits of an operant-based contingency management treatment and a cognitive-based self-control treatment to an education support control group in the treatment of phobias. Graduated *in vivo* exposure was used in both the self-control and the contingency management conditions and, although graduated *in vivo* exposure was not prescribed for the education/support condition, it was not specifically proscribed. In the study, 81 phobic children between 6 and 16 years of age and their parents were evaluated using child, parent and clinician measures. The children were assigned randomly to one of the three 10-week manualized treatment conditions (i.e. self-control, contingency management or education support). Although all three conditions were found to impart improvement in the child's functioning as measured by the reports of children, parents and clinicians, clinically significant improvements were noted only in the two active treatment conditions. Specifically, on a measure of clinical distress at post-test, 80% of the participants in the self-control and 80% of the participants in the contingency management conditions reported very little or no distress compared to 25% in the education/support condition; moreover, 88% of the participants in the self-control condition no longer met diagnostic criteria at post-test compared to 55% in the contingency management and 56% in the education/support condition. Thus, on the basis of clinical improvement indices, results tended to favour the self-control condition and contingency management conditions over the education/support condition. These differential treatment gains were maintained in subsequent follow-ups at 3, 6 and 12 months.

In a second recent study, Öst *et al.* evaluated the effects of an integrated cognitive-behavioural approach labelled "one-session treatment" [99]. This treatment has been found to be highly effective for adults with phobias [100–102], but not heretofore examined with children. This treatment is called "one-session" because it involves a single session involving a combination of cognitive-behavioural techniques, *in vivo* graduated exposure, participant modelling and social reinforcement. In the session, the therapist actively challenges maladaptive cognitions underlying the phobic avoidance by the child. This is accomplished by having the child openly discuss his or her beliefs about the phobic stimulus with the therapist while in the presence of the phobic stimulus. Treatment begins with an initial functional analysis and the development of a fear hierarchy. Once actual treatment begins, the therapist and child are distanced from the stimulus; however, as the child's beliefs are confronted and disproved, the therapist and child move closer to the stimulus. The hallmark, then, of one-session treatment is a graduated, systematic, prolonged exposure to the phobic stimulus combined with the active dissuading and repair of faulty cognitions. Importantly, this treatment is all accomplished in a highly supportive and trusting manner: the child must give assent before going on to the next step in the hierarchy and subjective units of distress (SUD) ratings are continuously monitored and considered before moving up to the next level. Notably, this treatment has been designed to be maximally effective in one session, approximately three hours in length.

Results from pilot studies with children show that the treatment produces significant gains immediately after treatment [103] and they continue at 1-year follow-up [99]. Even more impressively, the treatment has been found to be comparable to other treatments, and perhaps superior to them. Currently, Ollendick and Öst have developed a manual and treatment programme to systematically examine the effects of one-session treatment on children in a controlled trial. In this ongoing randomized trial, 120 children in Sweden and 120 in the United States are being randomly assigned to one-session treatment, an education support condition, and a waiting list control condition. Initial findings suggest that the one-session treatment is superior to the waiting list and no-contact conditions and the children "tolerate" the intense treatment well. That is, the interactive nature of the intervention appears to hold their attention and to motivate them to succeed in treatment. Moreover, ample use of participant modelling and reinforcement for graduated steps in approaching and engaging the feared object appear instrumental in its efficacy. Moreover, the children seem to enjoy the sessions and to take pride and ownership in their newly acquired interactive skills and reduced levels of anxiety.

Summary

On the basis of this brief overview, a variety of behavioural and cognitive-behavioural interventions have been shown to be more effective in the treatment of childhood fears and phobias than waiting list control conditions. In addition, some of these interventions have been shown to be superior to placebo or other treatments. Imaginal desensitization, *in vivo* desensitization, filmed modelling, live modelling and self-instruction training all enjoy "probably efficacious" status. Moreover, participant modelling and reinforced practice enjoy "well-established" status. Emotive imagery, one-session treatment and self-control treatments, on the other hand, can only be described as "experimental" at this time.

Acute Treatment: Pharmacological Interventions

Unlike the state of affairs with psychosocial interventions, no randomized clinical controlled trials for the pharmacological treatment of phobias in children and adolescents have been completed at this time [104]. The lack of pharmacological treatment studies appears to be related to the common misconception, as we noted earlier, that fears and phobias are a part of normal experience and not a condition associated with impairment or in need of pharmacological intervention. Our findings and those of others suggest otherwise.

Approaches to the pharmacological treatment of anxiety disorders have shifted over the past 10 years, and significant advances may soon be evident [104]. Recent treatment trials for adults suggest use of selective serotonin reuptake inhibitors (SSRIs) as the medications of choice rather than benzodiazepines or tricyclic antidepressants for most anxiety disorders, including phobias. Still, there is little empirical data regarding the efficacy of the SSRIs for specific phobias. Only in the past few years have there been published reports of a controlled trial for specific phobias [105], as well as uncontrolled case reports supporting their use [106,107].

Two pharmacological treatment trials deserve special mention. Benjamin et al. [105] recently completed a small ($n = 11$), 4-week double-blind placebo-controlled trial of paroxetine (up to 20 mg/day) for adults with specific phobias. The patients had been phobic for some time (10.9 ± 14 years) and only one had been offered a pharmacologic intervention in the past. Patients with symptom reduction $>50\%$ at endpoint were considered treatment responders. Of the patients on placebo, one of the six was considered a responder; in contrast, three of the six were considered responders to paroxetine. Although these results are promising, as can be noted, only 50% of the patients responded positively to paroxetine, and, of course, the sample was quite small.

Fairbanks et al. [108] completed a 9-week open trial of fluoxetine in children and adolescents aged 9–18 years with mixed anxiety disorders ($n = 16$). After not responding to brief psychotherapy, the patients were started on low-dose fluoxetine (5 mg/day), then increased weekly until side effects or improvement occurred to a maximum of 40 mg/day (children) and 80 mg/day (adolescents). Of the 16 patients enrolled, six had a phobia and four of these six responded favourably (67%).

Long-term pharmacological treatment trials for specific phobias are even less common. However, one long-term follow-up study of phobic adults indicated that 55% of responders to either pharmacotherapy or psychotherapy maintained their response at long-term follow-up (10–16 years) [109]. The other 45% experienced significant symptomatology, as did the non-responders in the original study. No long-term studies have been reported with children and adolescents.

Acute Treatment: Combined Psychosocial and Pharmacological Interventions

To date, no controlled clinical trials have examined the joint efficacy of psychosocial and pharmacologic treatments in children and adolescents with phobias. Given the independent promise of both treatments, however, there is reason to believe that synergistic effects may occur, as has been evidenced in the treatment of other anxiety disorders with children and adolescents, as well as with adults. Still, research into their combinatorial effects is needed before any reasonable conclusions can be drawn.

Continuation and Maintenance Treatments

Similar to other psychiatric and medical disorders, after achieving an adequate therapeutic response, it is important to continue the same treatment (cognitive-behavioural therapy and/or medications) to prevent relapse. During these phases, depending on the youngster's clinical state, she or he may need to be seen less frequently. Unfortunately, very little research in adults and none in youth regarding the continuation and maintenance treatment phases for phobias have been carried out. In adults with other anxiety disorders, it has been recommended to continue the medications for at least 12–18 months and, if the person is judged to be stable, to then reduce the medications slowly to avoid withdrawal side effects. It is conceivable that at least some children and adolescents will require treatment for years, consistent with findings from the adult literature [109].

DEVELOPING A TREATMENT STRATEGY

Based on our review, it seems that a series of logical steps might be followed in the acute treatment of phobias in children and adolescents. In most instances, behavioural and cognitive-behavioural treatments are called for, followed by the potential added use of pharmacologic interventions for the difficult-to-treat individual. We recommend the following progression of specific steps:

- *Step 1.* A sensible initial approach would consist of a thorough assessment, behavioural monitoring of the level of fear and its interference, delivery of knowledge about what we know about the nature of phobias, including their prevalence, onset and course, and the provision of support and encouragement for dealing with and overcoming the phobias. For mild cases of phobias, it is conceivable that they will remit relatively rapidly with this minimal intervention. Moderate to severe cases may require more intensive interventions.
- *Step 2.* At least some of the mild cases and most of the moderate to severe cases will not remit within a reasonable period of time (i.e. 4 weeks) under these minimal treatment conditions, and more intensive interventions

will be called for. Psychosocial interventions of the behavioural and cognitive-behavioural genre seem best suited for this purpose. In particular, interventions that include *in vivo* exposure, participant modelling, and reinforced practice are recommended. Such interventions can be effective in a relatively short period of time, conceivably even within one or two extended sessions or several shorter sessions spread out over a period of time.

- *Step 3.* Findings from the randomized controlled trials indicate that approximately 25% to 33% of phobic children and adolescents do not improve by the end of an appropriate clinical trial of psychosocial treatment (i.e. 8–10 sessions). Thus, patients should be continually monitored throughout treatment for behaviour change and more thoroughly after about 8–10 weeks to determine whether there has been an adequate response to treatment.
- *Step 4.* At this point in time, there are likely to be two groups who still need help: those who have partially responded but remain symptomatic and those who have failed to respond and may actually be getting worse. In both instances, efforts should be made to discover "why" the treatment is not working to its fullest, prior to abandoning the treatment strategy. For partial responders, frequently the solution is to fine-tune the treatment and to solicit greater involvement of the child and his or her parents in addressing whatever shortcomings exist. This is necessarily a highly idiosyncratic process and one requiring a careful functional analysis at the level of the specific patient.
- *Step 5.* For the refractory patient, the non-responder, it may be necessary to supplement the psychosocial intervention with pharmacological adjunctive therapy (e.g. paroxetine or fluoxetine). This may be especially so in severe cases of phobia, when the anxiety is so great that it interferes with the ability of the patient to benefit maximally from the psychosocial interventions. Rarely, however, should pharmacological intervention be used alone: there is simply no empirical data for recommending such at this time. In some instances, it might also be necessary to implement other concurrent psychosocial interventions as well, such as family therapy or perhaps even psychotherapy for the parents themselves to address issues related to the phobia in their child.

SUMMARY

Consistent Evidence

Specific phobias are present in about 3.5% of children from community settings and in about 15% of children and adolescents referred to clinic

PHOBIAS IN CHILDREN AND ADOLESCENTS: A REVIEW   273

settings. Although models of how children acquire phobias are diverse, treatments based on principles of exposure, participant modelling and positive reinforcement have become the treatments of choice and, for the most part, enjoy "well-established" status as effective interventions. Other interventions, including systematic desensitization, self-instruction training and non-participant modelling, are less well established, although evidence suggests that they are probably efficacious interventions as well. Still other treatments, such as emotive imagery and one-session treatment, appear promising but can only be viewed as experimental procedures at this point in time. Pharmacological interventions are notably lacking and few conclusions can be drawn about their use or their effectiveness.

Incomplete Evidence

Having noted generally positive outcomes for the psychosocial interventions, however, it should be quickly stated that even these procedures are in need of considerable additional empirical support. Although children were randomly assigned to treatment conditions in these studies, characteristics of the samples were only minimally specified (e.g. age, sex, diagnosis/ extent of fear) and adequate statistical power was notably lacking in some instances (the sample size was small in most studies). Moreover, much of the early support for these interventions has come from analogue studies which have been conducted in research or school settings and, not infrequently, with non-clinically referred children. As such, the children and the "treatment" in many of these studies may have differed substantially from that offered in clinic settings to clinic-referred children and their families [66,110,111]. Moreover, we were able to locate only one reasonably well-controlled study of pharmacotherapy with children and adolescents. Clearly, we have insufficient evidence on which to base any conclusions on its routine use in clinical practice.

Areas Still Open to Research

Although much is known about the nature of specific phobias in children and adolescents, much remains to be learned. For example, although various treatment strategies have been developed and shown to be effective, it is not clear how appropriate these interventions are for clinical practice or even if they are being used routinely in clinical practice settings. Issues such as these have been referred to as the "transportability" of efficacious assessment and treatment practices [66]. Moreover, we really know very little about the predictors of effective treatment. We need to know more about what treatments are effective for which children and "why" these treatments work or do not work for certain children. In pursuit of these questions, we will need to identify both the mediators and moderators of effective interventions.

REFERENCES

1. Ollendick T.H., Davis T.E. III, Muris P. (in press) Treatment of specific phobia in children and adolescents. In *Handbook of Interventions that Work with Children and Adolescents: Prevention and Treatment* (Eds P. Barrett, T.H. Ollendick). John Wiley & Sons, Chichester.
2. Ollendick T.H., Hagopian L.P., King N.J. (1997) Specific phobias in children. In *Phobias: A Handbook of Theory, Research and Treatment* (Ed. G.C.L. Davey), pp. 201–224. John Wiley & Sons, Chichester.
3. Ollendick T.H., King N.J., Muris P. (2002) Fears and phobias in children: phenomenology, epidemiology, and aetiology. *Child Adolesc. Ment. Health*, 7: 98–106.
4. Marks I.M. (1969) *Fears and Phobias*. Academic Press, New York.
5. King N.J., Hamilton D.I., Ollendick T.H. (1988) *Children's Phobias: A Behavioural Perspective*. John Wiley & Sons, Chichester.
6. Muris P., Merckelbach H. (2000) The etiology of childhood specific phobia: a multifactorial model. In *The Developmental Psychopathology of Anxiety* (Eds M.W. Vasey, M.R. Dadds), pp. 112–137. Oxford University Press, New York.
7. Ollendick T.H., King N.J., Yule W. (eds) (1994) *International Handbook of Phobic and Anxiety Disorders in Children and Adolescents*. Plenum Press, New York.
8. Ollendick T.H. (1979) Fear reduction techniques with children. In *Progress in Behavior Modification*, vol. 8 (Eds M. Hersen, R.M. Eisler, P.M. Miller), pp. 127–168. Academic Press, New York.
9. American Psychiatric Association (1994) *Diagnostic and Statistical Manual of Mental Disorders*, 4th edn. American Psychiatric Association, Washington, DC.
10. World Health Organization (1991) *International Classification of Mental and Behavioral Disorders, Clinical Descriptions and Diagnostic Guidelines*, 10th edn. World Health Organization, Geneva.
11. Ollendick T.H., Grills A.E., King N.J. (2001) Applying developmental theory to the assessment and treatment of childhood disorders: does it make a difference? *Child Psychol. Psychother.*, 8: 304–314.
12. Ollendick T.H., King N.J. (1991) Fears and phobias of childhood. In *Clinical Child Psychology: Social Learning, Development and Behavior* (Ed. M. Herbert), pp. 309–329. John Wiley & Sons, Chichester.
13. Ollendick T.H., Vasey M.W. (1999) Developmental theory and the practice of clinical child psychology. *J. Clin. Child Psychol.*, 28: 457–466.
14. Costello E.G., Angold A. (1995) Epidemiology. In *Anxiety Disorders in Children and Adolescents* (Ed. J.S. March), pp. 109–122. Guilford Press, New York.
15. Anderson J.C., Williams S., McGee R., Silva P.A. (1987) DSM-III disorders in preadolescent children. *Arch. Gen. Psychiatry*, 44: 69–76.
16. McGee R., Feehan M., Williams S., Partridge F., Silva P.A., Kelly J. (1990) DSM-III disorders in a large sample of adolescents. *J. Am. Acad. Child Adolesc. Psychiatry*, 29: 611–619.

17. Bird H.R., Canino G., Rubio-Stipec M., Gould M.S., Ribera J., Sesman M., Woodbury M., Huertas-Goldman S., Pagan A., Sanches-Lacay A. et al. (1988) Estimates of the prevalence of childhood maladjustment in a community survey in Puerto Rico. *Arch. Gen. Psychiatry*, **45**: 1120–1126.
18. Steinhausen H.-C., Metzke C.W., Meier M., Kannenberg R. (1998) Prevalence of child and adolescent psychiatric disorders: the Zurich epidemiological study. *Acta Psychiatr. Scand.*, **98**: 262–271.
19. Costello E.J., Stouthamer-Loeber M., DeRosier M. (1993) Continuity and change in psychopathology from childhood to adolescence. Presented at the Annual Meeting of the Society for Research in Child and Adolescent Psychopathology, Santa Fe, 19 March.
20. Essau C.A., Conradt J., Petermann F. (2000) Frequency, comorbidity, and psychosocial impairment of specific phobia in adolescents. *J. Clin. Child Psychol.*, **29**: 221–231.
21. Verhulst F.C., van der Ende J., Ferdinand R., Kasius M.C. (1997) The prevalence of DSM-III-R diagnoses in a national sample of Dutch adolescents. *Arch. Gen. Psychiatry*, **54**: 329–336.
22. Wittchen H.-U., Nelson C.B., Lachner G. (1998) Prevalence of mental disorders and psychosocial impairments in adolescents and young adults. *Psychol. Med.*, **28**: 109–126.
23. Silverman W.K., Kurtines W.M., Ginsburg G.S., Weems C.F., Rabian B., Serafini L.T. (1999) Contingency management, self-control, and education support in the treatment of childhood phobic disorders: a randomized clinical trial. *J. Consult. Clin. Psychol.*, **67**: 675–687.
24. Brady E.U., Kendall P.C. (1992) Comorbidity of anxiety and depression in children and adolescents. *Psychol. Bull.*, **111**: 244–255.
25. Last C.G., Strauss C.C., Francis G. (1987) Comorbidity among childhood anxiety disorders. *J. Nerv. Ment. Dis.*, **175**: 726–730.
26. Nottelmann E.D., Jensen P.S. (1995) Comorbidity of disorders in children and adolescents: developmental perspectives. In *Advances in Clinical Child Psychology*, vol. 17 (Eds T.H. Ollendick, R.J. Prinz), pp. 109–155. Plenum Press, New York.
27. Seligman L.D., Ollendick T.H. (1998) Comorbidity of anxiety and depression in children and adolescents: an integrative review. *Clin. Child Family Psychol. Rev.*, **1**: 125–144.
28. Menzies R.G., Clark J.C. (1993) The etiology of childhood water phobia. *Behav. Res. Ther.*, **31**: 499–501.
29. Rachman S. (1976) The passing of the two-stage theory of fear and avoidance: fresh possibilities. *Behav. Res. Ther.*, **14**: 125–134.
30. Rachman S. (1977) The conditioning theory of fear acquisition: a critical examination. *Behav. Res. Ther.*, **15**: 375–387.
31. McNally R.J., Steketee G.S. (1985) The etiology and maintenance of severe animal phobias. *Behav. Res. Ther.*, **23**: 431–435.
32. Öst L.G., Hugdahl K. (1981) Acquisition of phobias and anxiety response patterns in clinical patients. *Behav. Res. Ther.*, **19**: 439–447.
33. Öst L.G., Hugdahl K. (1985) Acquisition of blood and dental phobia and anxiety response patterns in clinical patients. *Behav. Res. Ther.*, **23**: 27–34.
34. Menzies R.G., Clarke J.C. (1995) The etiology of phobias: a nonassociative account. *Clin. Psychol. Rev.*, **15**: 23–48.
35. DiNardo P.A., Guzy L.T., Jenkins J.A., Bak R.M., Tomasi S.F., Copland M. (1988) Etiology and maintenance of dog fears. *Behav. Res. Ther.*, **26**: 241–244.

36. Menzies R.G., Clark J.C. (1993) The etiology of fear of heights and its relationship to severity and individual response patterns. *Behav. Res. Ther.*, **31**: 355–365.
37. Marks I.M. (1987) *Fears, Phobias, and Rituals.* Oxford University Press, New York.
38. Ollendick T.H., King N.J. (1991) Origins of childhood fears: an evaluation of Rachman's theory of fear acquisition. *Behav. Res. Ther.*, **29**: 117–123.
39. Seligman M.E.P. (1971) Phobias and preparedness. *Behav. Ther.*, **2**: 307–320.
40. Davey G.C.L. (1992) Classical conditioning and the acquisition of human fears and phobias: a review and synthesis of the literature. *Adv. Behav. Res. Ther.*, **14**: 29–66.
41. McNally R.J. (1987) Preparedness and phobias: a review. *Psychol. Bull.*, **101**: 283–303.
42. Muris P., Merckelbach H., de Jong P., Ollendick T.H. (2002) The etiology of specific fears and phobias in children: a critique of the non-associative account. *Behav. Res. Ther.*, **40**: 185–195.
43. Carey G. (1990) Genes, fears, phobias, and phobic disorders. *J. Counsel. Develop.*, **68**: 628–632.
44. Kendler K.S., Neale M.C., Kessler R.C., Heath A.C., Eaves L.J. (1992) The genetic epidemiology of phobias in women: the interrelationship of agoraphobia, social phobia, situational phobia, and simple phobia. *Arch. Gen. Psychiatry*, **49**: 273–281.
45. Stevenson J., Batten N., Cherner M. (1992) Fears and fearfulness in children and adolescents: a genetic analysis of twin data. *J. Child Psychol. Psychiatry*, **33**: 977–985.
46. Chess S., Thomas, A. (1977) Temperamental individuality from childhood to adolescence. *J. Am. Acad. Child Psychiatry*, **16**: 218–226.
47. Chess S., Thomas A. (1984) *Origins and Evolution of Behavior Disorders.* Brunner/Mazel, New York.
48. Kagan J. (1989) Temperamental contributions to social behavior. *Am. Psychol.*, **44**: 668–674.
49. Kagan J., Reznick J.S., Gibbons J. (1989) Inhibited and uninhibited types of children. *Child Develop.*, **60**: 838–845.
50. Kagan J., Reznick J.S., Snidman N. (1988) Biological bases of childhood shyness. *Science*, **240**: 167–171.
51. Ollendick T.H. (1986) Child and adolescent behaviour. In *Handbook of Psychotherapy and Behavior Change* (Eds S. Garfield, A. Bergin), pp. 525–564. John Wiley & Sons, New York.
52. Kagan J., Reznick J.S., Snidman N. (1987) The physiology and psychology of behavioral inhibition. *Child Develop.*, **58**: 1459–1473.
53. Biederman J., Rosenbaum J.F., Chaloff J., Kagan J. (1995) Behavioral inhibition as a risk factor. In *Anxiety Disorders in Children and Adolescents* (Ed. J.S. March), pp. 61–81. Guilford Press, New York.
54. Gray J.A. (1982) *The Neuropsychology of Anxiety.* Oxford University Press, Oxford.
55. Gray J.A., McNaughton N. (2000) *The Neuropsychology of Anxiety*, 2nd edn. Oxford University Press, Oxford.
56. Biederman J., Rosenbaum J.F., Hirshfeld D.R., Faraone V., Bolduc E., Gersten M., Meminger S., Reznick S. (1990) Psychiatric correlates of behavioral inhibition in young children of parents with and without psychiatric disorders. *Arch. Gen. Psychiatry*, **47**: 21–26.

57. Rosenbaum J.F., Biederman J., Gersten M., Hirshfeld D.R., Meminger S.R., Herman J.B., Kagan J., Reznick J.S., Snidman N. (1988) Behavioral inhibition in children of parents with panic disorder and agoraphobia: a controlled study. *Arch. Gen. Psychiatry*, **45**: 463–470.
58. Hirshfeld D.R., Rosenbaum J.F., Biederman J., Bolduc E.A., Faraone S.V., Snidman N., Reznick J.S., Kagan J. (1992) Stable behavioral inhibition and its association with anxiety disorder. *J. Am. Acad. Child Adolesc. Psychiatry*, **31**: 103–111.
59. Barrett P.M., Rapee R.M., Dadds M.R., Ryan S.M. (1996) Family enhancement of cognitive style in anxious and aggressive children: threat bias and the FEAR effect. *J. Abnorm. Child Psychol.*, **24**: 187–203.
60. Dadds M.R., Barrett P.M., Rapee R.M., Ryan S.M. (1996) Family process and child anxiety and aggression: an observational analysis. *J. Abnorm. Child Psychol.*, **24**: 715–734.
61. Siqueland L., Kendall P.C., Steinberg L. (1996) Anxiety in children: perceived family environments and observed family interactions. *J. Clin. Child Psychol.*, **25**: 225–237.
62. Whaley S.E., Pinto A., Sigman M. (1999) Characterizing interactions between anxious mothers and their children. *J. Consult. Clin. Psychol.*, **67**: 826–836.
63. Fonagy P., Target M. (1994) The efficacy of psychoanalysis for children with disruptive disorders. *J. Am. Acad. Child Adolesc. Psychiatry*, **33**: 45–55.
64. Weisz J.R., Weiss B., Alicke M.D., Klotz M.L. (1987) Effectiveness of psychotherapy with children and adolescents: a meta-analysis for clinicians. *J. Consult. Clin. Psychol.*, **55**: 542–549.
65. Weisz J.R., Donenberg G.R., Han S.S., Weiss B. (1995) Bridging the gap between laboratory and clinic in child and adolescent psychotherapy. *J. Consult. Clin. Psychol.*, **63**: 688–701.
66. Chambless D.L., Ollendick T.H. (2001) Empirically supported psychological interventions: controversies and evidence. *Ann. Rev. Psychol.*, **52**: 685–716.
67. Wolpe J. (1958) *Psychotherapy by Reciprocal Inhibition*. Stanford University Press, Stanford, CA.
68. Kondas O. (1967) Reduction of examination anxiety and "stage fright" by group desensitization and relaxation. *Behav. Res. Ther.*, **5**: 275–281.
69. Mann J., Rosenthal T.L. (1969) Vicarious and direct counterconditioning of test anxiety through individual and group desensitization. *Behav. Res. Ther.*, **7**: 359–367.
70. Barabasz A.F. (1973) Group desensitization of test anxiety in elementary school. *J. Psychol.*, **83**: 295–301.
71. Miller L.C., Barrett C.L., Hampe E., Noble H. (1972) Comparison of reciprocal inhibition, psychotherapy, and waiting list control for phobic children. *J. Abnorm. Psychol.*, **79**: 269–279.
72. Ollendick T.H., King N.J. (1998) Empirically supported treatments for children with phobic and anxiety disorders. *J. Clin. Child Psychol.*, **27**: 156–167.
73. Ollendick T.H., King N.J. (2000) Empirically supported treatments for children and adolescents. In *Child and Adolescent Therapy: Cognitive-Behavioral Procedures*, 2nd edn (Ed. P.C. Kendall), pp. 386–425, Guilford Press, New York.
74. Ultee C.A., Griffioen D., Schellekens J. (1982) The reduction of anxiety in children: a comparison of the effects of "systematic desensitization in vitro" and "systematic desensitization in vivo". *Behav. Res. Ther.*, **20**: 61–67.
75. Kuroda J. (1969) Elimination of children's fears of animals by the method of experimental desensitization: an application of learning theory to child psychology. *Psychologia*, **12**: 161–165.

76. Lazarus A.A., Abramovitz A. (1962) The use of "emotive imagery" in the treatment of children's phobias. *J. Ment. Sci.*, **108**: 191–195.
77. Cornwall E., Spence S.H., Schotte D. (1997) The effectiveness of emotive imagery in the treatment of darkness phobia in children. *Behav. Change*, **18**: 19–37.
78. King N., Cranstoun F., Josephs A. (1989) Emotive imagery and children's nighttime fears: a multiple baseline design evaluation. *J. Behav. Ther. Exp. Psychiatry*, **20**: 125–135.
79. Ollendick T.H., Cerny J.A. (1981) *Clinical Behavior Therapy with Children*. Plenum Press, New York.
80. Bandura A. (1971) *Psychological Modelling: Conflicting Theories*. Aldine-Atherton, Chicago, IL.
81. Bandura A. (1969) *Principles of Behavior Modification*. Holt, Rinehart & Winston, New York.
82. Bandura A., Grusec J.E., Menlove F.L. (1967) Vicarious extinction of avoidance behavior. *J. Pers. Soc. Psychol.*, **5**: 16–23.
83. Bandura A., Menlove F.L. (1968) Factors determining vicarious extinction of avoidance behavior through symbolic modelling. *J. Pers. Soc. Psychol.*, **3**: 99–108.
84. Hill J.H., Liebert R.M., Mott D.E.W. (1968) Vicarious extinction of avoidance behavior through films: an initial test. *Psychol. Rep.*, **22**: 192.
85. Lewis S. (1974) A comparison of behavior therapy techniques in the reduction of fearful avoidance behavior. *Behav. Ther.*, **5**: 648–655.
86. Ritter B. (1968) The group desensitization of children's snake phobias using vicarious and contact desensitization procedures. *Behav. Res. Ther.*, **6**: 1–6.
87. Bandura A., Blanchard E.B., Ritter B. (1969) Relative efficacy of desensitization and modelling approaches for inducing behavioral, affective, and attitudinal changes. *J. Pers. Soc. Psychol.*, **13**: 173–199.
88. Blanchard E.B. (1970) Relative contributions of modelling, informational influences, and physical contact in extinction of phobic behavior. *J. Abnorm. Psychol.*, **76**: 55–61.
89. Murphy C.M., Bootzin R.R. (1973) Active and passive participation in the contact desensitization of snake fear in children. *Behav. Ther.*, **4**: 203–211.
90. King N.J., Ollendick T.H. (1997) Annotation: treatment of childhood phobias. *J. Child Psychol. Psychiatry*, **38**: 389–400.
91. Obler M., Terwilliger R.F. (1970) Pilot study on the effectiveness of systematic desensitization with neurologically impaired children with phobic disorders. *J. Consult. Clin. Psychol.*, **34**: 314–318.
92. Leitenberg H., Callahan E.J. (1973) Reinforced practice and reduction of different kinds of fears in adults and children. *Behav. Res. Ther.*, **11**: 19–30.
93. Sheslow D.V., Bondy A.S., Nelson R.O. (1983) A comparison of graduated exposure, verbal coping skills, and their combination in the treatment of children's fear of the dark. *Child Family Behav. Ther.*, **4**: 33–45.
94. Beidel D.C., Turner S.M. (1988) Comorbidity of test anxiety and other anxiety disorders in children. *J. Abnorm. Child Psychol.*, **16**: 275–287.
95. Warren M.K., Ollendick T.H., King N.J. (1996) Test anxiety in girls and boys: a clinical-developmental analysis. *Behav. Change*, **13**: 157–170.
96. Kanfer F.H., Karoly P., Newman A. (1975) Reduction of children's fear of the dark by competence-related and situational threat-related verbal cues. *J. Consult. Clin. Psychol.*, **43**: 251–258.

97. Graziano A.M., Mooney K.C. (1980) Family self-control instruction for children's nighttime fear reduction. *J. Consult. Clin. Psychol.*, **48**: 206–213.
98. Graziano A.M., Mooney K.C. (1982) Behavioral treatment of "nightfears" in children: maintenance of improvement at 2½- to 3-year follow-up. *J. Consult. Clin. Psychol.*, **50**: 598–599.
99. Öst L.G., Svensson L., Hellstrom K., Lindwall R. (2001) One-session treatment of specific phobias in youths: a randomized clinical trial. *J. Consult. Clin. Psychol.*, **69**: 814–824.
100. Öst L.G. (1989) A maintenance program for behavioral treatment of anxiety disorders. *Behav. Res. Ther.*, **27**: 123–130.
101. Öst L.G., Brandberg M., Alm T. (1997) One versus five sessions of exposure in the treatment of flying phobia. *Behav. Res. Ther.*, **35**: 987–996.
102. Öst L.G., Ferebee I., Furmark T. (1997) One-session group therapy of spider phobia: direct versus indirect treatments. *Behav. Res. Ther.*, **35**: 721–732.
103. Muris P., Merckelbach H., Holdrinet I., Sijsenaar M. (1998) Treating phobic children: effects of EMDR versus exposure. *J. Consult. Clin. Psychol.*, **66**: 193–198.
104. Ginsburg G.S., Walkup J.T. (2003) Treatment of specific phobias. In *Handbook of Interventions that Work with Children and Adolescents: Prevention and Treatment* (Eds P. Barrett, T.H. Ollendick). John Wiley & Sons, Chichester.
105. Benjamin J., Ben-Zion I.Z., Karbofsky E., Dannon P. (2000) Double-blind placebo-controlled pilot study of paroxetine for specific phobia. *J. Psychopharmacol.*, **149**: 194–196.
106. Abene M.V., Hamilton J.D. (1988) Resolution of fear of flying with fluoxetine treatment. *J. Anxiety Disord.*, **12**: 599–603.
107. Viswnatha R., Paradis C. (1991) Treatment of cancer phobia with fluoxetine. *Am. J. Psychiatry*, **148**: 1090.
108. Fairbanks J.M., Pine D.S., Tancer N.K., Dummit III E.S., Kentgen L.M., Asche B.K., Klein R.G. (1997) Open fluoxetine treatment of mixed anxiety disorders in children and adolescents. *J. Am. Acad. Child Adolesc. Psychiatry*, **7**: 17–29.
109. Lipsitz J.D., Markowitz J.C., Cherry S., Fyer A.J. (1999) Open trial of interpersonal psychotherapy for the treatment of social phobia. *Am. J. Psychiatry*, **156**: 1814–1816.
110. Kazdin A.E. (1997) A model for developing effective treatments: progression and interplay of theory, research, and practice. *J. Clin. Child Psychol.*, **26**: 114–129.
111. Weisz J.R., Weiss B., Alicke M.D., Klotz M.L. (1987) Effectiveness of psychotherapy with children and adolescents: a meta-analysis for clinicians. *J. Consult. Clin. Psychol.*, **55**: 542–549.

Commentaries

5.1
Childhood Phobias: More Questions Than Answers
Michael Rutter[1]

The epidemiological and developmental study of children's fears goes back many years [1,2]. As a result, it is known that the various types of phobia differ in their usual age of onset. Thus, animal and insect phobias almost always begin in the preschool years, social phobias most often begin in adolescence, and agoraphobia may be first manifest from any time between late childhood to middle life [3–5]. However, age of onset apart, there appear to be few clearly differentiary features among phobias, at least as standard in adult life [6], with the single interesting exception of blood phobia, which is physiologically distinctive in being associated with a sudden drop in blood pressure and hence often with consequential fainting [7].

Simple (specific) phobias stand out among anxiety disorders in childhood in two key respects. First, they are particularly common: in the Virginia Twin Study of 8- to 16-year-olds, the prevalence was 212 per 1000, compared with 108 for overanxious disorder. Second, remarkably few were associated with functional impairment: 21% as compared with 41% for overanxious disorder and 93% for major depression [8]. It was also noteworthy that comorbidity was very low for phobias not associated with impairment, although it was high if impairment was present. In the National Comorbidity Survey, it was also striking that only 10% of adults with a phobia disorder had sought help in the past year, as compared with approximately half of those with a panic disorder [9]. Accordingly, to a much greater extent than with other forms of psychopathology, it is necessary to ask not only about the etiology of the phobias, but also about the factors that predispose to impairment.

Despite the long-standing interest in the origins of phobias, our understanding of the causal processes is decidedly limited. As Ollendick et al.'s authoritative review emphasizes, the main demonstrated risk factor is the temperamental characteristic of behavioural inhibition, which is associated with a six-fold increase in the rate of phobic disorders compared

---
[1] *Institute of Psychiatry, De Crespigny Park, Denmark Hill, London SE5 8AF, UK*

with uninhibited children. It was notable, however, that the inverse did not apply to the half of the inhibited group whose temperamental inhibition was not stable over time—emphasizing that although the concept of temperament includes stability, the findings show only moderate temporal consistency.

Studies in adults have generally shown that genetic influences account for a smaller proportion of the population variance in the liability to simple phobias than is the case with agoraphobia. Nevertheless, twin studies in childhood have shown heritabilities of about 40% for specific fears and phobias [10,11]. More importantly, multivariate analysis in Eley et al.'s general population twin study of 4-year-olds showed that most (62%) of the association between specific fears and the temperamental characteristic of shyness/inhibition was due to shared genetic influences [10]. In other words, much (but not all) of the genetic effect on simple phobias seems to operate through temperamental inhibition. However, it has also been found that early anxiety shares a genetic liability with the later development of depression [12]. Research findings are beginning to be informative on the crucial question of how genetic influences operate. Molecular genetic findings, when they become available, should be even more helpful.

All the evidence indicates an important role for environmental influences—probably on the persistence of phobias and the association with impairment as much as on the basic predisposition to develop a phobia, or on the specific phobia that is acquired. However, as Ollendick et al.'s review brings out, although fears can arise as a result of some unpleasant encounter, many do not have such an identifiable onset. Evolutionary factors also play a role in determining which fears are most readily acquired. As Susan Mineke's elegant monkey studies showed, it is easy to induce a fear of snakes but the same methods will not induce a fear of flowers [13]. Anxiety-fostering styles of parent–child interaction may also be influential, although the available research is weak [14]. Cognitive bias for threat has been considered another link factor for anxiety, but studies with adults suggest that the bias is mainly an accompaniment of symptoms, which disappears with symptom remission, making it less likely that the bias represents a predisposing individual trait [15]. Much remains to be learned!

Ollendick et al. provide a systematic evaluation of psychological interventions for phobias, concluding that several (including desensitization, modelling and cognitive self-instruction training) are probably efficacious. That is certainly encouraging but, as Weersing and Weisz's review [16] notes, scarcely any studies have shown *how* the interventions work. Not only do most not determine whether the therapy affects specific mechanisms, but scarcely any test whether the postulated mediating mechanism accounts for the therapeutic benefits. That is an important lack, because the various psychological interventions are supposed to operate through rather disparate routes. Over a quarter of a century ago, it was concluded that the essential elements in the treatment of phobias seemed to be a combination of exposure to the phobic stimuli plus some means of enabling the child to learn to master the situation, with the specific means of doing so of secondary importance [17]. We have made some progress since then, particularly in the development of cognitive-behavioural approaches, but we are not much further forward in identifying the big elements in therapeutic efficacy, or in understanding the causes of the individual differences in response to treatment.

In a real sense, phobias constitute one of the most apparently understandable mental disorders, as well as one of those most responsive to intervention. Despite this, large questions remain on the basic neurobiology, and on the psychological mechanisms in causation at response to treatment.

REFERENCES

1. Jersild A.T., Holmes F.B. (1935) *Children's Fears*. Teachers College, Columbia University, New York.
2. Lapouse R., Monk M. (1959) Fears and worries in a representative sample of children. *Am. J. Orthopsychiatry*, **29**: 803–818.
3. Marks I.M., Gelder M.G. (1966) Different ages of onset in varieties of phobia. *Am. J. Psychiatry*, **123**: 218–221.
4. Öst L.-G. (1987) Age of onset in different phobias. *J. Abnorm. Psychol.*, **96**: 223–229.
5. Rutter M., Tizard J., Whitmore K. (eds) (1970) *Education, Health and Behaviour*. Longman, London.
6. Fyer A.J. (1998) Current approaches to etiology and pathophysiology of specific phobia. *Biol. Psychiatry*, **44**: 1295–1304.
7. Rachman S.J. (1990) *Fear and Courage*. Freeman, New York.
8. Simonoff E., Pickles A., Meyer J., Silberg J.L., Maes H.H., Loeber R., Rutter M., Hewitt J.K., Eaves L.J., Lindon J. (1997) The Virginia Twin Study of Adolescent Behavioral Development: influences of age, sex, and impairment on rates of disorder. *Arch. Gen. Psychiatry*, **54**: 801–808.
9. Kessler R.C., Walters E.E. (1998) Epidemiology of DSM-III-R major depression and minor depression among adolescents and young adults in the national comorbidity survey. *Depress. Anxiety*, **7**: 3–14.
10. Eley T.C., Bolton D., O'Connor T.G., Perrin S., Smith P., Plomin R. (2003) A twin study of anxiety-related behaviours in pre-school children. *J. Child Psychol. Psychiatry*, **44**: 945–960.
11. Lichtenstein P., Annas P. (2000) Heritability and prevalence of specific fears and phobia in childhood. *J. Child Psychol. Psychiatry*, **41**: 927–937.
12. Silberg J.L., Neale M.C., Rutter M., Eaves L. (2001) Genetic and environmental influences on the temporal association between earlier anxiety and later depression in girls. *Biol. Psychiatry*, **49**: 1040–1049.
13. Ohman A., Mineke S. (2001) Fears, phobias and preparedness: toward an evolved model of fear and fear learning. *Psychol. Rev.*, **108**: 483–522.

14. Wood J.J., McLeod B.D., Sigman M., Hwang W.-C., Chu B.C. (2003) Parenting and childhood anxiety: theory, empirical findings, and future directions. *J. Child Psychol. Psychiatry*, **44**: 134–151.
15. Klein R.G., Pine D.S. (1990) Anxiety disorders. *Child Adolesc. Psychiatry*, **4**: 486–509.
16. Weersing V.R., Weisz J.R. (2002) Mechanisms of action in youth psychotherapy. *J. Child Psychol. Psychiatry*, **43**: 3–29.
17. Rutter M. (1976) *Helping Troubled Children*. Plenum Press, New York.

5.2
Fear, Anxieties and Treatment Efficacy in Children and Adolescents
Rachel G. Klein[1]

A key theoretical issue is whether fear in children reflects a unitary psychological phenomenon—that is, whether "the result" is the same whether fear is learned or preprogrammed. That the function of "normal" fear is to alert the organism to danger seems clear. It is viewed as a built-in adaptive signal. Can we assume that other fear-like experiences, such as watching scary movies, or pathological fear (i.e. phobias) and anxiety (i.e. separation or generalized anxiety disorder) represent similar processes? The answer to these questions has relevance to our approaches in the study of anxiety disorders. For one, can studying the neurobiology of normal fear inform on the mechanisms underlying distinct anxiety disorders? A body of well-accepted experimental work assumes such similarity [1], but other work suggests that neurobiological pathways of conditioned fear may be distinct from those of other fearful states [2]. The distinctions and similarities between "normal" fear and pathological anxiety have implications for our clinical understanding of childhood anxiety disorders.

Our beliefs about the importance of childhood phobias largely come from retrospective studies of adults with anxiety disorders. The findings from two large epidemiological studies, that adults with anxiety disorders reported onsets in childhood, highlighted the possible importance of childhood anxiety disorders [3,4]. In addition, the observation that anxiety disorders were the most common mental disorders in adults gave these disorders special prominence, especially with regard to specific phobias, since they mostly accounted for the high prevalence of anxiety diagnoses. In addition, panic disorder has been found to have greater familial loading among patients with specific phobias in childhood than those without such

---
[1] *New York University Child Study Center, 215 Lexington Avenue, New York, NY 10016, USA*

a history [5]. Finally, among adults with depression, a recalled history of anxiety disorders is significantly more frequent in women. It has been proposed that this sex difference in early anxiety accounts for the relative excess of depression in women, since early anxiety disorders are predictors of later depression [6]. Findings from these retrospective studies have been influential, but they can only be considered heuristic and suggestive, in view of the well-known limitations of restrospective recall. This is especially the case for previous anxiety symptoms, since their recall has been found to be particularly unreliable [7].

Unfortunately, longitudinal studies of children with anxiety disorders are scarce, but findings consistently show a modicum of stability for anxiety disorder from childhood to adolescence in girls, but not boys [8–10]. A prospective longitudinal follow-up of a general population of children and adolescents is also strongly suggestive that specific phobias and social phobia are distinct conditions. Specific phobias in either childhood or adolescence were exclusively predictive of specific phobias in adulthood. The course of social phobia was similarly specific, since it presaged only social phobia later on [11]. The sex difference in course and the diagnostic specificity of some childhood anxiety disorders over time argue against the notion that pathological anxiety and ordinary non-specific fear share similar underlying mechanisms.

It is tempting to assume similarities between specific phobias and social phobia, since both are treated with behavioural treatment, specifically exposure. However, this therapeutic commonality can be misleading. When extended to psychopharmacology, it would imply (probably erroneously) that selective serotonin reuptake inhibitors (SSRIs) are effective in specific phobias. SSRI studies in children with anxiety disorders have included specific phobias, but these co-occurred with other anxiety disorders, and were not the primary treatment target. To assume efficacy of SSRIs for specific phobias may not be justified.

Commendable efforts have been made to develop systematic treatments for childhood anxiety disorders, but, with a few exceptions, tests of their efficacy have fallen short of rigour. The vast majority of studies have relied on waiting list controls. However, these do not indicate whether the specific intervention was effective, only whether it is better than no treatment. Even this minimal hope of benefit remains dubious, since it is possible that placing anxious children who come for clinical services on a waiting list might be deleterious. Credible treatment controls are necessary to estimate the value of interventions. That this type of control is essential is highlighted by findings from two studies that found no difference in efficacy between a special cognitive-behavioural treatment package and a control treatment in children with anxiety disorders [12,13].

REFERENCES

1. Ledoux J. (1998) Fear and the brain: where have we been, and where are we going? *Biol. Psychiatry*, **44**: 1229–1238.
2. Kandel E. (2003) Genes, synapses, and long-term memory. Presented at the 93rd Annual Meeting of the American Psychopathological Association, New York, 7 March.
3. Robins L.N., Regier D. (1995) *Psychiatric Disorders in America: The Epidemiological Catchment Area Study*. Free Press, New York.
4. Curtis G.C., Magee W.J., Eaton W.E., Wittchen H.U., Kessler R.C. (1998) Specific fears and phobias: epidemiology and classification. *Br. J. Psychiatry*, **173**: 212–217.
5. Fyer A.J., Mannuzza S., Chapman T.F., Martin L.Y., Klein D.F. (1995) Specificity in familial aggregation of phobic disorders. *Arch. Gen. Psychiatry*, **52**: 564–573.
6. Breslau N, Chilcoat H.D., Peterson E., Schultz L. (2000) Gender differences in major depression: the role of anxiety. In *Gender and its Effects on Psychopathology* (Ed. E. Frank), pp. 132–149. American Psychiatric Press, Washington, DC.
7. Fendrich M., Weissman M.M., Warner V., Mufson L. (1990) Two-year recall of lifetime diagnoses in offspring at high and low risk for major depression. *Arch. Gen. Psychiatry*, **47**: 1121–1127.
8. Costello E.J., Angold A., Keeler G. (1999) Adolescent outcomes of childhood disorders: the consequences of severity and impairment. *J. Am. Acad. Child Adolesc. Psychiatry*, **38**: 121–128.
9. McGee R., Feehan M., Williams S., Anderson J. (1992) DSM-III disorders from age 11 to age 15 years. *J. Am. Acad. Child Adolesc. Psychiatry*, **31**: 50–59.
10. Rueter M.A., Scaramella L., Wallace I.E., Conger R.D. (1999) First onset of depressive or anxiety disorders predicted by the longitudinal course of internalizing symptoms and parent–adolescent disagreements. *Arch. Gen. Psychiatry*, **56**: 726–732.
11. Pine D.S., Cohen P., Gurley D., Brook J., Ma Y. (1998) The risk for early adulthood anxiety and depressive disorders in adolescents with anxiety and depressive disorders. *Arch. Gen. Psychiatry*, **55**: 56–64.
12. Last C., Hansen C., Franco N. (1998) Cognitive-behavioral treatment of school phobia. *J. Am. Acad. Child Adolesc. Psychiatry*, **7**: 404–411.
13. Silverman W.K., Kurtines W.M., Ginsburg G.S., Weems C.F., Rabian B., Serafini L.T. (1999) Contingency management, self-control, and education support in the treatment of childhood phobic disorders: a randomized clinical trial. *J. Consult. Clin. Psychol.*, **67**: 675–687.

5.3
Where Are All the Fearful Children?
Gabrielle A. Carlson and Deborah M. Weisbrot[1]

Who and where are all the fearful children? Much attention in the literature has been directed to the fears of "normal" childhood and the differentiation

---

[1] *Child and Adolescent Psychiatry, State University of New York at Stony Brook, Stony Brook, NY 11794-8790, USA*

of normal developmental fears from pathological fears [1]. Ironically, these concerns may not be the most salient issues encountered by the clinician in a typical child and adolescent psychiatry clinic.

These days, the child who presents to a typical child psychiatry clinic or private practice with classic symptoms of a phobia of dogs, water or snakes in isolation from other symptoms is rare. Perhaps symptoms resolve spontaneously during childhood or adolescence or continue to adulthood as subclinical phobic symptoms complicating other anxiety disorders. In fact, the degree of clinical relevance of treatment studies of phobic children which exclude subjects with other major psychiatric diagnoses remains to be seen.

Recently, we have become interested in studying children with complex, paralysing and intense fears that include "poltergeists", tidal waves, tornadoes, "Thomas the Tank Engine" videos, bathroom ceiling fans and a terrifying imaginary character called "Paper-cut man", to name a few. While ghost and monster fears are common in young children, these atypical children are older, and do not "fit" into any existing diagnostic category. Their concomitant symptoms of autism spectrum, atypical psychosis and severe anxiety and mood disorders defy current DSM classification. "Childhood-onset pervasive developmental disorder" (COPDD) was a designation used in DSM-III, that was discontinued for lack of empirical data. A research diagnosis derived from COPDD is "multiple complex developmental disorder" [2]. Criteria for this condition include problems with regulation of affective state and anxiety such as unusual fears and phobias, recurrent panic episodes, and high frequency of idiosyncratic anxiety reactions such as sustained periods of uncontrollable giggling, laughter or "silly" affect that is inappropriate in the context of the situation. Additionally, the syndrome is characterized by occasional irrational thinking, and impairments in social behaviour and sensitivity. Although such children have obviously been recognized for many years, there is little research on their fears, comorbidities and treatment. The need to understand the experiences of these children has become all the more important as effective treatment options for anxiety symptoms are now available.

Although we may know a great deal about childhood phobias based upon epidemiological studies, little is known about how phobic disorders present in children with complex comorbidities such as mood, anxiety or psychotic disorders. In a sample of children with pervasive developmental disorders (PDD), rates have been reported as high as 63.6% [4]. This is many times higher than rates in comorbid community samples. Whether this high rate is an expression of the general anxiety in this population or whether there is an impact of the change in how media depicts horror films, for instance, is not clear. Certainly science fiction and horror movies used to be kinder and gentler. The big, bad monster was killed by the hero in the end. Now, the monster lives to return for the sequel. Some children may be left with a sense that it can return at any time. Perhaps these vulnerable children develop phobias.

Phobias occur in other childhood comorbidities as well. The September 2001 bombing of the World Trade Center was more horrifying than our worst nightmare. As a part of the constellation of traumatic reactions, children may have experienced phobic symptoms, as well. We do not know who these children are, however, or what predicted their specific response.

Another area of under-recognized phobic symptoms occurs among hospitalized children and children who are medically ill [5]. Up to 25% of these children were found to have significant symptoms of anxiety, including a variety of phobias such as needle phobias and fears of dying. Clinical experience with children and adolescents who have epilepsy and multiple sclerosis suggests that a significant component of phobic anxiety exists and that treatment of such symptoms could potentially limit the distress experienced by these youngsters. Unfortunately, such symptoms are often dismissed as merely being inherent to having a severe medical illness and these children often do not receive treatment for their anxiety symptoms.

Finally, it is important to remind ourselves that often it may not be the phobic reaction which leads the parent to bring the child for treatment. More likely, behavioural difficulties, a depressive episode or symptoms of school refusal are the primary concerns. We do find that treatment of phobias based upon techniques such as exposure, systematic desensitization and positive reinforcement, among others, is highly effective, but attention must be paid to treatment for the comorbid disorders [6].

To really appreciate the multiple dimensions of childhood phobias, we must think "outside the DSM box". What emerges when we do that is that there are a number of children whose phobic symptoms are part of complex developmental constellations of cognitive, affective and anxiety symptoms. An appreciation of comorbidity and the complexities of how anxiety symptoms present in childhood remains critical to both the understanding and treatment of phobias in childhood.

REFERENCES

1. Freeman J.B., Garcia A.M., Leonard H.L. (2002) Anxiety disorders. In *Child and Adolescent Psychiatry: A Comprehensive Textbook* (Ed. M. Lewis), pp. 821–834. Lippincott, Williams and Wilkins, Philadelphia, PA.
2. Towbin K.E., Dykens E.M., Pearson G.S., Cohen D.J. (1993) Conceptualizing "borderline syndrome of childhood" and "childhood schizophrenia" as a developmental disorder. *J. Am. Acad. Child Adolesc. Psychiatry*, **32**: 775–782.

3. Buitelaar J.K., van der Gaag R.J. (1998) Diagnostic rules for children with PDD-NOS and multiple complex developmental disorder. *J. Child Psychol. Psychiatry*, **39**: 911–919.
4. Muris P., Steerneman P., Merckelback H., Holdrinet I., Meesters C. (1998) Comorbid anxiety symptoms in children with pervasive developmental disorders. *J. Anxiety Disord.*, **12**: 387–393.
5. Ettinger A.B., Weisbrot D.M., Vitale S.V., Gadow K.D., Nolan E.E., Lenn N.J., Andriola M.R., Hermann B.P., Novak G.P. (1998) Anxiety and depression in pediatric epilepsy patients. *Epilepsia*, **39**: 595–599.
6. Kendall P.C., Aschendbrand S.G., Hudson J.L. (2003) Child-focused treatment of anxiety. In *Evidence-Based Psychotherapies for Children and Adolescents* (Eds A.E. Kazdin, J.R. Weisz), pp. 81–100. Guilford Press, New York.

5.4
Etiology and Treatment of Childhood Phobias
Deborah C. Beidel and Autumn Paulson[1]

The etiology of childhood phobias is not completely understood. Various theories exist, one of which is direct conditioning. Although some attribute the onset of their fears to a specific traumatic event, such a pathway is neither necessary nor sufficient to explain the etiology of phobias. In one study, 56% of those with a specific phobia reported the existence of a traumatic conditioning event versus 40% of those with generalized social phobia versus 20% of those without a disorder [1]. These data have two important implications. First, despite the substantial number of individuals with phobic disorders who report traumatic events, a virtually equal number do not. Although it is possible that patient recall is faulty, other factors may be at play. For example, there is an interesting phenomenon known as cumulative conditioning (e.g. [2]), whereas phobias develop not as a result of one single, traumatic conditioning event but through a series of smaller, accumulating events. These small events could serve to sensitize a child for a future, more traumatic, event, ultimately leading to development of a phobia.

A second important implication from Stemberger *et al.* [1] is that some individuals who report the occurrence of traumatic events do not develop a phobic disorder. Again, mitigating factors, such as prior experience with the object or event, might distinguish those who develop a phobia from those who do not. Studies of fear inoculation in rhesus monkeys [3] and children with dental fears [4] demonstrate that prior experience (e.g. observing a non-fearful model) may "immunize" against the development of a phobia.

---

[1] *Maryland Center for Anxiety Disorders, University of Maryland, College Park, MD 20742, USA*

As these studies illustrate, a cognitive model of negative schemata and distorted expectations surrounding a fearful event or situation is not the only alternative to consider when trying to understand etiological pathways other than direct conditioning. In many instances, conditioning and social learning models still provide a more parsimonious explanation.

In addition to conditioning events, parental anxiety may be a risk factor for the development of phobias in children. In one study, children of parents with anxiety disorders were five times more likely to have an anxiety disorder than children of parents without an anxiety disorder [5]. However, these results do not necessarily need to invoke a genetic explanation. During unstructured, non-conflictual play situations, compared to normal controls, anxious parents remained distant from their children in the play setting. They also reported more worry about their child's engagement in typical child activities such as attending camps or riding a bicycle [6]. Children may perceive parental heightened apprehension and worrying, which, in turn, may influence how they respond to potentially stressful situations.

Among the different available interventions to treat childhood phobias, the strongest support is for those involving exposure to the feared stimulus. In fact, the limited pharmacological data on the treatment of specific phobias in children may result from the overwhelming efficacy of exposure interventions. Consistent with the data, guidelines from the National Institute of Mental Health Research Conference [7] do not support pharmacological interventions for treating specific phobias. Thus, resources may be put to better use in improving the available behavioural interventions.

REFERENCES

1. Stemberger R.T., Turner S.M., Beidel D.C., Calhoun K.S. (1995) Social phobia: an analysis of possible developmental factors. *J. Abnorm. Psychol.*, **104**: 526–531.
2. Mineka S., Zinbarg R. (1995) Conditioning and ethological models of social phobia. In *Social Phobia: Diagnosis, Assessment, and Treatment* (Eds R.G. Heimberg, M.R. Liebowitz, D.A. Hope, F.R. Schneier), pp. 134–162. Guilford Press, New York.
3. Mineka S., Cook, M. (1986) Immunization against the observational conditioning of snake fear in rhesus monkeys. *J. Abnorm. Psychol.*, **95**: 307–323.
4. Melamed B.G., Yurcheson R., Fleece E.L., Hutcherson S., Hawes R. (1978) Effects of film modelling on the reduction of anxiety-related behaviors in individuals varying in level of previous experience in the stress situation. *J. Consult. Clin. Psychol.*, **46**: 1357–1367.
5. Beidel D.C., Turner S.M. (1997) At risk for anxiety: I. Psychopathology in the offspring of anxious parents. *J. Am. Acad. Child Adolesc. Psychiatry*, **36**: 918–924.

6. Turner S.M., Beidel D.B., Roberson-Nay R., Tervo K. (2003) Parenting behaviors in parents with anxiety disorders. *Behav. Res. Ther.*, **41**: 541–554.
7. NIMH Research Conference (1993) Research recommendations for anxiety disorders and ADHD. *J. Am. Acad. Child Adolesc. Psychiatry*, **32**: 1099–1101.

5.5
From Development Fears to Phobias
Sam Tyano and Miri Keren[1]

Ollendick *et al.* provide us with a comprehensive and extended overview of phobias in children and adolescents, including the clinical picture and differential diagnosis, epidemiology and comorbidity, etiology, principles and methods of treatment. In this discussion, we propose to add the dimension of attachment security, first as having a possible role in making a developmental fear into a clinical disorder, such as phobia, and second as an important mediator in psychosocial treatments of phobias, especially in young children.

The link between attachment security and fears is contingent to the key role of anxiety in attachment theory [1,2]. Indeed, by definition, the attachment system is aroused by situations perceived by the child as dangerous; this in turn leads to "attachment behaviours", i.e. a whole set of proximity-seeking behaviours aimed at bringing the child close to the parental figure, supposedly a protective figure. This is a biologically based system aimed at survival, not very far from the concept of "fight or flight" responses to danger. The fear/wariness system describes the human infant's monitoring of and responses to social and non-social fearful cues. Therefore, this system is closely linked to the attachment system through shared activators, as fear is a major activator of the attachment system. As Ollendick *et al.* point out, fear is a normal part of life. As long as we feel basically protected, we find ways to "shake" these fears off, and they do not become phobias.

What makes developmental fears, such as fear of darkness or of snakes, become a phobia? As Ollendick *et al.* point out, the phobic child has "always been afraid of the phobic object", without having necessarily a history of exposure. The understanding of the importance of relational influences on the normal and abnormal development of the child has led to looking at the link between attachment research and clinical disorders [3]. Greenberg [4] as well as Zeanah and Boris [5] have shown the role of

---

[1] *Geha Mental Health Center, Tel-Aviv University Sackler School of Medicine, Petach-Tikvah, 49100 Israel*

attachment theory in the origin, maintenance and remediation of anxiety disorders, social withdrawal and inhibition, childhood depression and conduct disorders. Disturbed caregiving relationships are often one of the etiologic features that, together with other risk factors, contribute to the development of these clinical disorders. In the light of these, one may argue that the parent's reaction to the developmental fear may be one of the factors that determine whether a developmental fear will become a phobia. Parental communication that focuses on the phobic symptom and their concern, reinforcement of dependent and anxious behaviour in the attachment relationship, and maternal anxiety could then impact as mediating factors. Ollendick et al.'s review emphasizes the role of the perception, more than the actual experience, of the stimulus as potentially harmful. No need to say that the younger the child is, the more he/she is dependent on the parental perception of the environment.

In spite of these sound theoretical arguments, no study, to our best knowledge, has specifically looked at the link between the development of phobias and the security of attachment of young children. Interestingly enough, Shear [6] has provided a potential model of the role of attachment in the development of both agoraphobia and panic, in adults though. While waiting for such a study with young phobic children, Ollendick et al.'s report of a study comparing systematic desensitization, psychotherapy and waiting list control may give us a hint about the role of the parental impact on their young child's phobic disorder: contrary to the authors' expectations, the two treatments were found equally effective in reducing phobic behaviours! Their explanation lay in the fact that parents in both groups received training to help manage the children's behaviour, or in more psychodynamic terms, to contain their child's anxiety while exposing them to the feared stimulus. The specific modality of treatment that the child himself/herself received did not matter: both helped. The authors conclude that the parent intervention was a confounding factor. Instead, we suggest understanding their finding as an indirect argument for the crucial mediating role of the child's perception of his/her parent as a protective figure while he/she is exposed to the feared situation. We therefore would suggest adding to the thorough assessment recommended by Ollendick and his colleagues, an evaluation of the quality of the parent–child relationship, including attachment security.

REFERENCES

1. Bowlby J. (1999) *Attachment and Loss*, vol. 2 *Separation*, 2nd edn. Basic Books, New York.

2. Cassidy J. (1995) Attachment and generalized anxiety disorder. In *Rochester Symposium on Developmental Psychopathology*, vol. 6. *Emotion, Cognition and Representation* (Eds D. Cicchetti, S.L. Toth), pp. 343–370. University of Rochester Press, Rochester.
3. Thompson R.A. (2002) Attachment theory and research. In *Child and Adolescent Psychiatry: A Comprehensive Textbook* (Ed. M. Lewis), pp. 164–172. Lippincott Williams & Wilkins, Philadelphia, PA.
4. Greenberg M.T. (1999) Attachment and psychopathology in childhood. In *Handbook of Attachment: Theory, Research and Clinical Applications* (Eds J. Cassidy, P.R. Shaver), pp. 469–496. Guilford Press, New York.
5. Zeanah C.H. Jr, Boris N.W. (2000) Disturbances and disorders of attachment in early childhood. In *Handbook of Infant Mental Health* (Ed. C.H. Zeanah Jr), pp. 353–368. Guilford Press, New York.
6. Shear K.M. (1996) Factors in the etiology and pathogenesis of panic disorder: revising the attachment–separation paradigm. *Am. J. Psychiatry*, **153**: 125–136.

5.6
Assessment and Treatment of Phobic Disorders in Youth

John S. March[1]

Phobic disorders have received less attention than other anxiety disorders in childhood, perhaps because they present less commonly to clinical practitioners. Furthermore, our empirical nomenclature for better or worse is a categorical one, while children live in a dimensional universe where fears of bugs, snakes and the dark may be an intrinsic part of separation anxiety rather than something discrete [1]. Thus, Berkson's bias—the fact that a tendency to identify a disorder is heightened in the presence of comorbidity—may account in part for the differences between the prevalence rates in epidemiological (lower) and clinical (higher) samples.

The DSM-IV probably does not carve nature at developing joints and, as importantly, does not precisely track the hierarchically distributed neural networks that mediate these phenomenon at the level of neural substrate [2]. So, we have much to learn about the reciprocal relationships between fear-based information processes, behaviour and environmental contingencies.

Ollendick *et al.* highlight the importance of linking theory, intervention and outcome. As a statistically minded researcher, I would have preferred to have seen the treatment section of their review framed in terms of a measurement model that distinguishes moderator variables from mediational mechanism [3], since the assertion that empirical demonstration of

---

[1] *Department of Psychiatry and Behavioral Sciences, Duke Child and Family Study Center, 718 Rutherford Street, Durham, NC 27705, USA*

the mechanisms by which treatments work their magic is the centrepiece of the treatment literature is actually not well supported in the adult or paediatric literature. Nowhere is this more true than in the controversy regarding the "active ingredient" of cognitive and behavioural treatments [4]. Since desensitization, the various versions of modelling, and reinforced practice all involve behavioural experiments that are also embedded in the outcome (namely an increase in approach and decrease in escape avoidance behaviours), I would argue that hierarchy-based exposure to the phobic stimulus in the absence of real threat with resultant habituation to the phobic stimulus is common to all our evidence-based interventions. Until we have dismantling studies and mediational research—which are demonstrably hard to do given the primacy of exposure—the role of treatment components and change mechanisms must remain an open question.

In a perfectly evidence-based world, selecting an appropriate treatment regimen for the phobic child from among the many possible options would be reasonably straightforward. In the complex world of clinical practice, choices are rarely so clear cut [5]. Experts often recommend the combination of medication and psychosocial treatment as offering the best chance of normalization, but the hypothesis is only now being tested in the current generation of large comparative treatment trials. Psychosocial treatments usually are combined with medication for one of three reasons. First, in the initial treatment of the severely ill child, two treatments provide a greater "dose" and, thus, may promise a better and perhaps speedier outcome. For this reason, many patients with obsessive–compulsive disorder (OCD) opt for combined treatment even though cognitive-behavioural therapy (CBT) alone may offer equal benefit. Second, comorbidity frequently but not always requires two treatments, since different targets may require different treatments. For example, treating an 8-year-old who has attention-deficit/hyperactivity disorder and mild separation anxiety disorder with a psychostimulant and CBT is a reasonable treatment strategy [6]. Even within a single anxiety disorder, important functional outcomes may vary in response to treatment. For example, anticipatory anxiety in the acutely separation anxious child may be especially responsive to a benzodiazepine, and the critical functional outcome, reintroduction to school, to gradual exposure [7]. Third, in the face of partial response, an augmenting treatment can be added to the initial treatment to improve the outcome in the symptom domain targeted by the initial treatment. For example, CBT can be added to a selective serotonin reuptake inhibitor (SSRI) for OCD to improve OCD-specific outcomes. In an adjunctive treatment strategy, a second treatment can be added to a first one in order to positively impact one or more additional outcome domains. For example, an SSRI can be added to CBT for OCD to handle comorbid depression or panic disorder. Each of these assertions forms a testable hypothesis at a clinical decision node in a stage of treatment framework: initial treatment, partial response, treatment resistance and, not mentioned, maintenance treatment and treatment discontinuation [8].

Looking back from this review to Thomas Ollendick's early work on the assessment and treatment of phobic children [9,10], it is not too strong a statement to say that he and his students gave birth to the study of phobic disorders as an empirical discipline in much the same way that Michael Liebowitz gave birth to social anxiety disorder. While, as is plain for all to see, there are plenty of unanswered questions to keep the next generation of researchers more than busy, the field is indebted to him for pointing us in the right direction.

REFERENCES

1. March J., Parker J., Sullivan K., Stallings P., Conners C. (1997) The Multi-dimensional Anxiety Scale for Children (MASC): factor structure, reliability and validity. *J. Am. Acad. Child Adolesc. Psychiatry*, **36**: 554–565.
2. Pine D.S. (2003) Developmental psychobiology and response to threats: relevance to trauma in children and adolescents. *Biol. Psychiatry*, **53**: 796–808.
3. Kraemer H.C., Wilson G.T., Fairburn C.G., Agras W.S. (2002) Mediators and moderators of treatment effects in randomized clinical trials. *Arch. Gen. Psychiatry*, **59**: 877–883.
4. Foa E.B., Kozak M.J. (1991) Emotional processing: theory, research, and clinical implications for anxiety disorders. In *Emotion, Psychotherapy and Change* (Eds J. Safran, L. Greenberg), pp. 21–49. Guilford Press, New York.
5. March J., Wells K. (2003) Combining medication and psychotherapy. In *Pediatric Psychopharmacology: Principles and Practice* (Eds A. Martin, L. Scahill, D.S. Charney, J.F. Leckman), pp. 326–346. Oxford University Press, London.
6. March J.S., Swanson J.M., Arnold L.E., Hoza B., Conners C.K., Hinshaw S.P., Hechtman L., Kraemer H.C., Greenhill L.L., Abikoff H.B. et al. (2000) Anxiety as a predictor and outcome variable in the multimodal treatment study of children with ADHD (MTA). *J. Abnorm. Child Psychol.*, **28**: 527–541.
7. Kratochvil C.J., Kutcher S., Reiter S., March J. (1999) Pharmacotherapy of pediatric anxiety disorders. In *Handbook of Psychotherapies with Children and Families* (Eds S. Russ, T. Ollendick), pp. 345–366. Plenum Press, New York.
8. March J., Frances A., Kahn D., Carpenter D. (1997) Expert consensus guidelines: treatment of obsessive–compulsive disorder. *J. Clin. Psychiatry*, **58** (Suppl. 4): 1–72.
9. Ollendick T.H. (1983) Reliability and validity of the Revised Fear Surgery Schedule for Children (FSSC-R). *Behav. Res. Ther.*, **21**: 685–692.
10. Ollendick, T.H., Gruen, G.E. (1972) Treatment of a bodily injury phobia with implosive therapy. *J. Consult. Clin. Psychol.*, **38**: 389–393.

5.7
Phobias: From Little Hans to a Bigger Picture
Gordon Parker[1]

Ollendick et al.'s detailed, thoughtful and lucid review invites few challenges or quibbles. It is clear that Freudian interpretations of childhood phobias no longer inform us. For those whose psychiatric education preceded DSM-III, childhood phobias were interpreted as reflecting unconscious oedipal fears, with Freud's Little Hans projecting oedipal thoughts as a fear of horses. Symptom remission required addressing the "real" source of anxiety ("horses for courses" or "courses for horses" paradigms) rather than addressing anxiety *per se*.

Turning to the current review, we are informed that anxiety disorders are more prevalent in girls—but does this hold for all phobias in pre-pubescent groups? If so, why? Is there a differential gender effect across the anxiety disorders? If so, why?

The authors identify but do not speculate on an interesting phenomenon whereby phobic disorders are more likely to be associated with comorbid conditions in clinical than community samples. It may well be that seeking clinical attention is determined more by the "comorbid" condition or by a greater severity associated with multiple coterminous conditions. Irrespective of interpretation, we should suspect that treatment modality and therapeutic success will be influenced by the presence or absence of comorbid disorders.

Etiological considerations by the authors are intriguing and informative. Exposure to conditioning or triggering events does not appear salient (in not being over-represented in phobic children), so that we must presume a weighting to the diathesis factor in any diathesis–stress model. For the seemingly sizeable percentage of children not reporting a specific fear stimulus, a phobic diathesis is again to be suspected. It is disappointing then that the authors judged that any consideration of the intriguing notion of "inherited phobia proneness" was beyond the scope of their review. Treatment is not always informed by etiological knowledge, but the latter is rarely irrelevant.

The authors note work by Kendler and colleagues suggesting that genetic factors have only a modest role in the etiology of phobias. However, expecting close genetic links to state disorders (i.e. phobias) may be unwise. A clearer genetic influence on a broader "upstream" diathesis platform such as "propensity to fearfulness"—as explicated by the authors—is

---

[1] *School of Psychiatry, University of New South Wales, High Street, Randwick 2031, Sydney, Australia*

theoretically more plausible for pursuing genetic underpinning. This leads the authors into consideration of temperament as a vulnerability factor. They note that responses or initial reactions to unfamiliar people and novel situations have variably been described as "shyness versus sociability", "introversion versus extroversion" and "withdrawal versus approach". The possibility that such terms are essentially synonymous is strong. In one of our (unpublished) data sets we have observed strong associations between measures of behavioural inhibition, shyness, introversion and avoidant personality style (presumably trait characteristics) as well as social phobia (putatively a symptom state). Thus, while axis I states and axis II personality styles are conceptually and theoretically worlds apart, an integrative "spectrum concept" may provide a better model for allowing a predispositional temperament bedrock both disposing to and shaping symptomatic phobic avoidance.

The authors reference one paper suggesting that it remains unresolved whether behavioural inhibition is under genetic influence. We have (as yet unreported) data from a twin study suggesting moderate hereditability to both child and adult expression of behavioural inhibition. Whether genetically determined or not, behavioural inhibition is thus a strong candidate for the temperamental bedrock effecting a diathesis to early-onset phobic behaviour. Yet, even if it exerts a direct, powerful and continuing effect, epigenesis allows various surface manifestations and varying expressions over developmental stages. As observed by Rutter and Rutter [1], we must concede that just as a butterfly looks nothing like a caterpillar, "behaviours may change in *form* while still reflecting the same *process*".

Again as noted by the authors, family and developmental influences may modulate any temperament-based shy or sociable style. In a case-controlled Oxford, UK, study [2] using the Parental Bonding Instrument (PBI), socially phobic patients were distinctly more likely to assign their parents to the "affectionless control" quadrant of parental low care/high protection, while agoraphobic patients were more likely to report over-representation of parental "affectionate constraint" (i.e. high care and overprotection). To what extent such parental influences are causal, risk-modifying, iterative or responses to the early expression of vulnerability in children remains unestablished.

The authors' review of psychosocial treatments is highly informative although, as Gertrude Stein might now say, "CBT is CBT is CBT". When they conclude that a variety of behavioural and cognitive-behavioural treatments are effective, few of their detailed treatments appear pure in application. As for lickety-split, so-called "one-session" therapy (so what's the hurry?), most of the identified psychosocial treatments described by the authors are clearly pluralistic and multi-modal.

In terms of the pharmacological interventions, the authors proceed beyond the very limited database and their earlier cautious tone. Whatever gets you well should be continued while, given the "independent promise" of psychosocial and pharmacological acute treatments, they see no reason why "synergistic effects" should not be expected—although research is needed before any "reasonable conclusions can be drawn". Prudence returns, however, in their concluding paragraphs.

In essence, Ollendick *et al.* have produced an informed and informing overview respecting the complexities of the topic.

REFERENCES

1. Rutter M., Rutter M. (1993) *Developing Minds: Challenges and Continuity across the Life Span*. Penguin, Harmondsworth.
2. Parker G. (1979) Reported parental characteristics of agoraphobics and social phobics. *Br. J. Psychiatry*, **135**: 555–560.

5.8
Phobias in Childhood and Adolescence: Implications for Public Policy

E. Jane Costello[1]

In their elegant synthesis of what is known about childhood phobias, Ollendick *et al.* make several points whose significance for policy and public health deserves further emphasis.

First, phobias begin early in life. The National Comorbidity Survey (NCS) of over 8000 people aged 15–54 [1] asked participants for their age at the onset of their first episode of several DSM-III-R phobic disorders. The mean ages were 14.2 (SD 10.1) for simple phobia, 15.0 (SD 8.0) for social phobia and 18.8 (SD 10.1) for agoraphobia (with or without panic disorder). Thus, the majority of phobic individuals reported having their first episode in childhood or adolescence. This makes Ollendick *et al.*'s review perhaps the most important one in this book. Not only will successful treatments for children and adolescents relieve suffering among the young, they may also reduce relapse rates and therefore the number of episodes of phobic disorders throughout the rest of life.

In fact, children and adolescents with phobic disorders may well have had their first episode considerably earlier than suggested by the NCS.

---

[1] *Department of Psychiatry and Behavioral Sciences, Duke University Medical School, Box 3454 DUMC, Durham, NC 27710, USA*

There is a well-known tendency for people, when interviewed about their history of illness of any kind, to forget how early their illness began. In our longitudinal study of mental illness in children and adolescents, the Great Smoky Mountains Study (GSMS) [2], we found that the mean ages of onset for cases of DSM-IV phobia beginning by age 16 were 6.3 (SD 5.2) for specific phobias, 7.3 (SD 4.1) for social phobia and 9.5 (SD 3.6) for agoraphobia (with or without panic). Thus, among children and adolescents with phobic disorders, the majority will have their first episode before puberty.

This raises the question of whether children with phobic disorders will, without treatment, grow up to be phobic adults, or whether the two are different groups of people. Certainly, the idea that children will "grow out of" their early terrors is grounded in folk wisdom and parental experience. Clinicians may tell a different story, but it is dangerous to generalize about the life course of an illness from clinical samples, which tend to be biased in many ways [3,4]. So we need longitudinal studies of phobias in the general population to answer the question.

Unfortunately, such studies have not yet been carried out. The longitudinal studies that cover the period from childhood to adulthood have not yet given us detailed information about individual anxiety disorders. In GSMS we can so far follow subjects only to age 21. We used lagged analyses to test whether the occurrence of a phobic disorder in any wave of the data predicted the same disorder at a later wave. There was no prediction from one episode of specific phobia to another one, and agoraphobia was too rare in childhood to show significant continuity. Social phobia, however, showed strong continuity in girls (odds ratio (OR) 5.2, 95% confidence interval (CI) 1.3–21.6, $p<0.001$), though none in boys. Also, girls with social phobia were highly likely to have had a previous episode of depression (OR 11.2, 95% CI 1.6–77.0, $p<0.05$). These analyses suggest that children were indeed "growing out of" their specific phobias, but that girls with social phobias, in contrast, were likely to show persistent problems.

Ollendick et al.'s review devotes much attention to the effectiveness of a range of treatments for children and adolescents with phobias. This work is very encouraging, and also (and very importantly), it is programmatic. The review makes it quite clear which studies need to be done next, and which are the most promising areas of exploration for both pharmaceutical and behavioural treatments. But there are two aspects to successful treatment: it has to work, and it has to be available to those who need it. The review places emphasis on the first aspect, but the other is equally important.

How many children with phobic disorders actually receive treatment? In GSMS, only 29% of children with a history of phobias had *ever* seen a mental health professional, and we cannot say whether that contact was for treatment of phobia. This means that the children who reached the clinics that might have conducted the studies reviewed in Ollendick et al.'s paper represent only one in three of the children in the community who suffer from phobias.

In summary, everything that we know makes the case for the importance of *early* identification and treatment of phobias. As we learn more about them, it becomes ever more clear that early attention to these debilitating problems is necessary if we are to prevent suffering and disability that can sometimes last a lifetime.

REFERENCES

1. Kessler R.C., McGonagle K.A., Zhao S., Nelson C.B., Hughes M., Eshleman S., Wittchen H.U., Kendler K.S. (1994) Lifetime and 12-month prevalence of DSM-III-R psychiatric disorders in the United States: results from the National Comorbidity Study. *Arch. Gen. Psychiatry*, 51: 8–19.
2. Costello E.J., Angold A., Burns B.J., Stangl D.K., Tweed D.L., Erkanli A., Worthman C.M. (1996) The Great Smoky Mountains Study of Youth: goals, designs, methods, and the prevalence of DSM-III-R disorders. *Arch. Gen. Psychiatry*, 53: 1129–1136.
3. Berkson J. (1946) Limitations of the application of fourfold table analysis to hospital data. *Biometrics Bull.*, 2: 47–52.
4. Kleinbaum D.G., Kupper L.L., Morgenstern H. (1982) *Epidemiologic Research: Principles and Quantitative Methods*. Van Nostrand Reinhold, New York.

5.9
Phobias in Children and Adolescents: Data from Brazil

Heloisa H.A. Brasil[1] and Isabel A.S. Bordin[2]

Findings from population-based studies reveal that childhood phobias are moderately stable and relatively "pure". However, in clinical samples, comorbidity with other psychiatric disorders tends to be more common among phobic children. Since most of the data available in the literature come from industrialized countries, we consider this a great opportunity to present some unpublished data on phobias from two Brazilian studies.

In a consecutive sample of children and adolescents (6–14 years) scheduled for first appointment at the mental health outpatient clinic of the Federal University of Rio de Janeiro ($n = 78$, response rate $= 75\%$), rates of specific phobia (16.7%) and social phobia (11.5%) were obtained based on DSM-IV criteria [1]. Eleven types of specific phobias were identified, and

---

[1] *Instituto de Psiquiatria, Universidade Federal do Rio de Janeiro, Brazil*
[2] *Departamento de Psiquiatria, Universidade Federal de São Paulo, Brazil*

the most common situations were fear of heights (46.1%), seeing blood (38.5%) and being in the dark (30.8%). Interestingly, a great number of children (69.2%) had more than one type of specific phobia, and fears of animals, including insects, were less frequent (23.1%). Although the median age of the total sample was 10 years, 77.0% of children with specific phobia and 77.8% of children with social phobia were older than 9 years. As expected, a lower rate of specific phobia was reported in a population sample of Brazilian children of similar age. In a stratified community sample of children from the southeast region of Brazil ($n = 1251$, 7–14 years), the prevalence rate of simple (i.e. specific) phobia was 1.0% (confidence interval 95% = 0.29–1.80) [2].

In the Brazilian clinical sample, 23.1% of children with specific phobia and 22.2% of children with social phobia did not meet criteria for other psychiatric disorders. Considering the group of children with specific phobia, 69.2% had more than one type of specific phobia, 69.2% had at least one other anxiety disorder, 38.5% had attention deficit hyperactivity disorder and 15.4% were diagnosed with a disruptive disorder. It is noteworthy that 30.8% of children with specific phobia also had social phobia, and 44.4% of children with social phobia also had specific phobia.

Although there was distress and/or intense anxiety due to specific or social phobias in the Brazilian clinical sample, referrals were usually motivated by the presence of comorbidity. Children were better informants of phobic symptoms than mothers, who tended to minimize their impact on the child's functioning.

In the Brazilian clinical sample, the Child Behavior Checklist (CBCL) identified high rates of internalizing (68.0%) and externalizing behaviour problems (60.3%). "Pure" internalizing (23.1%) and "pure" externalizing cases (15.4%) were less frequent than cases with both types of behaviour problems (44.9%) [1].

Ollendick *et al.* review in detail different behavioural and cognitive-behavioural procedures used to treat phobic disorders in youth. Effective psychotherapy procedures according to randomized clinical trials and pharmacological interventions are discussed. However, future research is needed to clarify the usefulness of a variety of interventions in different settings and cultures. Effective short-time interventions would be of special interest for mental health outpatient clinics in world regions where financial resources are very scarce.

REFERENCES

1. Brasil H.H.A. (2003) Development of the Brazilian version of K-SADS-PL and study of its psychometrics properties. Doctoral thesis, Department of Psychiatry, Universidade Federal de São Paulo, Escola Paulista de Medicina.

2. Fleitlich-Bilyk B.W. (2002) The prevalence of psychiatric disorders in 7–14 year olds in the South East of Brazil. Doctoral thesis, Department of Child and Adolescent Psychiatry, Institute of Psychiatry, University of London.

5.10
Phobias: A View from the South Seas
John Scott Werry[1]

The main message to take from Ollendick et al.'s review is how comparatively little interest anxiety disorders in general and phobias in particular in children have attracted until recently. One might well ask why, given that in the period 1920–1939 there was more interest in what we would now call internalizing disorders than in externalizing ones. It will be recalled for example that the mental hygiene movement was obsessed with the shy withdrawn child, in sharp contrast to the staggering absorption of the past thirty years with attention-deficit/hyperactivity disorder. Interestingly, it is not just phobias that have lost favour to the stellar attention-deficit/hyperactivity disorder, but also conduct disorder, despite its huge cost to society and its oblique presentation in psychiatric clinics as comorbid disorders (including anxiety disorders).

Part of this neglect is the equally worrying lack of good studies of treatment. Only behaviour therapy seems to have provided any usable information here and even that is too scant to be sheeted home as definitive. This situation is little different from that of psychotherapy with children in general. Despite this lack of evidence for psychotherapies other than behavioural types, they continue to be taught and practised widely, leaving any consumer wondering what is wrong with child psychiatry and child psychology that it can tolerate such disdain for evidence of efficacy, efficiency and safety. Some of this no doubt stems from Freud's intolerance of dissent and insistence on the apostolic method of transmission, but in the 21st century funders of services should be more insistent on proof and not simply shell out monies for the modern equivalent of bleeding and purging.

I do not know for sure but I suspect that, in the US at least, pharmacotherapy is a front line of treatment for phobias and, dare I say it, I often use it myself, though the results are in general disappointing. It is sad to see this treatment as deficient in controlled trials as psychotherapy and, given that such trials are on the whole much better established as *de rigueur* for pharmacotherapy, we must ask why. Some of the problem lies with

---
[1] 19 Edenvale Crescent, Mt. Eden, Auckland 1003, New Zealand

pharmaceutical companies, which usually exclude children because they have not done the studies in this group required for approval. This is partly because of economics, as the market is perceived as not worth the trouble, and partly due to the lack of sufficient investigators in child and adolescent psychiatry. Whatever the cause, children and adolescents are often cut off from developments in pharmacotherapy and those of us not cowed by the threat of litigation are forced to use extrapolation from adult studies. We all know that such extrapolation without trial is hazardous, as target systems in the brain are immature and less often pharmacokinetics also show notable differences. In the end, children and adolescents are shut out and discriminated against.

The only other comment I would like to make is that in Ollendick *et al.*'s review there is no mention of Asperger's disorder as an important differential diagnosis to consider in children and adolescents who have marked social phobic anxiety. These patients often get diagnosed as having attention-deficit/hyperactivity disorder, but giving them stimulants which does help their hyperactivity may aggravate their phobic and other anxiety. For some reason, Asperger's disorder has attracted even less good research in treatment than phobic disorders, though assertions and evanescent miracle cures abound.

All this leads a reviewer to conclude that though most countries boast about their children and youth being their future and how much they value them, in reality, children and youth come a very poor second to narcissistic old men who eat too much, smoke too much, drink too much and exercise too little and whose health problems and other self-indulgences take from children and adolescents what is rightfully theirs.

CHAPTER

6

Social and Economic Burden of Phobias: A Review

Koen Demyttenaere, Ronny Bruffaerts and Andy De Witte
Department of Psychiatry, University Hospital Gasthuisberg, Herestraat 49, B-3000 Leuven, Belgium

INTRODUCTION

According to the *Global Burden of Disease* survey [1], anxiety disorders and major depression will be the most prevalent and disabling mental disorders by the year 2020. Among anxiety disorders, phobias are very common and place a significant burden on patients, family, caregivers and providers of health services. Although phobic symptoms may be temporarily reduced by selective avoidance of fearful situations, untreated phobias are unremitting and chronic, and this magnifies their long-term psychosocial and economic burden [2].

Despite the increased clinical and scientific attention, phobias are still largely under-recognized in primary care and more specialized clinical settings [3–5]. Of those who are diagnosed with a phobic disorder, only a minority seek treatment for their mental problems [6]. Phobic complaints are also viewed as trivial clinical conditions by several mental health professionals [2]. Prevalence rates of phobias have therefore been largely underestimated. It is only recently, in the Epidemiologic Catchment Area (ECA) study [7] and the National Comorbidity Survey (NCS) [8], that prevalence rates of phobias have become more accurate. Moreover, it is only since the introduction of the DSM-III that phobias were delineated into major and discrete categories and thus more likely to be the subject of theoretical and clinical research [6].

Nowadays, lifetime prevalence estimates of any phobia vary from around 10.0% to 13.0% [9]. Magee *et al.* [10] found lifetime prevalence rates of 11% and 13% for simple and social phobia, respectively, and 7% for

---

Phobias. Edited by Mario Maj, Hagop S. Akiskal, Juan José López-Ibor and Ahmed Okasha.
©2004 John Wiley & Sons Ltd: ISBN 0-470-85833-8

agoraphobia. In a Canadian community sample, Offord *et al.* [11] reported one-year prevalence rates of 6.7%, 6.4% and 1.6% for social phobia, simple phobia and agoraphobia, respectively. In recent community research, estimated lifetime prevalence rates for phobias are as high as 13–18% [3,12].

Until recently, little attention has been paid to the epidemiology of phobias in clinical settings. In the few available studies, phobias were found to be widespread in clinical settings, for example up to 8% current prevalence for any phobia [13]. Other recent studies found a current prevalence estimate of 8% and 14% lifetime prevalence in primary healthcare clinics [2,4].

One should also take into account that the prevalence of phobic disorders varies largely depending on the threshold used to determine distress or impairment and the number of types of possible phobic situations [14]. For instance, prevalence studies seldom investigate the concept of "clinical significance", one of the main inclusion criteria of many DSM disorders [15]. Indeed, despite the predominance of this criterion in diagnosing mental disorders, it is seldom assessed in surveys.

Due to the dramatic change in the organization and provision of mental health care over the past two decades, attention has been called to cost-effective solutions and decisions in organizing and delivering mental health services. It is argued that decision making should be grounded in a more rational, efficient and scientific evidence-based utilization of (limited) mental health resources [16]. The increasing awareness of the prevalence and clinical significance of phobias has emphasized the need for information on the clinical impairment associated with these disorders. The under-recognition, undertreatment and suboptimal mental health service use of people suffering from phobic disorders raise the question to what extent these disorders have an economic impact on the management of a mental health care delivery system. This confluence of events has called attention to the need for information on the personal, social, societal and economic burden of phobias. By reviewing the available evidence on this burden, clinicians and health care administrators can make decisions and recommendations that are appropriate, rational, effective and evidence-based in the management of phobias.

THE USE OF HEALTH SERVICES IN PHOBIAS

Despite the widespread availability of effective treatment for phobias, only a minority of subjects suffering from these disorders receive adequate treatment. Among major mental disorders, only substance abuse disorders have lower treatment rates [17]. In the ECA study, about 17% of the respondents with a phobic disorder reported a mental health outpatient visit in the last year [6]. Of those phobic individuals from the ECA study who sought professional help, about 70% did so for physical health reasons solely [6]. In only 5–6% of social phobics without comorbid depression, psychological problems were the main reason for seeking help [4,17,18]. Somewhat higher rates of help seeking were found by Wittchen *et al.* [19], who found that about one in five social phobics sought professional help for their emotional problems.

Determinants of Service Use

Help-seeking behaviour has been found to be dependent upon different factors: sociodemographic characteristics, the type of phobia, the presence of comorbid mental disorders, and, in the case of social phobia, generalized conditions.

Social phobics who seek help are more likely to be older, of higher socio-economic status, more educated, white and divorced or separated [17,20].

Investigating the data obtained in the NCS (Figure 6.1), Magee *et al.* [10] found that individuals with agoraphobia were more likely to seek help (41.0%), compared to individuals with simple (30.2%) and social (19.0%) phobia. Individuals with agoraphobia were also more likely to be taking medication (21.6%), compared to individuals with simple (6.0%) or social (6.2%) phobia. Comparable with these results, agoraphobia appeared to have the highest rate of service use, followed by social and simple phobia

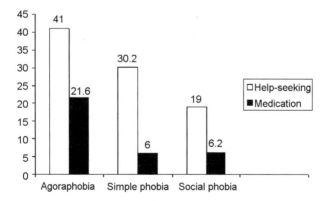

Figure 6.1 Help seeking and use of medication in agoraphobia, simple phobia and social phobia. Reproduced from Magee *et al.* [10] by permission of the American Medical Association

[21]. Friends and relatives were the main sources of help seeking, although phobic complaints are not the main reason for seeking help [5,22]. About 36% sought help of friends or relatives and non-psychiatric medical doctors. Private psychotherapists, clergy and social service agencies were consulted by 16–17% of social phobic individuals. A remarkable finding was, however, that only about 3–5% of individuals with pure social phobia sought outpatient psychiatric help [5,17].

The proportion of individuals seeking treatment is also dependent upon the presence of comorbid mental disorders. This has a considerable impact on help seeking, for example leading to an increase of 10% of the amount spent on utilization of services and an increase of about 25% of the number of outpatient visits [2]. Patel *et al.* [23] investigated five different sources of help seeking in individuals with social phobia. They found that, for every source investigated, social phobics with comorbid mental disorders, compared to those without such comorbidity, consulted more inpatient services (20.6% versus 1.8%), had more outpatient episodes (61.7% versus 53.1%), had more home visits by health and social services (19.5% versus 2.1%) had more therapy contacts (13.0% versus 6.6%) and finally had more contacts with general practitioners in the 12 months preceding the interview (37.1% versus 19.0%). Moreover, a statistical interaction between the presence of a comorbid disorder on the one hand and the source of help seeking on the other was not found: medical doctors were more likely to be consulted (13.3%) than other mental health professionals (8.9%), independent of the presence of a comorbid mental disorder. Similar results were obtained by Schneier *et al.* [17] and Davidson *et al.* [22]. These findings are very similar to those of Wittchen *et al.* [19] (Figure 6.2), who reported that the mean proportion of help-seeking individuals was significantly higher in the comorbid than in the pure condition of social phobia (28.0% versus 12.3%). The finding that comorbidity increases the odds of help-seeking behaviour does not, however, imply better management and outcome of the phobic disorder. Indeed, the presence of a comorbid disorder may obscure the identification of social phobia as such, and thus blur accurate recognition and treatment by the health professional. This conclusion, however, should be interpreted with great caution, since studies investigating the reasons for help seeking in social phobia with comorbidity remain somewhat indecisive on this topic. While some authors suggest that comorbidity leads to higher odds of reporting other complaints than the phobia [18], others conclude that phobic complaints are more likely to be reported when a comorbid disorder is present [4,19].

The proportion of individuals seeking help also varied upon generalized versus non-generalized forms of social phobia. The lowest mean proportion of help-seeking behaviour was found in non-generalized forms of social phobia (Figure 6.2): about 13% of persons with non-generalized social

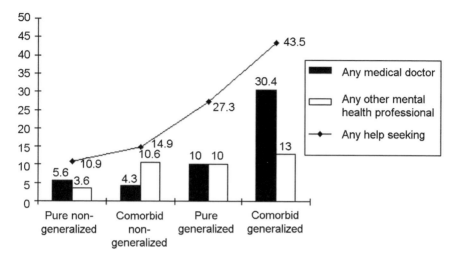

Figure 6.2 Proportion of help seeking in individuals with social phobia. Reproduced from Wittchen et al. [19] by permission of Cambridge University Press

phobia sought help in the six months preceding the interview, compared to slightly more than 40% in the generalized social phobia condition. Moreover, although we may say that generalized social phobia as well as the presence of a comorbid mental disorder may increase the odds of help seeking, it does so only for seeking help of medical doctors and not of non-medical mental health professionals [19].

Barriers to Treatment

The systemic model of Goldberg and Huxley [24] has been successful in identifying obstructions to help-seeking and inappropriate service use. Their model conceptualizes help-seeking pathways as a progression through a serious of levels, each separated by permeable filters. For example, starting from community-based prevalence rates (level 1), decreasing proportions of individuals make progress to the filter of primary care (level 2), conspicuous primary care morbidity (level 3), formal mental health services (level 4) and psychiatric inpatient care (level 5). A way of viewing the problem of a low service use is thus to consider various "hurdles" on the path from level 1 to level 5. Following this systemic model, it is conceivable that an optimal use of services is hampered by patient and doctor filtering barriers.

Patient-Filtering Barriers to Treatment

A recent study by Olfson et al. [5] investigated treatment barriers relating to social phobia. The authors simply asked individuals why they did not seek treatment for their problems. About one in five reported that "fear of what others might think" was a major barrier to treatment, since that is the core problem of social phobia. Furthermore, more than one in four individuals with social phobia was not seeking help because they "could handle the situation on their own". The finding that self-management is preferred over professional treatment is in line with findings from other studies [25–27]. Another hurdle is that phobic individuals are not likely to interpret their emotional problems in mental health terms [28]. Following the early age of onset, phobic behaviour can therefore be interpreted as a normal behavioural standard and not as deviating. Phobic patients often see their phobic complaints as caused by cautiousness rather than a mental disorder [10]. It looks as if the majority of individuals suffering from phobic disorders may have learned to live with their phobic fears and consider their lifestyle as normal, since it is the presence of a comorbid disorder (e.g. depression, other anxiety disorders or substance use disorders) that urges the individual to seek help. In this light, psychoeducation should be essential in dealing with the phobic patient [3]. In this light, we can also explain the finding that the proportion of help-seeking varies considerably depending upon the type of phobia. That agoraphobics have the highest rate of help-seeking behaviour could be explained by the hypothesis that these individuals are more likely to interpret their problems in mental health terms, for example because the age of onset of agoraphobia is much later in life than that of simple and social phobia [10].

A second barrier to treatment of phobic disorders lies in financial obstructions. As Olfson et al. [5] pointed out, a significant proportion of social phobic individuals reported that a lack of insurance (17%) and an inability to afford treatment (25%) were main reasons for not seeking professional help for their phobic complaints. However, the finding that economic considerations are barriers to treatment is questionable. Indeed, these findings were not supported by the German Early Developmental Stages of Psychopathology (EDSP) study [19]. The treatment rate was not dependent upon financial considerations such as inability to afford treatment, since the German health care system offers almost everybody free health care.

A third factor that may be a barrier to seeking help for phobic disorders is the lack of information about available treatment services. Almost 40% of the respondents who screened positive for social phobia said that "being unsure where to go for help" was the main reason for not seeking help [5]. In line with previous studies [22,29], we suggest that an increased awareness of social phobia may yield an increased knowledge of possible treatment services in the society.

Doctor-Filtering Barriers to Treatment

Poor recognition and referral are to some extent understandable, since most general practitioners have had little formal psychiatric training and have had their training in settings where emotional problems were of minor attention [28]. Many general practitioners are also likely to attribute social phobic complaints to nothing more than an extreme form of shyness [18]. They might also fear alienating patients if a mental disorder is diagnosed. It is therefore conceivable that general practitioners do not inquire systematically into the mental status of the patient presenting with somatic symptoms [18]. Moreover, most consultations in a general practice last about 15 minutes, and different problems are often presented. It is understandable that emotional problems are considered rather late in a consultation [28]. The topic of educating general practitioners in order to improve the interface with specialized mental health facilities has been the subject of much discussion in the literature [30,31]. It was found that the recognition of mental disorders in a general practice will be more accurate when the general practitioner adopts an empathic style, is trying to address psychological issues in the interview with the patient, and tries to avoid closed-ended questions and interrupting the patient [28].

THE BURDEN OF PHOBIAS

Phobias often lead to serious functional impairment in different areas of daily life. Numerous epidemiological studies, both in the general population and in clinical samples [2,10,12,17], have clearly shown that phobic disorders do not merely exact personal costs from persons who experience the disorder, but also impose costs on their environment (e.g. family members and communities) in terms of finances, social role functioning, disability and quality of life. Phobias may interfere with the normal development of social and personal relationships, and may thus have a long-term effect on the social, familial and working lives of sufferers. By disrupting schooling in adolescence, a time when social skills and academic attainment are of particular importance, the disorder limits educational training and career progression. Throughout the working lives of patients, continuing functional impairment also has an economic impact, reflected in the loss of working days due to illness and reduced work performance. Productivity is significantly reduced in at least one third of subjects with social phobia. Demographic data show that people with social phobia are less likely to be in the highest socio-economic group and have lower employment rates and household income compared to those with no psychiatric history [23].

The burden of phobias can be subdivided into three major areas. Direct costs include the expenses of treatment (medication, hospitalization, physician and nursing fees). Indirect costs include effects on work productivity, hourly wages, educational attainment and occupational choice of phobic patients. The concept of health-related quality of life refers to role functioning, sexual functioning, substance abuse, suicidality and daily impairments.

Direct Costs

In a report of the US National Advisory Mental Health Council (NAMHC), it is estimated that the 1990 total cost (direct and indirect and related costs) for all mental disorders was US$148 billion. For severe mental disorders (schizophrenia, bipolar disorder, major depression, anxiety disorders), it was US$74 billion. Four per cent of the total US direct health care costs are represented by these severe mental disorders [32]. Several cost-of-illness studies showed that all anxiety disorders have been estimated to cost $46.6 billion annually in the US [33]. These economic costs are higher than any other class of mental disorder and consume 30% of the money allocated for mental health in the United States. The annual cost of anxiety disorders in 1990 was estimated at approximately $42.3 billion (the contributions of generalized anxiety disorder and other anxiety disorders were not specified) [21]. Hospitalization is associated with the greatest direct cost and pharmacological therapy is a marginal contributor to overall costs [34].

In the Australian model used by Andrews [35], the total direct treatment costs of all anxiety disorder cases was approximately the same as that for all the schizophrenia cases. Although the cases of schizophrenia cost four times as much as anxiety disorders to treat (A$9700 per schizophrenia case versus A$2600 per anxiety disorder case), the prevalence of anxiety disorders is much greater than that of schizophrenia. Moreover, UK researchers Croft-Jeffreys and Wilkinson [36] estimated the total direct and indirect cost of all neuroses in UK general practice to be £373 million in 1984–85.

The use and the costs of medical resources of individuals with social phobia are higher compared to those of people without this condition, particularly in individuals with a comorbid condition. In the ECA survey, about 50% of the individuals with a social phobia with a comorbid condition attended an outpatient facility compared with only 15% of the non-affected population [17]. Total annual average health care costs were found to increase from £379 in a psychiatrically well population to £452 in individuals with pure social phobia, and almost doubled in those with social phobia and a comorbid disorder (£752), for the following sources investigated: costs of general practitioner (GP) visits, costs of inpatient and outpatient treatment, and costs of home visits [23].

In another interesting study, Katzelnick et al. [2] investigated the costs associated with social phobia in a managed care setting. For a 12-month period preceding the study, they investigated the number of ambulatory outpatient visits as well as the actual dollar amount spent on medical care of subjects with generalized social phobia, subjects with pure major depression and subjects with no diagnosis. In general, subjects with generalized social phobia, compared to subjects with pure major depression, have a similar number of annual outpatient visits and dollar amount spent (Figure 6.3). In more detail, persons with pure generalized social phobia spent about $2536 per year on total healthcare utilization, whereas the expenditure of patients with pure major depression was $3132 per year. Another important issue that needs to be addressed is the finding that contacts with the medical system are often unsatisfactory and patients may seek therapy on a number of separate occasions without receiving appropriate treatment for the primary, underlying cause. This has

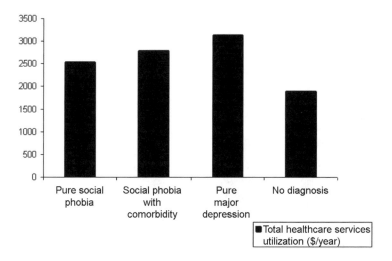

Figure 6.3 Healthcare service utilization of subjects with pure social phobia, social phobia with comorbid psychopathology and pure major depression, and people with no diagnosis. Reproduced from Katzelnick et al. [2] by permission of the American Psychiatric Association

important health cost implications, with significantly higher costs for general practitioner contacts [37].

Indirect Costs

It is obvious that the consequences of phobic disorders are far-reaching and likely related to wider personal and societal short- and long-term costs, such as low educational attainment, decreased work productivity, work impairment, economic inactivity and financial dependency. Another consistent finding is that indirect costs are significantly higher in comorbid cases of social phobia [2,19,38]. Due to the early age of onset, it is not surprising that the presence of a phobic condition is associated with academic difficulties. In general, we may say that phobia is consistently related to a lower educational attainment, compared to individuals without a phobic disorder. For example, higher social phobia severity scores (as measured with the Liebowitz Social Anxiety Scale, LSAS) were significantly associated with a lower probability of earning a college degree, and being in a managerial, technical or professional occupation (Figure 6.4) [23]. Or, viewed from a different angle, every 10-point decrease of the LSAS was related to a 1.8% lower probability of graduating from college [2]. Although no considerable differences were found in the highest educational attainment between those with social phobia and those without, fewer individuals with social phobia were of the highest socio-economic status [23].

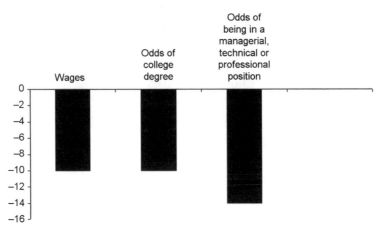

Figure 6.4 Percentage difference in wages, the odds of earning a college degree, and the odds of being in a managerial, technical or professional position between individuals with and without social phobia. Reproduced from Patel *et al.* [23] by permission of Elsevier

The presence of social phobia has also been associated with a range of work difficulties, such as decreased productivity, lower employment rates and financial dependency. Using the baseline data of the EDSP study, young people (aged between 14 and 24 years old) with social phobia had a significantly decreased work productivity: about 28% of the cases were not able to perform as normal in at least two days of the month preceding the interview [19]. Disability days were especially increased in social phobia with a depressive comorbid disorder [38]. Social phobics were also repeatedly late or absent [22]. Decreased work productivity was not limited to young age alone, as Patel et al. [23] have clearly shown in their secondary analysis of the 1994–95 Surveys of Psychiatric Morbidity, a community-based epidemiological study in Britain. It was striking that a significant proportion reported missing work as a direct result of social phobic complaints. For example, 16% reported that they took between 14 and 27 days in the past year, and, somewhat surprisingly, this figure was more pronounced in those with pure social phobia. It was also found that about 25% of all social phobics reported that they had quit a job in the past year, due to emotional, mental or nervous problems, compared to only 5% in those without psychiatric disorders [23].

The highest percentage of work impairment was found in social phobia with a comorbid disorder (ranging between 34% and 43%), followed by cases with pure social phobia (about 17%) [2,19]. These proportions were significantly increased, compared with a non-phobic population (about 10%), but lower than the percentage work impairment in pure major depression (about 38%). Different domains of work productivity used in the 1999 Wittchen et al. study have been soldered together in the Work Productivity Index, focusing on work productivity in the past seven days [39]. Their results were similar to those of their previous study [19], but they also revealed that the presence of a comorbid disorder yielded a higher level of long-term unemployment. There was also agreement upon the relationship between the presence of comorbidity and the proportion of economic inactivity.

Independently from comorbid disorders, it can be said that social phobia is strongly associated with lower rates of employment. Not even one in three was employed full-time, about one in five was unemployed, and about 40% of all social phobics were economically inactive [23]. In this light, the presence of social phobia was also associated with financial dependency and lower household income [17,23,40]. These people were also found to be repeatedly fired [22]. For example, about one in five individuals with pure or comorbid social phobia appeared to be on social welfare at the moment of the study, compared with only 10.6% of those without a disorder. There was, however, no difference in financial dependency between pure and comorbid social phobia.

Health-Related Quality of Life

Despite the high prevalence found for phobic disorders, only a few studies concentrate specifically on aspects of the quality of life in phobia. In large part this might be due to the long-standing truism that the costs of human suffering simply cannot be measured. However, this truism might no longer be accurate since, throughout decades, a certain degree of consensus has been developed with regard to the concept of quality of life [41]. This does not imply that the relationship between phobic disorders and associated quality of life can be assessed easily. An accurate measurement is mainly obstructed by, first, a lack of well-defined psychometrically validated scales for systematic evaluation of the burden of phobic disorders [42]. In the case of social phobia, most rating scales focus on particular symptoms rather than effects caused by the disease [43]. Second, the lack of systematic studies on the quality of life of phobia sufferers has also to do with the nature of the concept itself. Studying impairment, burden and costs of phobias could be approached in several ways. In a holistic perspective, one should not only focus on clinical severity of a particular disorder, but also take into account impairments that might cause behavioural dysfunctions ("disabilities"). Moreover, when effects of phobias are assessed from the perspective of subjective well-being, the quality of life is measured as perceived by the persons themselves. In short, we can conclude that different measures with different thresholds are currently applied with regard to the assessment of quality of life in phobias. It is therefore obvious to conclude that there is no "gold standard" for assessing costs and burden or associated symptom severity of phobias. As shown in Table 6.1, instruments could be systematically subdivided according to generic and specific domains that are assessed, such as clinical severity, functional disability and quality of life [44–46]. Moreover, some of the measures are self-rated while others are rated by the clinician. Consequently, it is almost redundant to say that the widespread availability and use of different rating scales hamper accurate measurement of quality of life.

Anyhow, from a clinical point of view, it is understandable that the quality of life in individuals with phobia is significantly impaired. First, the considerable comorbidity of phobia is in itself a significant impairing factor of individuals suffering from this condition. Second, the reported young age of onset (ranging between 10 and 15 years) places an additional burden on the quality of life. It has been proposed that the early age of onset may develop a nidus around which other pathological processes and complications can be formed [22]. The early onset of phobia may thus interfere with the development of personal, sexual, social and intellectual functioning.

TABLE 6.1 Rating scales measuring quality of life, disability and impairment in phobic disorders (adapted from Bobes [45] by permission of Physicians Postgraduate Press, Inc.)

Clinical severity
Generic measures
  Clinical Global Impression—Severity of Illness Scale*
  Clinical Global Impression—Improvement Scale*
  Hamilton Rating Scale for Anxiety*
  Hamilton Rating Scale for Depression*
Specific measures
  Liebowitz Social Anxiety Scale*
  Social Avoidance and Distress Scale*
  Fear Questionnaire**
  Duke Brief Social Phobia Scale**
  Social Phobia and Anxiety Inventory**
Functional disability
Generic measures
  Global Assessment of Functioning*
  Social and Occupational Functioning Assessment Scale*
  World Health Organization Disability Assessment, Schedule 2*
  Sheehan Disability Scale*
  Disability Profile*
  Quality of Life Enjoyment and Satisfaction Questionnaire**
  Quality of Life Index**
Specific measures
  Liebowitz Self-Rated Disability Scale**
  Reilly Work Productivity and Impairment Questionnaire**
Quality of life
Generic measures
  World Health Organization Quality of Life—100**
  World Health Organisation Quality of Life—BREF**
  Quality of Life Interview**
  Wisconsin Quality of Life Index**
  Quality of Life Inventory**
  Short Form 36-Items Scale*
  Short Form 12-Items Scale*

*Clinician-rated
**self-rated

Functioning and Impairment

Phobias in general place a considerable obstacle in the way of regular social interactions with others. When looking at different types of phobic disorders, agoraphobic individuals appear to have the least perceived role impairment (about 26%), whereas individuals with simple or social phobia are more likely to report role impairment (about 33%) [10]. This finding could in part be related to the most common age of onset of social phobia, mid-adolescence, interfering with the development of social skills in puberty and adolescence [19,22,47]. The effect of early experiences of illness may adversely influence the ongoing psychological and social development, especially the formation of intimate relationships. The consequences of this interference are reflected in the finding that phobic individuals are more likely to have dysfunctional relationships compared to normal individuals. Social phobics reported current impairment in social contacts and the relationship with the partner [19]. This figure was even more elevated in the presence of a comorbid disorder (26.7%), and even more when individuals suffered from a generalized form of social phobia (39.1%). Role impairment was also reflected in the finding that social phobia is related to having fewer social contacts and friends. Almost 30% of social phobic individuals were never married, compared to 21% of individuals without social phobia [23]. Social phobics were almost twice as likely to be divorced compared to normal subjects (11.2% versus 6.0%). These findings were, however, countered by Weiller et al. [4], who did not find differences in marital status in social phobics and normal individuals. Moreover, social phobic individuals are almost three times more likely to have feelings of dissatisfaction with their family life (odds ratio, $OR = 2.8$; confidence interval, $CI = 1.71–4.46$) and almost six times more likely to have these feelings with friends ($OR = 5.9$; $CI = 2.5–14.2$) [12]. Similar results were obtained by Katzelnick et al. [2]. It has also been suggested that children of parents with social phobia have increased odds for developing psychiatric disorders in their lives [48]. This disaffiliative behaviour may lead to one of the core problems of dysfunctional social relationships in social phobia: the inability to initiate and maintain intimate and romantic relationships [49,50]. The impaired social life may also become part of a vicious circle, in which difficulties with phobic and/or social situations make it difficult to develop new social relationships or meet new potential partners.

Schneier et al. [43] examined the nature of impairment of functioning in persons with social phobia. Impairment and disability caused by the phobia symptoms were assessed using the (clinician-rated) Disability Profile and the (self-rated) LSAS. Both the current (in the past 2 weeks) and most severe (lifetime) impairment caused by the social phobia symptoms were investigated. A common finding was that, for more than 50% of the subjects, social phobia was associated with at least moderate impairment in mood regulation, whereas activities such as personal care and shopping were less reported. The highest level of disability was found in individuals with comorbid social phobia, followed by individuals with pure major depression, individuals with pure social phobia and normal controls [2]. Furthermore, social phobics with a comorbid major depression reported over twice as many disability days in the past 30 days (5.4), compared to normal individuals (2.3) [38]. This finding is conceivable since social phobics were more depressed than normals, independent of the presence of a comorbid disorder. Comparing individuals with social phobia to patients with a chronic physical illness (i.e. chronic herpes infection), those with social phobia were more likely to be markedly impaired, as assessed by the Short Form-12 [51].

Sexual Functioning

In investigating the presence of sexual dysfunctions in social phobics, Leary and Dobbins [49] pointed to the fact that social phobics may be at risk for being involved in fewer relationships that include a sexual dimension. A more recent contribution was made by Figueira et al. [52]. Using the Structural Clinical Interview for DSM-IV [53], they retrospectively investigated the sexual function in male and female patients who attended the Anxiety and Depression Program of the Federal University of Rio de Janeiro. The following characteristics of sexual functioning were assessed in patients who were diagnosed with either social phobia or panic disorder: virginal status, age of first sexual relationship, with whom they had this first relationship, frequency of intercourse, masturbatory practices, current presence of sexual partner, sexual orientation, and occurrence of panic attacks during sexual intercourse. Compared to normal controls and individuals with any panic disorder, it is striking that social phobia is more likely to have a greater negative impact on sexual functioning, especially in male patients. About one in three male social phobics did not have a sexual partner at the time of the study, and 58% had their first sexual experience with a prostitute. Another finding was that 48% reported having (had) premature ejaculation. This figure was considerably increased compared to the prevalence of premature ejaculation both in community (about 21%) [54] and clinical (about 30%) [55] studies.

Suicidality

Suicidal thoughts and suicidal behaviour are often present in individuals with phobias. Suicide rates (suicide attempts and completed suicides) were found to be significantly increased in individuals with social phobia [5,17,56,57], in some cases as common as in depression [2]. In the data from the National Anxiety Disorders Screening Day ($n = 10\,637$), about 22% of those with social phobia had (had) thoughts of committing suicide in the past 30 days, compared to 8.6% of those without social phobia. After controlling for sociodemographic and psychiatric characteristics, social phobia was still associated with a 1.4 times greater risk of having suicidal thoughts. Other studies revealed that roughly between 20% and 33% of individuals with social phobia have had suicidal ideas or behaviour [17,58]. In more detail, thoughts about death appeared to be most common among social phobic patients (about 40%), followed by feeling so low that one wanted to commit suicide (about 24%), feelings of wanting to be dead (18%), and having had one or more suicide attempts in the past (about 8%) [17]. Another study found that about 70% of individuals with social phobia felt hopeless in the past 30 days prior to the interview [5]. Although suicidal thoughts are frequent in both uncomplicated and comorbid social phobia, it is suggested that suicidal behaviour (i.e. suicide attempts) is especially increased in individuals with comorbid social phobia [56,57]. For example, a previous suicide attempt was present in about 1% of those with pure social phobia, and almost 16% of those with a comorbid social phobia [17]. The occurrence of a comorbid disorder might thus be a determinant of a suicide attempt in individuals suffering from social phobia [22,43]. Thus, in the presence of another psychiatric disorder, social phobia may represent an additional risk factor for suicidal behaviour.

This conclusion should be interpreted with great caution, since other studies clearly contradict these findings. In this light, Davidson et al. [22] pointed to the fact that increased suicide risk among individuals with social phobia still exists after controlling for comorbid mental disorders, such as major depression. In line with Schneier et al. [17], these authors stated that preoccupying thoughts of death can be found in comparable numbers of both pure and comorbid social phobia. They suggested that social phobia in itself may cause suicidal ideas [22]. A French household study [58] pointed to the fact that the risk of suicidal thoughts and suicidal behaviour was increased solely in social phobic women without comorbid disorder.

Alcohol and Drug Abuse

High rates of alcohol and drug abuse can be found among individuals with phobic disorders. The association between the occurrence of social phobia and alcohol or drug abuse has been investigated in a number of studies, leading to the consistent finding that alcohol and drug use or dependence is higher among individuals with social phobia, compared to non-phobic subjects [10,17,22]. As early as the 1980s, Smail et al. [59] reported that more than 50% of individuals with alcohol dependence were either agoraphobic, social phobic or both. They also found a linear association between the severity of the phobic complaints and the severity of the alcohol dependence. Self-medication with alcohol or drugs was reported in more than 40% of cases to control anxieties and fears [59,60]. Bibb and Chambless [61] examined 254 agoraphobic outpatients with the Michigan Alcoholism Screening Test [62], finding that about one in five individuals scored more

SOCIAL AND ECONOMIC BURDEN OF PHOBIAS: A REVIEW 319

than 5 and were thus likely to be alcohol dependent. In general, older studies were more likely to conclude that high vulnerability to alcohol dependence primarily exists among individuals with agoraphobia and social phobia, and low vulnerability among individuals with simple phobia [61,63]. In the ECA survey [7], a DSM-III diagnosis of phobia was more than twice as frequently associated with a substance abuse disorder compared to normal individuals [64]. In more recent studies, Wittchen et al. [19,39,65] found that young adults with social phobia smoked significantly more cigarettes compared to healthy controls (Figure 6.5). They also had higher rates of nicotine dependence. Moreover, a higher proportion of social phobics were alcohol dependent, and alcohol intake was higher compared to healthy individuals.

However, the extent to which an anxiety disorder causes alcohol or drug abuse or vice versa remains somewhat speculative. For anxiety disorders in general and phobias in particular, there has been extensive research showing that alcohol dampens fear and stress responses [59] and reduces tension and clinical anxiety [66,67]. Social phobic individuals with a comorbid drug abuse disorder were asked which came first, the social

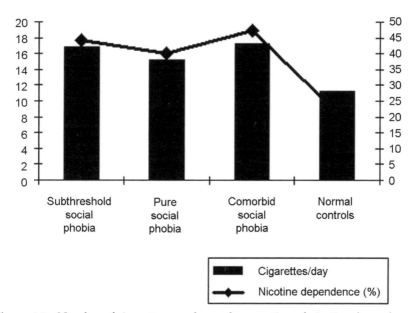

Figure 6.5 Number of cigarettes per day and proportion of nicotine dependence in individuals with subthreshold social phobia, pure social phobia, comorbid social phobia and normal controls. Reproduced from Wittchen et al. [65] by permission of Cambridge University Press

phobia or the comorbid disorder. Social phobia was the primary diagnosis for 71.4% of the individuals while for the others the comorbid disorder was preceding (14.3%) or concurrent with the social phobic disorder (14.3%) [2]. Especially persons suffering from the generalized form of social phobia tend to reduce their fears and anxieties by taking alcohol or drugs [57].

A particular problem in the comorbidity between phobic disorders and alcohol or drug abuse may lie in the long interval between the time of onset of phobia and the time of onset of the drug abuse. Time intervals between one and nine years have been reported between the onset of social phobia and the onset of alcohol or substance use disorders [38,68,69]. A possible explanation for this long interval could be that the phobic disorder remains subclinical for a long time. This interpretation is illustrated by an interesting follow-up study using data from the ECA study [7]. It was not only concluded that social phobia was a potential risk factor for developing alcohol abuse or dependence, but also that individuals with subclinical social phobia (i.e. individuals with an unreasonable fear of a social situation not meeting the criteria of avoidance or impairment) were more than twice as likely to develop alcohol abuse or dependence emerging later [70]. Thus, even individuals without clinically significant avoidance or impairment could be at risk for severe alcohol conditions, and therefore a potential focus of preventive efforts. While some studies have produced evidence that social phobia precedes the onset of alcohol disorders [10], other studies have emphasized a bidirectional or reciprocal relationship between social phobia and alcohol disorders [71]. Anyway, concomitant alcohol disorders place an additional burden on the quality of life of phobic persons. It is indeed conceivable that these patients will seek help only in the later course of their comorbid alcohol use.

ECONOMIC ASPECTS OF TREATMENT OF PHOBIC DISORDERS

Little is known about the economic impact of the treatment of phobias. Cost-minimization analyses to determine the cheapest intervention are lacking. Although it is common to compare treatments in randomized controlled trials, until recently it has been rare for such trials to include an economic evaluation. Our literature search in the Medline, Psychlit and Ovid databases failed to find any such published studies related to treating phobias. Likewise, published cost-effectiveness or cost-utility analyses were not found in the literature. Cost-benefit analysis predicts that the increased costs associated with the diagnosis and effective treatment may be offset by savings due to increased productivity among treated persons.

As we have described earlier, several studies have been conducted to identify different domains that need to be assessed when measuring quality of life. We have also shown that no gold standard exists among different measures of quality of life (Table 6.1). The time seems to be ripe for researchers and clinicians to reach a consensus to be adopted in new treatment studies on phobic disorders. First, there is general agreement on the idea that not only statistically (quantitative) significant changes over time are important, but also clinically significant (qualitative) changes should be taken into account in order to define treatment outcome [72–74]. Second, when investigating treatment outcome in terms of qualitative changes, it may be redundant to say that it is necessary to use measures with reliable levels of validity to highlight these changes. Since no scale used to evaluate treatment outcome in phobic disorders (Table 6.1) has been fully validated or adapted to different culture or language situations [45], psychometric validity testing is limited. Third, it might be questioned to what extent a change in phobic symptomatology is to be interpreted as improved functioning. For example, in evaluating the use of different validated measures for social phobia [75], it was suggested that the LSAS is not an accurate instrument for measuring improved social functioning, although it is recommended as a standard outcome measure [45]. This should be taken into account in the evaluation of different treatment options for phobic disorders, since most studies are likely to use the LSAS as an outcome measure [75,76].

We suggest that treatment outcome should also be evaluated using composite outcome measures, such as the Social Phobia Endstate Functioning Index (SPEFI) [77] or the Index of Social Phobia Improvement (ISPI) [78]. The SPEFI was developed to compare the level of functioning after treatment with that of controls, while the ISPI was developed to assess the degree of improvement between pre- and post-treatment evaluation. Combining these measures with more commonly used instruments, such as the Clinical Global Impression, the Hamilton Rating Scale for Anxiety, the Fear Questionnaire and the LSAS, we may be employing a multiaxial system yielding a more accurate treatment evaluation of relevant domains of phobic disorders, such as fear, distorted beliefs, anticipatory anxiety, avoidance behaviour and autonomic symptoms [79].

Clinicians as well as researchers still view cognitive-behavioural therapy (CBT) as the most effective intervention in phobias. In cases of social phobia, there is general agreement that CBT group sessions yield similar effects to individual sessions [80]. From an economic point of view, one could thus argue that no therapeutic efficacy would be lost in more cost-effective CBT group sessions. Bruce and Saeed [3] suggest a group CBT (consisting of management skills, social skills training, cognitive restructuring and exposure) lasting for 16 to 24 sessions. Average costs of 16 to 24 sessions are estimated to be in the range of US$750 to US$2000, depending upon the type of provider. It may be argued that such high costs may be prohibitive for some patients and thus may lead to a suboptimal treatment. This, however, is not in line with research performed both in the United States and Europe. Most third-payers in the United States are likely to cover 50–80% of the costs of treatment of phobic disorders on condition that therapy is delivered by a licensed professional [3]. Furthermore, as we have described earlier, treatment rates were independent of the costs of mental health facilities [19].

Although CBT group sessions are seen as standard treatment, a pilot study reports that the application of interpersonal psychotherapy may be as effective for social phobia as CBT [81]. However, a comparison between different psychotherapeutic treatment options in terms of health-economic aspects was not feasible.

Despite the large number of trials comparing different pharmacological treatments for social phobia, there appears to be a vacuum about their comparative costs and benefits. Although a number of pharmacoeconomic studies have reported that direct health care expenditures for initiating treatment with selective serotonin reuptake inhibitors are comparable or even lower than expenditures for patients who initiate treatment with a tricyclic antidepressant, there appears to be a lack of comparative research on economic aspects of phobic disorders [82].

SUMMARY

Consistent Evidence

It is nowadays well established that the service use of individuals with phobia is far from optimal. This may be due to several structural and attitudinal barriers that hamper optimal service delivery. A major structural barrier to treatment seems to be the poor recognition in primary care. In a significant part, this has to do with the phobic condition itself, since individuals seldom present phobic complaints when visiting a health professional. Consequent on this, improving GPs' knowledge and diagnostic capacities may yield a better interface between primary care and specialized mental health facilities. There is also insufficient knowledge of the available treatment for phobic disorders. Another important barrier to treatment lies in the fact that many individuals do not interpret their phobias as mental health problems. Due to the early onset of the disorder, many phobic individuals may have learned to live with their problem, despite the fact that it goes along with a high burden of impairment in personal, social and professional life.

The direct costs of phobic disorders tend to be high, being comparable to those of depressive disorders. Phobic disorders may yield several indirect costs, such as decreased educational attainment, decreased work productivity, economic inactivity and financial dependency. The considerably impaired quality of life is related to the frequent comorbidities. The early age of onset may also interfere with the development of personal, sexual, social and intellectual functioning. Phobic disorders have been associated with higher rates of suicidality and alcohol or drug abuse. It is conceivable that the impairment in these domains places a considerable burden not only at the personal, but also at the societal and economic level.

Incomplete Evidence

Although there is some evidence that the use of psychotherapeutic and/or psychopharmacological agents is effective in treating phobic disorders, valid outcome measures assessing therapeutic change are lacking. We have stressed the need for a multiaxial system exploring treatment changes on different domains of phobic disorders, such as fear, distorted beliefs, anticipatory anxiety, avoidance behaviour and autonomic symptoms, but also assessing changes in emotional functioning, and interpersonal and working relationships.

Areas Still Open to Research

The vast majority of research in this area deals almost exclusively with social phobia. There seems to be a lack of scientific interest in burden and impairments related to other phobic conditions. An important direction for future research may thus be the development of a scientific interest in agoraphobia and simple phobia on nearly every domain we have addressed in this review: the use of health services, direct and indirect costs, health-related quality of life, and measuring treatment outcome with regard to quality of life.

REFERENCES

1. Murray C.J.L., Lopes A.D. (eds) (1996) *The Global Burden of Disease: A Comprehensive Assessment of Mortality and Disability from Diseases, Injuries, and Risk Factors in 1990 and Projected to 2020.* Harvard School of Public Health, Cambridge, MA.

2. Katzelnick D.J., Kobak A., Deleire T., Henk H.J., Greist J.H., Davidson J.R.T., Schneier F.R., Stein M.B., Helstad C.P. (2001) Impact of generalised social anxiety disorder in managed care. *Am. J. Psychiatry*, **158**: 1999–2007.
3. Bruce T.J., Saeed S.A. (1999) Social anxiety disorder: a common, under-recognized mental disorder. *Am. Fam. Physician*, **60**: 2311–2322.
4. Weiller E., Bisserbe J.C., Boyer P., Lépine J.P., Lecrubier Y. (1996) Social phobia in general health care: an unrecognized, untreated, disabling disorder. *Br. J. Psychiatry*, **168**: 169–174.
5. Olfson M., Guardino M., Struening E., Schneier F.R., Hellman F., Klein D.F. (2000) Barriers to the treatment of social anxiety. *Am. J. Psychiatry*, **157**: 521–527.
6. Eaton W.W., Dryman A., Weissman M.M. (1991) Panic and phobia. In *Psychiatric Disorders in America: The Epidemiologic Catchment Area Study* (Eds L.N. Robins, D.A. Regier), pp. 155–179. Free Press, New York.
7. Robins L.N., Regier D.A. (1991) *Psychiatric Disorders in America*. Free Press, New York.
8. Kessler R., McGonagle K.A., Zhao S., Nelson C.B., Hughes M., Eshleman S., Wittchen H.U., Kendler K.S. (1994) Lifetime and 12-month prevalence of DSM III-R psychiatric disorders in the United States: results from the National Comorbidity Survey. *Arch. Gen. Psychiatry*, **51**: 8–19.
9. Federoff I.C., Taylor S. (2001) Psychological and pharmacological treatments of social phobia: a meta-analysis. *J. Clin. Psychol.*, **21**: 311–324.
10. Magee W.J., Eaton W.W., Wittchen H.U., McGonagle K.A., Kessler R.C. (1996) Agoraphobia, simple phobia, and social phobia in the National Comorbidity Survey. *Arch. Gen. Psychiatry*, **53**: 159–168.
11. Offord D.R., Boyle M.H., Campbell D., Goering P., Lin E., Wong M., Racine Y.A. (1996) One-year prevalence of psychiatric disorders in Ontarians 15 to 64 years of age. *Can. J. Psychiatry*, **41**: 559–563.
12. Stein M.B., Kean Y.M. (2000) Disability and quality of life in social phobia: epidemiologic findings. *Am. J. Psychiatry*, **157**: 1606–1613.
13. Olfson M., Fireman B., Weissman M.M., Leon A.C., Sheehan D.V., Kathol R.G., Hoven C., Farber L. (1997) Mental disorders and disability among patients in a primary care group practice. *Am. J. Psychiatry*, **154**: 1734–1740.
14. Pélissolo A., André C., Moutard-Martin F., Wittchen H.U., Lépine J.P. (2000) Social phobia in the community: relationship between diagnostic threshold and prevalence. *Eur. Psychiatry*, **15**: 25–28.
15. American Psychiatric Association (1994) *Diagnostic and Statistical Manual of Mental Disorders*, 4th edn. American Psychiatric Association, Washington, DC.
16. Kesteloot K. (2001) Hervormingen in de gezondheidszorg. Economische achtergronden en ethische implicaties. In *Moeten, mogen, kunnen. Ethiek en wetenschap. Lessen voor de eenentwinstigste eeuw* (Eds B. Raymaekers, A. van de Putte, G. van Riel). Leuven: Universitaire Pers/Davidsfonds, Leuven.
17. Schneier F.R., Johnson J., Hornig C.D., Liebowitz M.R., Weissman M.M. (1992) Social phobia: comorbidity and morbidity in an epidemiologic sample. *Arch. Gen. Psychiatry*, **49**: 282–288.
18. Bisserbe J.C., Weiller E. (1999) Social anxiety disorder in primary care: extent of recognition and prescribed treatments. In *Focus on Psychiatry: Social Anxiety Disorder* (Eds H.G.M. Westenberg, J.A. den Boer), pp. 207–213. Syn-Thesis, Amsterdam.
19. Wittchen H.-U., Stein M.B., Kessler R.C. (1999) Social fears and social phobia in a community sample of adolescents and young adults: prevalence, risk factors, and co-morbidity. *Psychol. Med.*, **29**, 309–323.

20. Gallo J.J., Marino S., Ford D., Anthony J.C. (1995) Filters on the pathway to mental health care: II. Sociodemographic factors. *Psychol. Med.*, **25**: 1149–1160.
21. Greenberg P.E., Sisitsky T., Kessler R.C., Finkelstein S.N., Berndt E.R., Davidson J.R., Ballenger J.C., Fyer A.J. (1999) The economic burden of anxiety disorders in the 1990s. *J. Clin. Psychiatry*, **60**: 427–435.
22. Davidson J.R.T., Hughes D.L., George L.K., Blazer D.G. (1993) The epidemiology of social phobia: findings from the Duke Epidemiological Catchment Area study. *Psychol. Med.*, **23**: 709–718.
23. Patel A., Knapp M., Henderson J., Baldwin D. (2002) The economic consequences of social phobia. *J. Affect. Disord.*, **68**: 221–233.
24. Goldberg D.P., Huxley P. (1980) *Mental Illness in the Community: Pathways to Psychiatric Care*. Tavistock, London.
25. Issakidis C., Andrews G. (2002) Service utilisation for anxiety in an Australian community sample. *Soc. Psychiatry Psychiatr. Epidemiol.*, **37**: 153–163.
26. Wells J.E., Robins L.N., Bushnell J.A., Jarosz D., Oakley-Browne M.A. (1994) Perceived barriers to care in St Louis (USA) and Christchurch (NZ): reasons for not seeking professional help for psychological distress. *Soc. Psychiatry Psychiatr. Epidemiol.*, **29**: 155–164.
27. Meltzer H., Bebbington P., Brugha T., Farrell M., Jenkins R., Lewis G. (2000) The reluctance to seek treatment for neurotic disorders. *J. Mental Health*, **9**: 335–343.
28. Ellen S.R., Norman T.R., Burrows G.D. (2000) Assessing anxiety and depression in primary care. *Med. J. Aust. Practice Essentials*, 14–19.
29. Marks I. (1991) Phobias and related anxiety disorders. *Br. Med. J.*, **302**: 1037–1038.
30. Bland R.C., Newman S.C., Orn H. (1997) Help-seeking for psychiatric disorders. *Can. J. Psychiatry*, **42**: 935–942.
31. Ormel J., van den Brink W., Koeter M.W., Giel R., Van Der Meer K., Van De Willige G., Wilmink F.W. (1990) Recognition, management, and outcome of psychological disorders in primary care: a naturalistic follow-up study. *Psychol. Med.*, **20**: 909–923.
32. The National Advisory Mental Health Council Health Care Reform for Americans with Severe Mental Illnesses: Report of the National Advisory Mental Health Council. *Am. J. Psychiatry*, **150**: 1447–1465.
33. DuPont R.L., Rice D.P., Miller L.S., Shiraki S.S., Rowland C.R., Harwood H.J. (1996) Economic costs of anxiety disorders. *Anxiety*, **2**: 167–172
34. Souetre E., Lozet H., Cimarosti I., Martin P., Chignon J.M., Ades J., Tignol J., Darcourt G. (1994) Cost of anxiety disorders: impact of comorbidity. *J. Psychosom. Pes.*, **38** (Suppl. 1): 151–160.
35. Andrews G. (1991) *The Tolkien Report: A Description of a Model Mental Health Service*. Clinical Research Unit for Anxiety Disorders, Sydney.
36. Croft-Jeffreys C., Wilkinson G. (1989) Estimated costs of neurotic disorder in UK general practice 1985. *Psychol. Med.*, **19**: 549–558.
37. Ballenger J.C., Davidson J.R.T., Lecrubier Y., Nutt D.J., Bobes J., Beidel D.C., Ono Y., Westenberg H.G. (1998) Consensus statement on social anxiety disorder from the International Consensus Group on Depression and Anxiety. *J. Clin. Psychiatry*, **59** (Suppl. 17): 54–60.
38. Lecrubier Y. (1998) Comorbidity in social anxiety disorder: impact on disease burden and management. *J. Clin. Psychiatry*, **59** (Suppl. 17): 33–37.

39. Wittchen H.U., Feutsch M., Sonntag H., Muller N., Liebowitz M. (2000) Disability and quality of life in pure and comorbid social phobia: findings from a controlled study. *Eur. Psychiatry*, **15**: 46–58.
40. Leon A.C., Portera L., Weissman M.M. (1995) The social costs of anxiety disorders. *Br. J. Psychiatry*, **166** (Suppl. 27): 19–22.
41. Mendlowics M.V., Stein M.B. (2000) Quality of life in individuals with anxiety disorders. *Am. J. Psychiatry*, **157**: 669–682.
42. Fayers P.M., Hand D.J., Bjordal K., Gronvold M. (1997) Causal indicators in quality of life research. *Quality of Life Res.*, **6**: 393–406.
43. Schneier F.R., Heckelman L.R., Garfinkel R., Campeas R., Fallon B.A., Gitow A., Street L., Del Bene D., Liebowitz M.R. (1994) Functional impairment in social phobia. *J. Clin. Psychiatry*, **55**: 322–331.
44. Rabkin J., Wagner G., Griffin K.W. (2000) Quality of life measures. In *Handbook of Psychiatric Measure*, pp. 135–150. American Psychiatric Association, Washington, DC.
45. Bobes J.B. (1998) How is recovery from social anxiety disorder defined? *J. Clin. Psychiatry*, **59** (Suppl. 17): 12–16.
46. Antony M.M. (1997) Assessment and treatment of social phobia. *Can. J. Psychiatry*, **42**: 826–834.
47. Lieb R., Wittchen H.-U., Höfler M., Fuetsch M., Stein M.B., Merikangas K.R. (2000) Parental psychopathology, parenting styles, and the risk of social phobia in offspring. *Arch. Gen. Psychiatry*, **57**: 859–866.
48. Mancini C., Van Am100ringen M., Szatmari P., Fugere C., Boyle M. (1996) A high-risk pilot study of the children of adults with social phobia. *J. Am. Acad. Child Adolesc. Psychiatry*, **35**: 1511–1517.
49. Leary M.R., Dobbins S.E. (1983) Social anxiety, sexual behaviour, and contraceptive use. *J. Pers. Soc. Psychol.*, **45**: 1347–1354.
50. Lecrubier Y., Wittchen H.-U., Faravelli C., Bobes J., Patel A., Knapp M. (2000) A European perspective on social anxiety disorder. *Eur. Psychiatry*, **15**: 5–16.
51. Wittchen H.U., Beloch E. (1996) The impact of social phobia on quality of life. *Int. Clin. Psychopharmacol.*, **11** (Suppl. 3): 15–24.
52. Figueira I., Possidente E., Marques C., Hayes K. (2001) Sexual dysfunction: a neglected complication of panic disorder and social phobia. *Arch. Sex. Behav.*, **30**: 369–377.
53. First M.B., Spitzer R.L., Gibbon M., Williams J.B.W. (1995) *Structural Clinical Interview for DSM-IV Axis I Disorders—Patient Edition*. New York State Psychiatric Institute, New York.
54. Laumann E.O., Paik A., Rosen R.C. (1999) Sexual dysfunction in the United States: prevalence and predictors. *JAMA*, **281**: 537–544.
55. Read S., King M., Watson J. (1997) Sexual dysfunction in primary medical care: prevalence, characteristics, and detection by the general practitioner. *J. Publ. Health Med.*, **4**: 387–391.
56. Lipsitz J.D., Schneier F.R. (2000) Social phobia: epidemiology and cost of illness. *Pharmacoeconomics*, **18**: 23–32.
57. Montgomery S. (1999) *SSRIs and Social Anxiety*. Science Press, London.
58. Lépine J.P., Lellouch J. (1995) Diagnosis and epidemiology of agoraphobia and social phobia. *Clin. Neuropharmacol.*, **18**: S15–26.
59. Smail P., Stockwell T., Canter S., Hodgson R. (1984) Alcohol dependence and phobic states. I. A prevalence study. *Br. J. Psychiatry*, **144**: 53–57.

60. Stravinsky A., Lamontagne Y., Lavallee Y.J. (1986) Clinical phobias and avoidant personality disorder among alcoholics admitted to an alcoholism rehabilitation setting. *Can. J. Psychiatry*, **31**: 714–719.
61. Bibb J., Chambless D. (1986) Alcoholism and alcohol abuse among diagnosed agoraphobics. *Behav. Res. Ther.*, **24**: 49–58.
62. Selzer M.L. (1971) The Michigan Alcoholism Screening Test: the quest for a new diagnostic instrument. *Am. J. Psychiatry*, **127**: 1653–1658.
63. Thyer B.A., Parrish R.T., Himle J., Cameron O.G., Curtis G.C., Nesse R.M. (1986) Alcohol abuse among clinically anxious patients. *Behav. Res. Ther.*, **24**: 357–359.
64. Regier D.A., Farmer M.E., Rae D.S., Locke B.Z., Keith S.J., Judd L.L., Goodwin F.K. (1990) Comorbidity of mental disorders with alcohol and other drug abuse. *JAMA*, **264**: 2511–2518.
65. Wittchen H.U., Stein B., Kessler R. (1999) Social fears and social phobia in a community sample of adolescents and young adults: prevalence, risk factors, and comorbidity. *Psychol. Med.*, **29**: 309–323.
66. Cappell H., Herman C.P. (1972) Alcohol and tension reduction: a review. *Q. J. Studies Alcohol*, **33**: 33–64.
67. Kusher M.G., Sher K.J., Erickson D.J. (1999) Prospective analysis of the relation between DSM-III anxiety disorders and alcohol use disorders. *Am. J. Psychiatry*, **156**: 723–732.
68. Mullaney J.A., Trippett C.J. (1979) Alcohol dependence and phobias: clinical description and relevance. *Br. J. Psychiatry*, **135**: 565–573.
69. Lecrubier Y. (1997) Implications of early onset social phobia on outcome. *Eur. Neuropsychopharmacol.*, **7** (Suppl. 2): S85.
70. Crum R.M., Pratt L.A. (2001) Risk of heavy drinking and alcohol use disorders in social phobia: a prospective analysis. *Am. J. Psychiatry*, **158**: 1693–1700.
71. Himle J.A., Abelson J.P., Haghightgou H., Hill E.M., Nesse R.M., Curtis G.C. (1999) Effect of alcohol on social phobia. *Am. J. Psychiatry*, **156**: 1237–1243.
72. Crits-Christoph P., Connolly M.B. (1997) Measuring change in patient following psychological and pharmacological interventions: anxiety disorders. In *Measuring Patient Changes* (Eds H.M. Strupp, L.M. Horowitz, M.J. Lambert), pp. 155–188. American Psychological Association, Washington, DC.
73. Jacobson N.S., Truax P. (1991) Clinical significance: a statistical approach to defining meaningful change in psychotherapy research. *J. Consult. Clin. Psychol.*, **59**: 12–19.
74. Jacobson N.S., Roberts L.J., Berns S.B., McGlinchey J.B. (1999) Methods for defining and determining the clinical significance of treatment effects. Description, application, and alternatives. *J. Consult. Clin. Psychol.*, **67**: 300–307.
75. Cox B.J., Ross L., Swinson R.P., Direnfeld D.M. (1998) A comparison of social phobia outcome measures in cognitive-behavioural group therapy. *Behav. Modif.*, **2**: 285–297.
76. Lampe L.A. (2000) Social phobia: a review of recent research trends. *Curr. Opin. Psychiatry*, **13**: 149–155.
77. Turner S.M., Beidel D.C., Long P.J., Turner M.W., Townsly R.M. (1993) A composite measure to determine the functional status of treated social phobics: the social phobia endstate functioning index. *Behav. Ther.*, **24**: 265–275.
78. Turner S.M., Beidel D.C., Wolff P.L. (1994) A composite measure to determine improvement following treatment for social phobia: the index of social phobia improvement. *Behav. Res. Ther.*, **32**: 471–476.

79. Figueira I., Jacques R. (2002) Social anxiety disorder: assessment and pharmacological treatment. *German J. Psychiatry*, **5**: 40–48.
80. Oosterbaan D.B., van Dyck R. (1999) Non-drug treatment for social anxiety disorder. In *Focus on Psychiatry: Social Anxiety Disorder* (Eds H.G.M. Westenberg, J.A. den Boer), pp. 191–205. Syn-Thesis, Amsterdam.
81. Lipsitz J.D., Markowitz J.C., Cherry S., Fyer A.J. (1999) Open trial of interpersonal psychotherapy for the treatment of social phobia. *Am. J. Psychiatry*, **156**: 1814–1816.
82. Iverson-Riddel J., Veenhuis P.E. (2000) *Clinical Guidelines Series for Area Programs. VI. Treatment of Anxiety Disorders in Adults.* Department of Health and Human Services, Raleigh, NC.

Commentaries

6.1
Burden of Phobias: Focus on Health-Related Quality of Life
Mark H. Rapaport, Katia K. Delrahim and Rachel E. Maddux[1]

According to the Anxiety Disorders Association of America (ADAA) and the National Institute of Mental Health (NIMH), anxiety disorders are the most common mental illness in the US, with 19.1 million (13.3%) of the adult population (ages 18–54) affected. Among anxiety disorders, phobias (including social, specific and agoraphobia) affect approximately 11.5 million (8%) adult Americans [1,2]. Although often under-recognized and under-treated, phobic disorder is a highly prevalent, chronic and disabling condition that results in marked functional impairment [3–7]. In addition, as is the case with many other psychiatric illnesses, there is a high comorbidity rate associated with anxiety disorders, specifically social phobia [5,8,9]. As Demyttenaere et al. state in their introductory paragraph, with a high prevalence rate and increased comorbidity, phobic disorder places a "significant burden" not only on suffering patients, but also on family members, caregivers and healthcare services.

Even though the burden associated with anxiety disorders has recently been documented in epidemiologic studies such as the Epidemiologic Catchment Area (ECA) study and the National Comorbidity Survey (NCS), neither the ECA nor the NCS provided extensive data on quality of life measures crucial in determining the impairment of daily functioning of suffering patients. Both studies demonstrated the disabling effect of anxiety disorders, illustrating that these disorders and specifically social phobia are associated with high rates of outpatient medical treatment fees and financial dependency, and are negatively related to level of education, socioeconomic status, and work productivity, leading to substantial economic burden and burden on the community [9–13]. These individuals were more likely to be frequent users of emergency medical services and were more likely to be hospitalized for physical problems than individuals without anxiety [10,11,13]. However, in order to truly capture the "burden"

---

[1] Department of Psychiatry and Mental Health, Cedars Sinai Medical Center, 8730 Alden Drive, Thalians Suite C301, Los Angeles, CA 90048, USA

of anxiety disorders, one needs to extend the focus beyond the *direct* and *indirect* costs to include the overall impairment of daily functioning.

Although signs and symptoms remain the defining characteristics of psychiatric nosology, there is increasing recognition that the scope of assessment should include broader dimensions such as daily functioning and quality of life related to health and health care [14,15]. This has led to a consensus that successful treatment must go beyond ameliorating signs and symptoms to address the broader issue of restoration of health. The 1948 World Health Organization definition of health as "a state of complete physical, mental, and social well-being and not merely the absence of disease" has resurfaced as an important touchstone for the evaluation of both mental and physical health treatment outcomes [16]. Demyttenaere *et al.* provide a comprehensive review of the societal and individual burden of phobic disorders. They delineate "burden" into three separate but not mutually exclusive categories: (1) direct costs, (2) indirect costs and (3) health-related quality of life. The thoughtful assessment of health-related quality of life for psychiatric patients and the impact of our treatment interventions on quality of life is emerging as one of the most important issues in the field of psychiatry [17,18].

The concept of health-related quality of life has been defined in a number of ways, and many measures exist for assessing the construct [15,19]. Most definitions explicitly state that the assessment of quality of life, as related to health and health care, should take into account the patient's subjective perception of his/her life circumstances [20]. This includes social relationships, physical health, functioning in daily activities, work and economic status, and overall sense of well-being [21]. However, there is a lack of psychometrically validated scales and systemic studies for the specific assessment of quality of life in phobic disorders. In fact, there is only a handful of empirical work looking at quality of life in anxiety disorders, and the majority of focus has been on social phobia rather than phobic disorders as a whole [3,4,8,15,22,23].

As psychiatrists move toward a comprehensive approach to treatment, the relationships between quality of life dysfunction and specific clinical features of phobic disorders need to be understood. Because definitions of quality of life emphasize the importance of an individual's perceptions of his/her life circumstances, it is important to consider how factors like increased comorbidity, early age of onset, or disease chronicity might alter one's perceptions [14]. More clinical research investigating functional impairment and quality of life will provide information that will improve treatment interventions and may facilitate more appropriate allocation of clinical resources. There is a need to examine the relative contribution of illness-specific factors (severity of symptoms, psychiatric comorbidity and duration of illness) and demographic factors on quality of life and functional disability across anxiety disorders [14].

REFERENCES

1. Narrow W.E., Rae D.S., Regier D.A. (1998) NIMH epidemiology note: prevalence of anxiety disorders. One-year prevalence best estimates calculated from ECA and NCS data. Population estimates based on US Census estimated residential population age 18 to 54. Unpublished manuscript.
2. Anxiety Disorders Association of America (2002) Anxiety Disorders Information. http://www.adaa.org/AnxietyDisorderInfor/index.cfm.
3. Stein M.B., Kean Y.M. (2000) Disability and quality of life in social phobia: epidemiologic findings. *Am. J. Psychiatry*, **157**: 1606–1613.
4. Simon N.M., Otto M.W., Korbly N.B., Peters P.M., Nicolaou D.C., Pollack M.H. (2002) Quality of life in social anxiety disorder compared with panic disorder and the general population. *Psychiatr. Serv.*, **53**: 714–718.
5. Lépine J.P., Pelissolo A. (2000) Why take social anxiety disorder seriously? *Depress. Anxiety*, **11**: 87–92.
6. Kessler R.C., McGonagle K.A., Zhao S., Nelson C.B., Hughes M., Eshleman S., Wittchen H.-U., Kendler K.S. (1994) Lifetime and 12-month prevalence of DSM-III-R psychiatric disorders in the United States: results from the National Comorbidity Survey. *Arch. Gen. Psychiatry*, **51**: 8–19.
7. Schneier F.R., Johnson J., Hornig C.D., Liebowitz M.R., Weissman M.M. (1992) Social phobia: comorbidity and morbidity in an epidemiologic sample. *Arch. Gen. Psychiatry*, **49**: 282–288.
8. den Boer J.A. (2000) Social anxiety disorder/social phobia: epidemiology, diagnosis, neurobiology, and treatment. *Compr. Psychiatry*, **41**: 405–415.
9. Patel A., Knapp M., Henderson J., Baldwin D. (2002) The economic consequences of social phobia. *J. Affect. Disord.*, **68**: 221–233.
10. Schneier F.R., Johnson J., Hornig C.D., Liebowitz M.R., Weissman M.M. (1992) Social phobia: comorbidity and morbidity in an epidemiological sample. *Arch. Gen. Psychiatry*, **55**: 322–331.
11. Kobak K.A., Schaettle S.C., Greist J.H., Jefferson J.W., Katzelnick D.J., Dottl S.L. (1998) Computer interview assessment of social phobia in a clinical drug trial. *Depress. Anxiety*, **7**: 97–104.
12. Creed F., Morgan R., Fiddler M., Marshall S., Guthrie E., House A. (2002) Depression and anxiety impair health-related quality of life and are associated with increased costs in general medical inpatients. *Psychosomatics*, **43**: 302–309.
13. Greenberg P.E., Sisitsky T., Kessler R.C., Finkelstein S.N., Berndt E.R., Davidson J.R., Ballenger J.C., Fyer A.J. (1999) The economic burden of anxiety disorders in the 1990s. *J. Clin. Psychiatry*, **60**: 427–435.
14. Rapaport M.H., Clary C., Fayyad R., Endicott J. (2002) Quality of life impairement in depressive and anxiety disorders. Presented at the Meeting of the American Psychiatric Association, Philadelphia, 18–23 May.
15. Mendlowicz M.V., Stein M.B. (2000) Quality of life in individuals with anxiety disorders. *Am. J. Psychiatry*, **157**: 669–682.
16. World Health Organization (1948) *Charter*. WHO, Geneva.
17. Katschnig H. (1997) How useful is the concept of quality of life in psychiatry? In *Quality of Life in Mental Disorders* (Eds H. Katschnig, H. Freeman, N. Sartorius), pp. 3–16. John Wiley & Sons, New York.

18. Staquet M.J., Hays R.D., Fayers P.M. (eds) (1998) *Quality of Life Assessment in Clinical Trials: Methods and Practice*. Oxford University Press, New York.
19. Gladis M., Gosch E., Dishuk N., Crits-Christoph P. (1999) Quality of life: expanding the scope of clinical significance. *J. Consult. Clin. Psychol.*, **67**: 320–331.
20. Mendlowicz M.V., Stein M.B. (2000) Quality of life in individuals with anxiety disorders. *Am. J. Psychiatry*, **157**: 669–682.
21. Patrick D.L., Erickson P. (1998) What constitutes quality of life? Concepts and dimensions. *Clin. Nutr.*, **7**: 53–63.
22. Safren S.A., Heimberg R.G., Brown E.J., Holle C. (1996) Quality of life in social phobia. *Depress. Anxiety*, **4**: 126–133.
23. Wittchen H.U., Beloch E. (1996) The impact of social phobia on quality of life. *Int. Clin. Psychopharmacol.*, **11** (Suppl. 3): 15–23.

6.2
Reducing the Burden of Phobias: Patient Factors, System Issues

Naomi M. Simon and Julia Oppenheimer[1]

Documenting the impairment and direct economic costs associated with the phobias has become necessary as a means to justify the expenditure of limited resources in healthcare systems for the diagnosis and treatment of these highly prevalent, yet under-diagnosed and under-treated, disorders. As the costs of healthcare have skyrocketed, and demands on physician time increased, research advances in the understanding and treatment of mood and anxiety disorders have not been adapted or disseminated in clinical settings in a systematic or consistent fashion. This is clearly the case for the phobias. Katzelick *et al.* [1] recently found that in a managed care setting where the rates of generalized social anxiety disorder were 8.2%, only 0.5% of patients were diagnosed, and fewer than a third of these diagnosed patients were treated. Further clarification of the direct, particularly economic and health system costs, and indirect costs associated with the phobias will enable improved cost–benefit analyses, with the hope that this will provide the impetus for greater investment by healthcare systems in appropriate detection and interventions. However, for the phobias in general, and social anxiety in particular, there is a complex interaction of disorder-related patient behaviours and systems issues that contribute to their under-diagnosis and under-treatment. Better understanding of these contributing factors is critical to systematically improve the diagnosis and appropriate treatment of these highly impairing disorders in general clinical practice settings.

---

[1] *Center for Anxiety and Traumatic Stress Related Disorders, Massachusetts General Hospital, 15 Parkman Street, Boston, MA 02114, USA*

The phobias in general, and social anxiety disorder in specific, are particularly problematic for patient self-referral for treatment. The very early onset of these disorders, with high overlap with trait-like features such as shyness and avoidance, frequently leads patients to conclude that "this is simply how I am and may always be". This lack of recognition of change from a formerly recalled experience of the self contributes to a lack of help-seeking behaviour, with many of the patients who do seek help presenting many years after disease onset. Schneier *et al.* [2] have proposed that patients with early onset social anxiety disorder may not be capable of providing meaningful answers to questions that require comparison of current function to an earlier time period of normal function.

Rates of treatment-seeking of patients with agoraphobia, as noted, are higher than those of social phobics, with 70.5% of patients with agoraphobia with self-reported role impairment seeking treatment [3]. Potentially contributing to this are the greater somatic symptoms, impairment in physical function, and physical health concerns associated with agoraphobia, particularly when panic attacks are present; we recently found support for this greater impairment associated with physical or somatic symptoms for a group of treatment-seeking patients with panic disorder compared with an age- and sex-matched group with social anxiety disorder [4]. For social anxiety disorder, however, the impairments may be less measurable. For example, many patients report that they would have taken alternate school or career paths had their symptoms not interfered at a critical age in their education, social and occupational development. These losses, such as the projected life course an individual may have followed without the disorder, are difficult to accurately project and may contribute to the lack of recognition of social phobia as a disorder by patients and families, as well as healthcare providers.

That being older, of higher socioeconomic status and of higher education are associated with treatment seeking [5] indirectly supports the notion that lack of education about the nature of phobias, and particularly social anxiety disorder, as treatable disorders serves as a significant barrier to help-seeking by individuals with these disorders. This concept has been recognized by the pharmaceutical industry in the United States where direct to consumer marketing for social anxiety has been initiated, and has brought many patients to the clinic, often stating "I had no idea this was something that could be treated". Although not all clinicians support the notion of direct to consumer pharmaceutical marketing, this serves as an example of the need for patient education and outreach to improve self-referral of patients with social anxiety disorder in particular, a disorder where patients by definition are fearful of the opinion of others, and of embarrassing themselves.

In addition to patient factors, there is still a significant need for physician education about the phobias, their treatment and their impact on patients and systems. A greater awareness about the common presenting symptoms may help diminish unnecessary medical tests, and increase suspicion about phobias or other anxiety disorders even when physician time is limited. Further, greater awareness of effective interventions, and improved data about their impact on direct and indirect costs, including potential reduction in comorbid disorders such as depression and alcohol abuse, for patients and healthcare systems, should motivate greater diagnosis and treatment within healthcare systems. Such critical work has been ongoing for patients with panic disorder in primary care, and serves as one model of system intervention and research. Katon *et al.* [6] developed a "collaborative care" intervention in primary care consisting of patient education, treatment with selective serotonin reuptake inhibitors, and psychiatric assessment on site, and found the intervention was more effective than usual care. Although the overall cost effectiveness, accounting for increased mental health costs and reduced other healthcare expenditures, was equivocal, the bulk of the associated costs were related to the medication, which they proposed should decrease with time as the number of medications available in generic form increases. These efforts in panic disorder serve as an excellent start towards the documentation of the direct cost savings, in addition to treatment benefits, of systematic intervention for anxiety disorders, and such work remains needed for the rest of the anxiety disorders. This work will be critical in providing motivation and guidance for the necessary expenditure of healthcare resources to improve the appropriate detection and treatment of phobias.

REFERENCES

1. Katzelick D.J., Kobak A., Deleire T., Henk H.J., Greist J.H., Davidson J.R.T., Schneier F.R., Stein M.B., Helstad C.P. (2001) Impact of generalized social anxiety disorder in managed care. *Am. J. Psychiatry*, **158**: 1999–2007.
2. Schneier F.R., Heckelman L.R., Garfinkel R., Campeas R., Fallon B.A., Gitow A., Street L., Del Bene D., Liebowitz M.R. (1994) Functional impairment in social phobia. *J. Clin. Psychiatry*, **55**: 322–331.
3. Magee W.J., Eaton W.W., Wittchen H.U., MgGonagle K.A., Kessler R.C. (1996) Agoraphobia, simple phobia, and social phobia in the National Comorbidity Survey. *Arch. Gen. Psychiatry*, **53**: 159–168.
4. Simon N.M., Otto M.W., Korbly N.B., Peters P.M., Nicolaou D.C., Pollack M.H. (2002) Quality of life in social anxiety disorder compared with panic disorder and the general population. *Psychiatr. Serv.*, **53**: 714–718.
5. Schneier F.R., Johnson J., Hornig C.D., Liebowitz M.R., Weissman M.M. (1992) Social phobia: comorbidity and morbidity in an epidemiologic sample. *Arch. Gen. Psychiatry*, **49**: 282–288.
6. Katon W.J., Roy-Byrne P., Russo J., Cowley D. (2002) Cost-effectiveness and cost offset of a collaborative care intervention for primary care patients with panic disorder. *Arch. Gen. Psychiatry*, **59**: 1098–1104.

6.3
Health-Related Quality of Life: Disease-Specific and Generic Dimensions in Social Phobia

Per Bech[1]

Health-related quality of life covers the three dimensions of physical, social and mental well-being outlined by the World Health Organization (WHO) [1]. As social phobia is defined as anxiety or phobic avoidance interfering with usual social activities and relationships, the health-related dimension of social well-being is a disease-specific quality of life measurement. On the other hand, mental or psychological well-being can be considered as a generic (disease-anonymous) quality of life dimension of social phobia and therefore of importance when comparing social phobia with other psychiatric or somatic disorders.

Only a few studies measuring social and psychological well-being in patients with social phobia have been published. Moreover, different quality of life scales have been used in these studies. In general, social well-being has been found to be decreased more than mental well-being in the epidemiological studies [2–4] as well as in the clinical studies [5–7].

Both Wittchen *et al.* [3] and Simon *et al.* [7] have used the Medical Outcome Studies (MOS) Short-form (SF-36) [8] in their studies. SF-36 is a multi-dimensional questionnaire including physical, social and mental well-being. In the epidemiological study by Wittchen *et al.* [3] and in the clinical study by Simon *et al.* [7], the subjects included had a mean age of 37 years, and the ratio between females and males was 2 to 1. In both studies the national scores are shown. Thus, in the study by Wittchen *et al.* [3] the German norms for SF-36 are given, and in the Simon *et al.* study [7] the US norms. The scores on the two subscales "social functioning" and "role limitation due to emotional problems" are lower than those on the subscale of mental well-being. However, the subscales included in the clinical study show higher impairment than those included in the epidemiological study.

In the longitudinal study by Yonkers *et al.* [9] on the clinical course of social phobia, the patients reported that they were around 39 years old when they first contacted a therapist, but that they were 14 years old at the onset of their illness. This early age of onset of social phobia has caused many problems when attempting to differentiate between the symptoms of social anxiety and shyness or avoidance behaviour personality. Most persons with social phobia consider their symptoms of anxiety as part of their habitual lifestyle behaviour. Therefore, personal construct trials have

---

[1] *Psychiatric Research Unit, Frederiksborg General Hospital, Dyrehavevej 48, DK-3400 Hillerød, Denmark*

indicated, as discussed by Bech [10], that individuals with social phobia consider their ideal self to be very close to their social introversion or avoidance behaviour. Even the most positive results with cognitive-behavioural therapy have shown that, although quality of life scores have improved during treatment, patients with social phobia remain clearly below those of normal controls [11]. The rather poor efficacy of cognitive therapy has been discussed in more detail by Hughes [12], who concluded that the outcome is only of clinical significance in those patients with most limited difficulties in quality of life.

Patients with social phobia are probably most accurately evaluated by use of health-related quality of life instruments covering both disease-specific (social) and generic (psychological) well-being. As the SF-36 subscale of mental well-being is a mixture of negative and positive items, the WHO-Five Well-Being Scale, which is a unidimensional psychological well-being scale, should be considered in future research as the most appropriate scale to be used in patients with social phobia [13].

REFERENCES

1. Bech P. (1998) *Quality of Life in the Psychiatric Patient*. Mosby-Wolfe, London.
2. Bech P., Angst J. (1996) Quality of life in anxiety and social phobia. *Int. Clin. Psychopharmacol.*, **11** (Suppl. 3): 16–20.
3. Wittchen H.U., Fuetsch M., Sonntag H., Muller N., Liebowitz M. (2000) Disability and quality of life in pure and comorbid social phobia: findings from a controlled study. *Eur. Psychiatry*, **15**: 46–58.
4. Stein M.B., Kean Y.M. (2000) Disability and quality of life in social phobia: epidemiologic findings. *Am. J. Psychiatry*, **157**: 1606–1613.
5. Schneier F.R., Heckelman L.R., Garfinkel R., Campeas R., Fallon B.A., Gitow A., Street L., Del Bene D., Liebowitz M.R. (1994) Functional impairment in social phobia. *J. Clin. Psychiatry*, **55**: 322–331.
6. Safren S.A., Helmberg R.G., Brown E.J., Holle C. (1997) Quality of life in social phobia. *Depress. Anxiety*, **4**: 126–133.
7. Simon N.M., Otto M.W., Korbly N.B., Peters P.M., Nicolaou D.C., Pollack M.H. (2002) Quality of life in social anxiety disorder compared with panic disorder and the general population. *Psychiatr. Serv.*, **56**: 714–718.
8. Ware J.E., Gandek B. (1994) The SF-36 health survey: development and use in mental health research and the IQOLA Project. *Int. J. Ment. Health*, **23**: 49–73.
9. Yonkers K.A., Dyck I.R., Keller M.B. (2001) An eight-year longitudinal comparison of clinical course and characteristics of social phobia among men and women. *Psychiatr. Serv.*, **52**: 637–643.
10. Bech P. (1999) Social anxiety disorder: the impact on quality of life. In *Focus on Psychiatry: Social Anxiety Disorder* (Eds H.G.M. Westenberg, J.A. den Boer), pp. 109–115. Syn-Thesis, Amsterdam.
11. Heimberg R.G. (2002) Cognitive-behavioral therapy for social anxiety disorder: current status and future directions. *Biol. Psychiatry*, **51**: 101–108.

12. Hughes I. (2002) A cognitive therapy model of social anxiety problems: potential limits on its effectiveness? *Psychol. Psychother.*, **75**: 411–435.
13. Bech P., Olsen L.R., Kjoller M., Rasmussen N.K. (2003) Measuring well-being rather than the absence of distress symptoms: a comparison of the SF-36 Mental Health subscale and the WHO-Five Well-Being Scale. *Int. J. Meth. Psychiatr. Res.*, **12**: 85–91.

6.4
What's So Different About Anxiety Disorders (Such as Phobias)?

Paul E. Greenberg, Howard G. Birnbaum and Tamar Sisitsky[1]

It is by now widely recognized that certain psychiatric disorders are just as costly to society from a social and economic perspective as major physical illnesses, such as cancer or heart disease. One reason for this profile is that anxiety/stress disorders are among the most commonly occurring chronic disorders in the general population, after back problems, arthritis and hypertension. In fact, anxiety disorders rival long-term physical illnesses like asthma and diabetes in terms of resulting impairment [1]. But, unlike the most widespread and disabling physical diseases, anxiety disorders are distinguished by their relatively young age of onset. According to the World Health Organization, in many Western countries, 50% of lifetime anxiety disorder sufferers will have experienced their first episode by the age of fifteen [2]. Only hay fever has a comparable lifetime prevalence and early age onset among physical conditions, and it tends to be active for only a small portion of each year.

Although the epidemiological characteristics of anxiety disorders are consistent with a widespread and deep societal problem, the health care response to this concern has been woefully incomplete. In fact, less than one in three anxiety disorder sufferers in the United States obtain treatment each year in the medical sector [3]. This reality underscores the importance of early outreach to reduce the risk for serious adverse life events from occurring during the anxiety sufferer's most formative years, including the possibility of lower educational attainment (i.e. high school dropout, lower rate of college attendance, non-completion of college), teenage childbearing, marital instability, poor career choice and unemployment. Since a number of these adverse life events are irreversible, the timing of treatment relative to an early age of onset is especially important.

Within the spectrum of anxiety disorders, phobias have certain specific features that are especially noteworthy in terms of their social and economic

---

[1] *Analysis Group, Inc., Boston, MA 02199, USA*

burden. Simple and social phobias, in particular, are highly prevalent in the US, affecting approximately 7–8% of the adult population each year and as much as 13% on a lifetime basis [4]. One of the characteristics of phobias that results in adverse impacts on role functioning and activities of daily living is the extent to which sufferers of these disorders impose self-limitations on the activities they are willing to undertake and accomplish. For example, an individual suffering from agoraphobia is likely to avoid situations that require travel, while a social phobia sufferer is likely to avoid interpersonal interactions. These responses can impose significant limitations on the range of productive contributions such individuals can make to society. In fact, it has been reported that social phobia, agoraphobia and simple phobia all result in excess work cutback, presumably for reasons such as these [5]. In addition to these responses, among those with phobias who are working, it has been found that the rate of employment and type of job obtained are adversely affected by the presence of these chronic conditions.

The profile of phobia sufferers sheds light on potential opportunities for cost offsets. Mania, major depression and dysthymia are especially likely among this group of individuals, in addition to both drug and alcohol abuse/dependence. Epidemiological evidence suggests that it is the phobia that tends to occur first, which is not surprising, given the early age of onset. While it may be the case that a particular phobia causally relates to later-onset psychiatric disorders, it is also possible that confounding factors (e.g. genetic, environmental) are the underlying causes of both conditions. In the case of substance abuse and dependence, however, it has been shown that early-onset anxiety disorders, including phobias, are significant predictors of subsequent substance disorders. This implies that more effective outreach to treat phobias at an early age could prevent a substantial number of drug and alcohol problems from arising later in life. Thus, the opportunities for substantial cost offsets from broader treatment are substantial in the case of phobias.

Less is known about patients' comorbidity patterns in terms of physical illnesses. It would be useful to assess the extent to which excess costs are incurred within the healthcare system as a result of phobia patients' elevated risk of physical disorders. This research has been well developed in the case of other psychiatric disorders. In a workplace-based study of employer claims data, for example, it was found that for every dollar spent treating depression itself, an additional dollar was spent treating comorbid physical illnesses, and an additional 50 cents was spent treating comorbid psychiatric disorders [6].

Phobias are a highly prevalent form of anxiety disorders, which are vastly under-treated and enormously burdensome. They often begin to take effect during an individual's formative years and can have long-term negative impacts. Not surprisingly, phobias can be extremely costly to society as the many adverse consequences of these disease characteristics take full effect. From a research perspective, a better understanding is needed of the cost–benefit proposition from earlier and more widespread outreach to effectively treat those directly affected by phobias. In addition, it would be useful to better document the hidden, family burden of phobias, which could include excess treatment for psychiatric care, as well as lost work time for caregivers who are employed.

REFERENCES

1. Kessler R.C., Greenberg P.E., Mickelson K.D., Meneades L.M., Wang P.S. (2001) The effects of chronic medical conditions on work loss and work cutback. *J. Occup. Environ. Med.*, **43**: 218–225.
2. Kessler R.C., Greenberg P.E. (2002) The economic burden of anxiety and stress disorders. In *Neuropsychopharmacology: The Fifth Generation of Progress* (Eds K.L. Davis, D. Charney, J.T. Coyle, C. Nemeroff), pp. 981–992. Lippincott Williams & Wilkins, Baltimore, MD.
3. Kessler R.C., Zhao S., Katz S.J., Kouzis A.C., Frank R.G., Edlund M., Leaf P. (1999) Past-year of outpatient services for psychiatric problems in the National Comorbidity Survey. *Am. J. Psychiatry*, **156**: 115–123.
4. Kessler R.C., McGonagle K.A., Zhao S., Nelson C.B., Hughes M., Eshleman S., Wittchen H.U., Kendler K.S. (1994) Lifetime and 12-month prevalence of DSM-III-R psychiatric disorders in the United States: results from the National Comorbidity Survey. *Arch. Gen. Psychiatry*, **51**: 8–19.
5. Kessler R.C., Frank R.G. (1997) The impact of psychiatric disorders on work loss days. *Psychol. Med.*, **27**: 861–873.
6. Birnbaum H.G., Greenberg P.E., Barton M., Kessler R.C., Rowland C.R., Williamson T.E. (1999) Cost analysis. Workplace burden of depression: a case study in social functioning using employer claims data. *Drug Benefit Trends*, **11**: 6–12.

6.5
Why Take Social Phobia Seriously?
Fiona Judd[1]

The approach to, and recognition of, the impact of phobic disorders have changed dramatically over the past 30 years. Marks, in his classic paper on classification [1], noted that phobias only achieved a separate diagnostic label in the American Psychiatric Association classification in 1952, and in

---

[1] *Centre for Rural Mental Health, Monash University and Bendigo Health Care Group, PO Box 126, Bendigo 3552, Australia*

the International Classification of Diseases in 1955. In his paper, in which he divides phobias of external stimuli (e.g. animal phobias), the agoraphobic syndrome and social phobias, Marks noted the need to know more about social phobias before definitely classifying them on their own. The review undertaken by Demyttenaere et al. clearly demonstrates the importance of work which has better identified and understood social phobia, clearly justifying a separate classification.

Historically, attention focused on the "visible" disorders. Marks [1] noted that the agoraphobic syndrome was the commonest and most distressing variety seen by psychiatrists; at that time it formed roughly 60% of all phobias at the Maudsley. By contrast, social phobic disorders formed 8% of those seen, and animal phobias were rare in hospital practice, representing about 3% of all phobics who came for treatment. By contrast, epidemiological studies have demonstrated social and simple phobias are more common than agoraphobia [2].

In 1985, Liebowitz and colleagues [3] subtitled their paper on social phobia "Review of a neglected anxiety disorder". They noted the absence of data regarding prevalence, severity and treatment. The statement by Demyttenaere et al. that the majority of research on burden and impairment is now found on social phobia rather than other phobic conditions is a stark contrast to this.

It is of note that data obtained from the National Comorbidity Survey indicates that both agoraphobia and social phobia cause economic burden [4], with agoraphobia being associated with greater utilization of psychiatric medical services and other specialist medical services than social phobia. By contrast, social phobia was associated with greater indirect cost resulting from work cutback days. Furthermore, the Global Burden of Disease [5] study ranked the disease burden, measured in Disability-Adjusted Life Years (DALYs) due to panic disorder, in the top 50. Social phobia was not included in this list for either the world or developed regions.

Why, then, has attention turned to social phobia? The review of Demyttenaere et al. provides a clear answer to this question. The disorder is common, there is often significant comorbidity, and the burden is high. Of note, burden is substantial in all three major areas of direct costs, indirect costs and health-related quality of life. Thus, it is of concern that Demyttenaere et al.'s review has demonstrated that only a minority of individuals with social phobia receive adequate treatment. Of note, Magee et al. [6] found social phobics were less likely to seek treatment than both agoraphobics and individuals with simple phobia.

Why do social phobics not receive adequate treatment? Demyttenaere et al. suggest this results from both patient filtering and doctor filtering barriers to treatment. The latter are of particular concern but also offer an opportunity for change. The differentiation of generalized and non-generalized social anxiety disorder [7] is an important one, which must be conveyed to those general practitioners who simply attribute social phobic complaints to an extreme form of shyness.

However, this differentiation into two subtypes, which has led to a focus on the generalized form, should be viewed with caution by clinicians. The generalized form is more common in psychiatric practice and is more often associated with a comorbid anxiety disorder [8]. As Demyttenaere et al. have noted, direct care costs for this group are comparable to those of subjects with pure major depression, and their rate of impairment in social contacts and relationship with partner is greater than that for the non-generalized form.

However, the non-generalized form, which is more common in non-clinical samples, does cause marked interference with work, social life or education, or marked distress to a significant number of those with the disorder [9]. It is essential that this group of individuals, like those with so-called simple phobia, are not neglected by clinicians and researchers.

REFERENCES

1. Marks I.M. (1970) The classification of phobic disorders. Br. J. Psychiatry, 116: 377–386.
2. Kessler R.C., McGonagle K.A., Zhao S., Nelson C.B., Hughes M., Eshleman S., Wittchen H., Kendler K. (1994) Lifetime and 12 month prevalence of DSM-IIIR psychiatric disorders in the United States: results from the National Comorbidity Survey. Arch. Gen. Psychiatry, 51: 8–19.
3. Liebowitz M.R., Gorman J.M., Fyer A.J., Klein D.F. (1985) Social phobia: review of a neglected anxiety disorder. Arch. Gen. Psychiatry, 42: 729–736.
4. Greenburgh P.E., Sisitsky T., Kessler R.C., Finkelstein S.N., Berndt E.R., Davidson J.R.T., Ballenger J.C., Fyer A.J. (1999) The economic burden of anxiety disorders in the 1990s. J. Clin. Psychiatry, 60: 427–435.
5. Murray C.J.L., Lopez A.D. (eds) (1996) The Global Burden of Disease: A Comprehensive Assessment of Mortality and Disability from Diseases, Injuries, and Risk Factors in 1990 and Projected to 2020. Harvard School of Public Health, Cambridge, MA.
6. Magee W.J., Eaton W.W., Wittchen H.U., McGonagle K.A., Kessler R.C. (1996) Agoraphobia, simple phobia, and social phobia in the National Comorbidity Survey. Arch. Gen. Psychiatry, 53: 159–168.
7. Ballenger J.C., Davidson J.R.T., Lecrubier Y., Nutt D.J. (1998) Consensus statement on social anxiety disorder. J. Clin. Psychiatry, 59 (Suppl. 17): 54–60.
8. Wittchen H.U., Nelson C.B., Kessler R.C. (1999) Social fears and DSM-IV. Social phobia in a community sample of adolescents and young adults: prevalence, risk factors and comorbidity. Psychol. Med., 29: 309–329.
9. Stein M.B., Walker J.R., Ford D.R. (1996) Public speaking fears in a community sample: prevalence, impact on functioning, and diagnostic classification. Arch. Gen. Psychiatry, 53: 169–174.

6.6
Phobias in Primary Care and in Young Children
Myrna M. Weissman[1]

Demyttenaere *et al.* provide a comprehensive review of the economic and social burdens of phobias. New studies in primary care and studies of children provide additional information.

Findings from a study of patients coming to primary care may help to clarify the under-utilization of services by patients with phobias. In a systematic sample of over 200 patients coming to an urban primary care practice, we found a 7% lifetime prevalence of blood–injection–injury phobias [1]. Patients with blood–injury phobias, as compared to those without, were significantly younger, more likely to have mood disorders and were highly socially impaired. The presence of a blood–injury phobia had a potentially serious impact on healthcare in that these patients, over the subsequent year, were *less* likely to have blood–injection-related procedures, such as glucose tests, serum cholesterol tests or flu shots. Blood–injury phobia was almost never diagnosed in the primary care setting, despite the fact that it was common. These patients seemed to be avoiding laboratory tests that involved blood drawing.

In the same study, we found the lifetime prevalence of social phobias was over 5% [2]. Patients with social phobias also seemed to avoid medical care. These patients were more likely to have other psychiatric disorders and to be functionally impaired. However, they made far *fewer* primary care visits per year when compared with patients with other psychiatric disorders or with controls. Their mental health utilization was at the same low level of the other psychiatric patients. Patients with social phobias had high rates of substance abuse but seemed to be avoiding going to their primary care physician for medical or for psychiatric care.

Finally, using a systematic sample of over 1000 primary care attenders in the same clinic, we found high rates of suicidal ideation in patients with panic disorder, or panic attacks, with and without agoraphobia. If the patient had both major depression and panic disorder, there was a 15-fold increased risk of having suicidal ideation. Again, neither the panic attacks, the agoraphobia nor the suicidal ideation was diagnosed and most of these people did not receive any psychiatric treatment [3].

Major depression has been a focus of most physician education and screening in primary care. Few studies have looked at the range of psychiatric disorders in patients coming to primary care. Few have concentrated on the phobias. These studies point out the need to broaden

---

[1] *New York State Psychiatric Institute, 1051 Riverside Drive, New York, NY 10032, USA*

both the screening and the physician education in primary care to include the anxiety disorders and suggest that the presence of an anxiety disorder has both mental and physical health consequences.

The social cost and burden of the phobias is also evident in studies of prepubertal children. There are now several epidemiologic [4–6] as well as clinical studies [6] showing that anxiety disorders, particularly phobias, before puberty are an early precursor of major depression. We have been following a group of depressed parents and normal controls and their offspring over 20 years. Now the third generation, the grandchildren, have been assessed. The major findings are strong familial aggregation of major depression across three generations (mood disorders in the grandparent were associated with mood disorder in the grandchildren, irrespective of the parental mood disorder), and the stability of the sequence of disorders spread across generations (specific phobias in childhood were followed by the emergence of major depression in adolescence). This increased risk of major depression, preceded by anxiety, was stable across three generations in the high-risk sample. Few prepubertal children who are phobic, shy and fearful ever receive treatment. The symptoms are often interpreted as being part of one's character and not a treatable state. As more treatment, both behavioural and pharmacological, becomes available for these disorders in children, possibly intervention studies will be developed. These findings suggest that the treatment of the phobic disorders in prepubertal adolescents could lead to the prevention of secondary depression. This is a hypothesis that has never been clinically tested.

Demyttenaere et al. note quite correctly that the majority of research of the phobias is on the social phobia, also known as social anxiety disorder. In addition to the epidemiological and clinical studies, data showing the high familial loading of the social phobias—over a three-fold increased risk in familial aggregation [7]—are also relevant to a discussion of burden. The more generalized social phobias characterized by fear and avoidance in a wide variety of social situations are specifically found in families. Based on the evidence for familial loading as well as evidence for moderate heritability from twin studies [8], there has been increased interest in attempting to determine the role of genetics. However, this work is still in its infancy [9].

REFERENCES

1. Gross R., Gameroff M.J., Olfson M., Feder A., Weissman M.M. (2002) Blood–injection–injury phobia in primary care. Presented at the American Psychiatric Association Annual Meeting, Philadelphia, 18–23 May.

2. Gross R., Olfson M., Gameroff M.J., Feder A., Weissman M.M. (2001) Social anxiety disorder in primary care. Presented at the American Psychiatric Association Annual Meeting, New Orleans, 5–10 May.
3. Goodwin R., Olfson M., Feder A., Fuentes M., Pilowsky D.J., Weissman M.M. (2001) Panic and suicidal ideation in primary care. *Depress. Anxiety*, **14**: 244–246.
4. Kessler R.C., Nelson C.B., McGonagle K.A., Edlund M.J., Frank R.G., Leaf P.J. (1996) The epidemiology of co-occurring addictive and mental disorders: implications for prevention and service utilization. *Am. J. Orthopsychiatry*, **66**: 17–31.
5. Pine D.S., Cohen P., Gurley D., Brook J., Ma Y. (1998) The risk for early-adulthood anxiety and depressive disorders in adolescents with anxiety and depressive disorders. *Arch. Gen. Psychiatry*, **55**: 56–64.
6. Weissman M.M., Warner V., Wickramaratne P.J., Nomura Y., Merikangas K., Bruder G., Tenke C.E., Grillon C. (2003) Offspring at high risk for anxiety and depression: preliminary findings from a three generation study. In *Fear and Anxiety: Benefits of Translational Research* (Ed. J. Gorman). American Psychiatric Association Press, Washington, DC.
7. Stein M.B., Chartier M.J., Hazen A.L., Kozak M.A., Tancer M.E., Lander S., Furer P., Chubaty D., Walker J.R. (1998) A direct interview family study of generalized social phobia. *Am. J. Psychiatry*, **155**: 90–97.
8. Kendler K.S., Neale M.C., Kessler R.C., Heath A.C., Eaves L.J. (1992) The genetic epidemiology of phobias in women: the interrelationship of agoraphobia, social phobia, situational phobia, and simple phobia. *Arch. Gen. Psychiatry*, **49**: 273–281.
9. Stein M.B., Chartier M.J., Kozak M.V., King N., Kennedy J.L. (1998) Genetic linkage to the serotonin transporter protein and $5HT_{2A}$ receptor genes excluded in generalized social phobia. *Psychiatry Res.*, **81**: 282–291.

6.7
Treatments Are Needed to Reduce the Burden of Phobic Illness
Peter P. Roy-Byrne and Wayne Katon[1]

Demyttenaere *et al.*'s review of the social and economic burden of phobias describes the health service use and determinants of use, barriers to obtaining treatment, prevalence and type of functional disability, types and amounts of associated costs, and impairment in quality of life, across a range of phobic disorders. The conclusions of this review are strikingly similar to those described by previous authors for depression: phobias are common, disabling, costly and associated with multiple impairments in quality of life. Despite this widespread burden of phobias on both the individual and society, stigma is high, perception of the problem as "psychiatric" by these individuals is infrequent, and help seeking is

---

[1] *Department of Psychiatry and Behavioral Sciences, University of Washington School of Medicine, Harborview Medical Center, 325 9th Avenue, Seattle, WA 98104, USA*

relatively low. The end result is that only a minority of patients with phobias receive effective treatment.

The gap between scientific knowledge about efficacious treatments for anxiety and depression, which is considerable, and the quality of care that these patients actually receive, which is poor, has been most frequently addressed for depression, with only a smattering of evidence for anxiety [1,2]. Strategies to increase the effective treatment of phobia in a variety of health care settings, especially primary care where many of these patients initially present for evaluation and treatment [3,4], are urgently needed. Such studies are crucial in order to reduce the substantial burden of illness. While no studies appear to have specifically addressed this issue with respect to the phobias, there may be things we can learn from closely related clinical areas.

Much of this review is focused on social phobia and the review concludes that relatively little data exists for the other phobic disorders. In contrast, there is a substantial amount of published information on panic disorder as it presents in a variety of health care settings, including information on quality of life, functional impairment, cost and quality of care [5,6]. Many panic disorder patients have substantial degrees of phobic avoidance and, even in the absence of agoraphobia, panic disorder is often construed as a "phobia" of internal bodily sensations [7]. Moreover, a review of this literature would lead to the same conclusions, i.e. panic is prevalent, disabling, costly, impairs quality of life and is infrequently treated despite the availability of treatment. What is available in the field of panic that could help address this interesting question about the gap between "efficacy" and "effectiveness"? Given the disappointing absence of cost studies in the phobia literature, is there data on cost of panic that might further inform the issue of effectiveness from this, as well as the clinical, perspective? As it turns out, there are a number of interesting studies of panic disorder that are relevant to these questions. Many of these studies focus on the primary care setting.

Our group tested the effectiveness of panic disorder pharmacotherapy embedded in the disease management framework of "collaborative care" by randomizing 115 patients to either this one-year intervention ($n = 57$) or care as usual by the primary care physician ($n = 58$) [8]. Intervention patients received selective serotonin reuptake inhibitors (SSRIs), videotape and pamphlet education, two psychiatrist visits and two phone calls in the first eight weeks and up to five follow-up phone calls over the year. Intervention patients had greater improvements in panic, anxiety, depressive, functional and quality of life measures (the latter measured with the Short Form-36) at three and six months and were more likely to receive effective pharmacotherapy (correct dose and type and duration). More importantly, this intervention was also shown to have a 70% probability of being a "dominant" intervention based on a greater number of anxiety-free days and lower total outpatient costs over a 12-month period in intervention compared to control patients. The added mental health costs of the intervention appeared to be offset by reduced direct medical care costs [9]. When the time off work to visit the doctor was considered, even more cost–benefit was seen for the intervention, since control patients had higher numbers of physician visits. About half of the mental health costs in intervention patients were costs of SSRIs. Given that fluoxetine is now off patent (with many other SSRIs to follow in 2003 and 2004), the cost of the collaborative intervention will decrease significantly further in the future.

This interesting finding is consistent with two other less well-designed studies of panic disorder costs in the specialty care setting. In the first study, Salvador-Carulla et al. [10] showed reduced medical care utilization among treated panic disorder patients in a 24 months pre-/post-design where patients were treated naturalistically with medication and psychotherapy by psychiatrists. When this was combined with savings from reduced indirect costs attributable to lost productivity (indirect costs were not measured in our study cited above), these savings were greater than the added mental health costs of the intervention. Finally, we used a managed formulary database and diagnostic codes to investigate in a pre-/post-design whether use of SSRIs in 120 panic disorder patients was associated with reductions in emergency room (ER) and laboratory visits, hypothesizing that these two measures would be most likely associated with overuse of medical care due to the dramatic physical manifestations of panic attacks [11]. The study showed significant reduction in ER and laboratory visits (40%) and costs (64%) compared with baseline. Total costs were still increased when medication and psychiatric visit costs were included. No indirect costs were considered in this analysis.

A larger three-site collaborative study investigating the effectiveness of a combined cognitive-behavioural therapy and pharmacotherapy approach to care as usual in 240 panic disorder over one year is now nearing completion [12]. Preliminary results of the first 6 months of this intervention show broad and highly significant effects across clinical, functional and quality of life measures [13]. Both direct and indirect costs will be considered in this analysis but have not yet been examined.

These findings suggest that anxiety disorder treatment is associated with broader effects on burden of illness than just symptomatic improvements (i.e. effects on functional status and quality of life), that these improvements may reduce direct medical and indirect (work and social function) costs, and that, even when the cost of treatment is considered, these treatments may be cost-effective, if not cost-neutral. Although our study showed that overall costs might be negligible, even modest costs would likely be associated with cost–benefit ratios that are traditionally seen as economically justifiable for other medical disorders. Future studies might extend these strategies to the group of phobic disorders discussed in this chapter, particularly social phobia and agoraphobia. Second-wave strategies that must also be pursued in this type of research with any of these disorders include investigating whether consideration of patient preference for different treatment modalities (e.g. medication, psychotherapy, group and individual formats etc.) before treatment assignment will improve patient recruitment (improving representativeness of study samples) as well as improving engagement in treatment and possibly cost-effectiveness; including broader measures of societal burden that span a more diverse set of stakeholders (family and employer have been inconsistently represented) in our outcome domains; designing treatments that can target multiple anxiety disorders rather than one because of the high rate of comorbidity between disorders; and determining how interventions need to be modified for culturally and economically disadvantaged populations. Consideration of these issues makes it clear that, although research on burden of illness has brought us part of the way toward the public health goal of understanding and ultimately treating these disorders, there is still a long way to go.

REFERENCES

1. Roy-Byrne P., Sherbourne C.D., Craske M.G., Stein M.B., Katon W., Sullivan G., Means-Christensen A., Bystritsky A. (2003) Moving treatment research from clinical trials to the real world: the design of a first-generation effectiveness study for panic disorder. *Psychiatr. Serv.*, **54**: 327–332.
2. Wells K.B. (1999) Treatment research at the crossroads: the scientific interface of clinical trials and effectiveness research. *Am. J. Psychiatry*, **156**: 5–10.
3. Stein M.B., McQuaid J.R., Laffaye C., McCahill E. (1999) Social phobia in the primary care medical setting. *J. Family Practice*, **49**: 514–519.
4. Spitzer R.L., Williams J.B., Kroenke K., Linzer M., deGruy F.V. III, Hahn S.R., Brody D., Johnson J.G. (1994) Utility of a new procedure for diagnosing mental disorders in primary care: the PRIME-MD 1000 study. *JAMA*, **272**: 1749–1756.
5. Roy-Byrne P.P., Stein M.B., Russo J., Mercier E., Thomas R., McQuaid J., Katon W.J., Craske M.G., Bystritsky A., Sherbourne C.D. (1999) Panic disorder in the primary care setting: comorbidity, disability, service utilization, and treatment. *J. Clin. Psychiatry*, **60**: 492–499.
6. Katon W. (1989) *Panic Disorder in the Medical Setting*. US Government Press, Washington, DC.
7. Reiss S., Peterson R.A., Gursky D.M., McNally R.J. (1986) Anxiety sensitivity, anxiety frequency and the predictions of fearfulness. *Behav. Res. Ther.*, **24**: 1–8.
8. Roy-Byrne P., Katon W., Cowley D., Russo J. (2001) A randomized effectiveness trial of collaborative care for patients with panic disorder in primary care. *Arch. Gen. Psychiatry*, **58**: 869–876.

9. Katon W., Roy-Byrne P., Russo J., Cowley D. (2002) Cost-effectiveness and cost offset of a collaborative care intervention for primary care patients with panic disorder. *Arch. Gen. Psychiatry*, **59**: 1098–1104.
10. Salvador-Carulla L., Segui J., Fernandez-Cano P., Canet J. (1995) Costs and offset effect in panic disorders. *Br. J. Psychiatry*, **27** (Suppl.): 23–28.
11. Roy-Byrne P.P., Clary C.M., Miceli R.J., Colucci S.V., Xu Y., Grudzinski A.N. (2001) The effect of SSRI treatment of panic disorder on emergency room and laboratory resource utilization. *J. Clin. Psychiatry*, **62**: 678–682.
12. Craske M.G., Roy-Byrne P.P., Stein M.B., Donald-Sherbourne C., Bystritsky A., Katon W.J., Sullivan G. (2002) Treating panic disorder in primary care: a collaborative care intervention. *Gen. Hosp. Psychiatry*, **24**: 148–155.
13. Roy-Byrne P., Craske M., Stein M., Sherbourne C., Bystrisky A., Katon W., Sullivan G. (2003) Improving care for panic disorder in primary care. In *Beyond the Clinic Walls: Expanding Mental Health, Drug and Alcohol Services Research Outside the Specialty Care System*. US Department of Health and Human Services, Washington, DC.

6.8
Early Diagnosis Can Reduce the Social and Economic Burden of Phobias

Antonio E. Nardi[1]

Phobic disorders are at the same time among the most disabling and the most prevalent of mental disorders. Often misdiagnosed and undertreated, they account for a staggering one-third of all costs related to mental disorders [1,2].

Agoraphobia is a severe disabling phobic syndrome, as it involves many ordinary daily situations and some patients can become restricted to their home. Economic, familial and social problems, together with low self-esteem and conjugal conflicts, are usually associated to agoraphobia, even of mild or moderate severity. The suicide risk is high and can be aggravated when comorbidity with major depression or drug abuse is present [3].

Social anxiety disorder patients commonly have educational underperformance [4]. They also have a lower probability of getting married and a higher chance of living with their parents, a lower economic status and a higher probability of losing their job. They are frequent users of the public health system [2,4]. All these problems can be worsened if the social anxiety disorder is accompanied by other mental disorders [2,4]. Comorbidity with somatic diseases, such as essential tremor or muttering, can also worsen the patient's quality of life [4]. The limitation of their lives and the economic

---

[1] *Institute of Psychiatry, Federal University of Rio de Janeiro, Rua Visconde de Piraja, 407/702, Rio de Janeiro 22410-003, Brazil*

and social problems are always underestimated, as the patients have never lived without the disorder.

Patients with social anxiety disorder identify the age of about 25 as the worst period of their lives. Perhaps this is due to the fact that around this age a shy teen behaviour cannot be sustained anymore, while the economic and social demands of adulthood cannot be postponed.

The low professional accomplishment due to social anxiety disorder is directly related to job instability, greater absenteeism or job changes [2]. There is a high percentage of jobless people among social anxiety disorder patients and in the USA more than 70% of social anxiety disorder patients are in the lowest economic group [2,5].

We studied in Brazil a social anxiety disorder sample ($n = 138$), compared with a control group of individuals without axis I disorders. We found that in men the rate of being out of the workforce was 61% in social phobic patients and 19% in the control group (a statistically significant difference). Among women, the corresponding figures were 45% and 34%. The mean number of years of education was 12.5 in the social anxiety disorder patients and 18.6 in the control group [6].

Some patients with phobic symptoms can work and try to adapt their life to their symptoms. However, there are losses that are very difficult to quantify. For example, the profession one desires can be made unaffordable by phobic symptoms, because it may require contact with the public. Patients become expert in avoiding feared situations like interviews or talks to a small group, even if this would be useful to their career. The early onset of symptoms in adolescence interferes with the acquisition of social abilities. The consequence is a social isolation pattern. Many phobic people are single, divorced or separated [2,5], and some only have contact with close relatives.

Specific phobias can also become a severe problem to patients, impairing dramatically their quality of life. Fear of medical procedures may delay necessary treatment of illnesses; fear of travelling may adversely affect a person's professional development; fears of gagging may restrict social life. The phobia of aeroplanes can limit careers and bring economic consequences.

Most of the costs of phobic disorders are not related to treatment but are the results of lost income and disability among people who are receiving no treatment for their phobic disorder. One of the astonishing things about working in the phobic disorders field is how media educational campaigns result in a dramatic increase of the number of treated patients with these conditions; patients often have symptoms for years, with no awareness that others have similar symptoms or that specific medical treatment exists. The consequences of an untreated phobic disorder can be devastating to the patient and his family. Education, information and knowledge leading to an early diagnosis and treatment are key elements in lowering the social and economic burden of phobias.

REFERENCES

1. DuPont R.L., DuPont C.M., Rice D.P. (2002) Economic costs of anxiety disorders. In *Textbook of Anxiety Disorders* (Eds D.J. Stein, E. Hollander), pp. 475–483. American Psychiatric Publishing, Washington, DC.
2. Schneier F.R., Heckelman L.R., Garfinkel R., Campeas R., Fallon B.A., Gitow A., Street L., Del Bene D., Liebowitz M.R. (1994) Functional impairment in social phobia. *J. Clin. Psychiatry*, **55**: 322–331.
3. Liebowitz M.R., Gorman J.M., Fyer A.J., Klein D.F. (1985) Social phobia: review of a neglected anxiety disorder. *Arch. Gen. Psychiatry*, **42**: 729–736.
4. Goisman R.M., Warshaw M.G., Steketee G.S., Fierman E.J., Rogers M.P., Goldenberg I., Weinshenker N.J., Vasile R.G., Keller M.B. (1995) DSM-IV and the disappearance of agoraphobia without a history of panic disorder: new data on a controversial diagnosis. *Am. J. Psychiatry*, **152**: 1438–1443.
5. Weiller E., Bisserbe J.C., Boyer P., Lépine J.P., Lecrubier Y. (1996) Social phobia in general health care: an unrecognized undertreated disabling disorder. *Br. J. Psychiatry*, **168**: 169–174.
6. Nardi A.E. (2000) *Transtorno de Ansiedade Social*. Medsi, Rio de Janeiro.

6.9
The High Cost of Underrecognition of Phobic Disorders

Julio Bobes[1]

Demyttenaere *et al.*, in their review, emphasize the significant social and economic burden that phobias produce in patients and their families. The recent interest in comprehensive outcome assessment, including aspects such as disability and quality of life, in the realm of phobic disorders [1–4] has contributed to a better understanding of these previously neglected disorders, especially social phobia and agoraphobia.

The European Study of the Epidemiology of Mental Disorders (ESEMeD-MHEDEA 2000) [5] aimed to evaluate various epidemiological aspects of depressive and anxiety disorders in the community in six European countries, including a total of 22 000 individuals representative of the non-institutionalized population aged 18 and over from Belgium, France, Germany, Italy, the Netherlands and Spain. These subjects were interviewed at home by using a computer-assisted personal interview (CAPI) including the most recent version of the Composite International Diagnostic

---

[1] C/Fuertes Acevedo 10-E, 2B, Oviedo, Spain

Interview (CIDI). Preliminary findings demonstrate that the prevalence of social anxiety disorder (SAD) ranges between 2% and 4%, being similar to that of post-traumatic stress disorder (PTSD) (2–3%) and generalized anxiety disorder (GAD) (1–4%). This disorder is inadequately treated and has an impact on quality of life greater than diabetes. Work days lost per year by people suffering from SAD (6.9) are similar to other phobic disorders, but lower than depressive disorders (8.4), GAD (8.7) and PTSD (10.5).

It can be concluded that, in spite of the progress made in the last decade, greater attention and educational efforts must be placed on phobic disorders, in order to improve their recognition and to provide adequate treatment.

There is a considerable need for studies in infants and adolescents. Early detection and intervention are extremely important. It is also necessary to highlight the "loss of opportunities" experience as a result of phobic disorders (work, education, social enrichment and social support networks).

It is clear that clinicians need to better understand this issue and to be able to intervene at an early stage. Cost-effectiveness and cost-utility studies need to be made in order to complete our current understanding.

REFERENCES

1. Bech P., Angst J. (1996) Quality of life in anxiety and social phobia. *Int. Clin. Psychopharmacol.*, **11** (Suppl. 3): 97–100.
2. Lecrubier Y. (1998) Comorbidity in social anxiety disorder: impact on disease burden and management. *J. Clin. Psychiatry*, **59** (Suppl. 17): 33–37.
3. Wittchen H.U., Fuetsch M., Sonntag H., Müller N., Liebowitz M. (2000) Disability and quality of life in pure and comorbid social phobia: findings from a controlled study. *Eur. Psychiatry*, **15**: 46–58.
4. Carpiniello B., Baita A., Carta M.G., Sitzia R., Macciardi A.N., Murgia S., Altamura A.C. (2002) Clinical and psychosocial outcome of patients affected by panic disorder with or without agoraphobia: results from a naturalistic follow-up study. *Eur. Psychiatry*, **17**: 394–398.
5. Alonso J., Ferrer M., Romera B., Vilagut G., Angermeyer M., Bernert S., Brugha T.S., Taub N., McColgen Z., De Girolamo G. et al. (2002) The European Study of the Epidemiology of Mental Disorders (ESEMeD/MHEDEA 2000) project: rationale and methods. *Int. J. Meth. Psychiatr. Res.*, **11**: 55–67.

6.10
Unanswered Questions on Phobias: What Can We Do to Meet the Need?
T. Bedirhan Üstün[1]

It is widely known that epidemiological data could be used to indicate the "need" either met or unmet in the community [1]. Perhaps using the scientific evidence may serve as the best advocacy: "we counted the people, they suffer from well-defined disorders, they are limited in their daily lives and overall productivity, there are treatments which are effective, acceptable and affordable; however, these people remain undiagnosed and untreated". These are very logical and powerful arguments against which the people responsible for providing treatments gasp with surprise and silence. Most often, however, no action follows to correct this situation.

The above schema applies to "phobias" as well as all other mental disorders. They are frequent, disabling, burdensome to people and to society, and use of interventions for these conditions seems to be far from optimal [2]. It seems that there is inertia in the face of evidence. The first question to answer is why there is inertia despite the presence of real disorders and effective treatments.

In general, the stigma associated with mental disorders both in the public and among professionals is a contributory factor to hindering the disclosure of such problems. In the case of phobias there may be additional factors related to the fear of stigma. The personal experience of this disorder may be regarded more as a trait (e.g. prudence, harm avoidance). Moreover, inability to express "fears" as emotions (i.e. a type of alexithymia) may be an underlying or coexisting feature. Evidently anxiety and phobic disorders start early in life: therefore coping mechanisms to deal with these disorders may gradually be engraved in the lifestyles of patients and it may therefore be difficult to uncover the signs of illness.

What we need, then, may be more mental health literacy efforts to enlighten the public about these disorders and possible interventions. Structured self-help programmes may be a good match for people with social phobia. Most importantly, given the "illness career" of these people with social phobia, it is essential that we intervene early in their lives, before any comorbidity with depression or substance abuse develops [3] and other negative life consequences take place. It is possible to design prevention programmes in at-risk children to manage fears and anxiety, distorted beliefs and dysfunctional behaviour.

The second question is about the nature of the need: do the head-counts in the epidemiological surveys really signify the need? What actually drives

---
[1] World Health Organization, 1211 Geneva 27, Switzerland

patients to treatment seeking is the distress or functional limitations in their lives. This issue has been addressed as "clinical significance" in DSM-IV, but has been poorly operationalized in surveys. The ICD uncouples disability from disease and uses the International Classification of Functioning, Disability and Health (ICF) to measure and classify associated disability. Such independent assessment of disease symptoms and functional limitations provides a good scientific approach to study the contribution of each component (i.e. disease and disability) separately in the resulting outcome: the need for treatment [4].

The final question is one of policy: what can be done to change the current practice? We should gather evidence in a comparative framework, including all diseases together so as to put mental disorders (including phobias) in "parity" with physical disorders. When one applies similar criteria to measure the burden, costs, effectiveness and other system outcomes, the glaringly unequal treatment for mental disorders becomes evident. Such comparative assessments should be made public to inform policy and shape health care provision. Both policy makers and practitioners are in need of good evidence to guide their decision making.

Evidence alone cannot change the world. It takes quite a long time until evidence is assimilated in daily practice. The gap between evidence and practice arises because of the complex systems challenges, which we are not especially well equipped to deal with. Bridging this gap may be facilitated by employing the learning tools that have emerged from systems thinking as it applies to quality improvement in health care [5]. This "pragmatic science" is a kind of operational research that identifies the Plan–Do–Study–Act (PDSA) method and the principles of its application to systems challenges. Using science and information technology we can speed up the dissemination and uptake of good practices [6].

REFERENCES

1. Üstün T.B. (2000) Unmet need for management of mental disorders in primary care. In *Unmet Need in Psychiatry: Problems, Resources, Responses* (Eds G. Andrews, S. Henderson), pp. 157–171. Cambridge University Press, London.
2. Üstün T.B., Sartorius N. (1995) *Mental Illness in General Health Care: An International Study*. John Wiley & Sons, Chichester.
3. Kessler R. (2003) The impairments caused by social phobia in the general population: implications for intervention. *Acta Psychiatr. Scand.*, **417** (Suppl.): 19–27.
4. Üstün T.B., Chatterji S., Rehm J. (1998) Limitations of diagnostic paradigm: it doesn't explain "need". *Arch. Gen. Psychiatry*, **55**: 1145–1146.
5. Berwick D.M., Nolan T.W. (1998) Physicians as leaders in improving health care. *Ann. Intern. Med.*, **128**: 289–292.
6. Berwick D.M. (2003) Disseminating innovations in health care. *JAMA*, **289**: 1969–1975.

Index

abuse and dependence liability 164
adolescents
  Brazilian studies 299–301
  effectiveness of treatment 298
  fear, anxieties and treatment efficacy 283–5
  implications for public policy 297–9
  internalizing/externalizing behaviour 300
  phobias in
    commentaries 280–302
    review 245–79
    psychosocial interventions 257–69
    treatment strategy for 271–2
adrenergic agents 127–8
affective disorders 50, 73–4
age effects 65
age of onset 11–12, 297
  identification of 90
agoraphobia 6–12, 16–19, 23, 25, 37, 46, 62, 109, 132, 147, 149
  age of onset 297
  and panic attacks 33–6, 55, 147, 171–2
  and panic disorder 243, 297–8
  see also panic disorder
  areas still open to research 200
  choice of treatment 168–9
  combined *in vivo* exposure and pharmacotherapy 181–2
  consistent evidence 198
  definitions 42
  diagnosis 40
  differential diagnosis 18–19
  drug trials for treatment 171
  economic burden 340
  evidence-based treatment guidelines 168
  future studies 347
  help seeking and use of medication 305
  in childhood 247
  in vivo exposure 34, 181–2, 186, 220–1
    basic components 180–1
    efficacy of 181

    methods of delivery 182–3
  incomplete evidence 199
  onset and discourse 17
  panics in 17–18
  pharmacotherapy of 128–9, 159, 167–70
  politicization of 36
  psychological treatment 228–9
  psychotherapeutic interventions 179–80
  rates of treatment-seeking 333
  social and economic burden 348
  targeted maintenance treatment 169
  without history of panic disorder 16–19
  without panic disorder 45, 144, 175, 297–8
agoraphobic syndrome 340
airport travellers 161
alcohol, hazards of 161
alcohol abuse 100, 161, 318–20, 334
alprazolam 118, 125, 129, 149
American Psychiatric Association 1
amitriptyline 13
animal models 96–7
animal phobia 7, 12, 24, 47
animal studies 151
anorexia nervosa 26
anticonvulsants 126–7, 153
antidepressants 39, 42, 120–1, 123, 128, 130, 147, 161–2, 168
  delayed action 169
  discontinuation of 169
  non-responders to 164
  panic disorder 128
antipanic drugs 36
antipanic medications 39
antipsychotics 100, 127
anxiety 11, 62
  and therapeutic relationship 240
  as manifestation of depressive illness 238
  epidemiological dissection 81
  meaning and etiology 239–40

anxiety (cont.)
  precipitant for onset of 239
anxiety disorders 7, 15, 35, 50, 59–60, 65, 71
  age of onset 337
  and affective disorders 70
  cognitive-behavioural therapy (CBT) 229
  comorbidity 66
  early intervention 113–15
  epidemiological aspects 337, 350
  gender effect in 295
  genetic epidemiology 83
  in acute studies 157
  in children 76
  late-life 107
  modes of acquisition (MOAs) 83
  prevalence in children 247–8
  psychodynamic therapy 238
  social and economic burden 337–9
  treatment of 143
    broader effects on burden of illness 346
  see also generalized anxiety disorder (GAD); social anxiety disorder (SAD)
Anxiety Disorders Association of America (ADAA) 329
anxiety neurosis 33
anxiolytics 149, 161
anxious personality disorder 54
assertiveness 53
atenolol 118, 127, 129
attachment security 290–1
attention-deficit/hyperactivity disorder 109
  in children 249, 301
attentional bias in social phobia 56
Australian National Mental Health Survey 67, 235
autonomic symptoms 117, 127–8
autonomous anxiety syndromes 238
aversions 55, 57
  disablement due to 29
  discomfort due to 29
  examples 29
avoidance, presence of 5
avoidance behaviour 117, 161
avoidance measures 53
avoidance problem 112
avoidance scale 111

avoidant personality disorder (APD) 12, 23, 37, 51, 54, 73–4, 93, 190
azapirones 126

barbiturate-assisted desensitization 125
barbiturates 129
behavioural desensitization 129
behavioural experimentation 223–6
  specific phobias 225
behavioural inhibition, genetic influences 296
behavioural toxicity of pharmacotherapeutic agents used in social phobia 172–4
benzodiazepines 97, 125–6, 129–31, 144, 146, 159, 161–2, 164, 169–70, 270
  adverse effects 126
beta-blockers 127–8, 159, 163
$beta_1$-blocker 129
$beta_1$-receptors 127
$beta_2$-blocker 129
$beta_2$-receptors 127
biological-constitutional factors 253
bipolar comorbidity in phobic patients 101
bipolar disorder 166
  and social phobia comorbidity 98–102
bipolar I disorder 104
bipolar II disorder 104
bird phobia 251
blood–injection–injury phobia 57, 194
blood–injury phobia 6, 12–13, 37, 44, 47
blood pressure 255
body dysmorphic disorder 19, 23, 130
breast cancer 27
Brief Social Phobia Scale 155
broad-spectrum effects 39
brofaramine 164
brofaromine 121
bromazepam 125, 170
bupropion 125
bupropion-SR 125
buspirone 126, 149

cardiorespiratory crisis 96
categorical approach 59–60
Child Behaviour Checklist (CBCL) 300
childhood-onset pervasive developmental disorder (COPDD) 286
childhood phobias 90, 342–4
  age of onset 280

INDEX 357

agoraphobia in 247
and retrospective studies of adults with anxiety disorders 283
anxiety disorders 76
assessment and treatment 292–4
attention-deficit/hyperactivity disorder 249, 301
Brazilian studies 299–301
causal processes 280
claustrophobia 251
cognitive-behavioural procedures 266–9
cognitive-behavioural therapy (CBT) 222
combined psychosocial and pharmacological interventions 270–1
commentaries 280–302
comorbidity 287, 293
consistent evidence 272–3
contingency management 265–6
continuation treatment 271
development fears to phobias 290–1
effectiveness of treatment 298
epidemiology 247–9
etiology 249–57, 288–90, 295
exposure therapy 289
fears, anxieties and treatment efficacy 283–8
gender factor 298
implications for public policy 297–9
importance of linking theory, intervention and outcome 292
incomplete evidence 273
increased rates of anxiety disorders and phobic disorders in parents 256
inhibited and uninhibited 254–5, 281
internalizing/externalizing behaviour 300
longitudinal studies 284
maintenance treatments 271
modelling techniques 262–5
overanxious disorder 249
pharmacological interventions 269–70, 297
prevalence of anxiety disorders 247–8
principles of treatment 257–71
psychological treatment 290–1
psychosocial interventions 257–69, 273, 281–2
review 245–79
separation anxiety disorder 249
small animal phobias 251
social anxiety 176
social cost and burden of phobias 343
social phobia 130, 247, 251
specific phobias 249, 272–3, 280
areas still open to research 273–4
SSRIs 124, 284
stable/unstable 255–6
systematic desensitization 258–62
treatment 288–90
treatment strategy 271–2
choking phobia 130
cholinergic gene expression 96
cholinergic receptor regulation 96
citalopram 42, 121, 124, 132, 147
classification 1–32, 43–5, 59–60
clusters in 47–9
commentaries 33–60
comorbidity in 47–9
context in 47–9
critical evaluation 38–40
politics and pathophysiology 36–8
purposes of 2–3
review 1–32
claustrophobia 7
in children 251
Clinical Global Impression 321
clinical severity measures 315
clinical significance of phobias 108
clinical theories and empirical findings 94–8
clomipramine 42, 121, 129
clonazepam 125–6, 144, 170
clonidine 127
clusters in classification 47–9
cognitive approach to phobias 55–9
cognitive-behavioural group treatment (CBGT) 190–2
cognitive-behavioural therapy (CBT) 92, 109, 132–3, 143–5, 156–7, 176, 185–7, 190, 293, 321–2
anxiety disorders 229
durability of 226–8
efficacy of 215–16, 242
in children 222, 266–9
vs. pharmacotherapy 191–2, 238
cognitive restructuring 189–90, 238
cognitive therapy 225
for panic disorder 34

collaborative care intervention in primary care 334
combined cognitive-behavioural therapy and pharmacotherapy approach, effectiveness 346
combined psychosocial and pharmacological interventions in children 270–1
combined treatments 156–7, 169, 216
  delayed action of antidepressants 169
comorbid depression 114, 132
comorbid disorders 215, 334
comorbid mood and anxiety disorders 113, 118
comorbid personality disorders 186
comorbid social phobia, work impairment 313
comorbid substance use, in social anxiety disorder 123
comorbid substance use disorders 132
comorbidity 35, 69–70, 111–12, 149
  and phobias 99
    diagnostic and therapeutic challenges 165–7
  and phobias and mood disorders, diagnostic and treatment implications 103–4
  and phobic disorders and alcohol or drug abuse 320
  and quality of life 348
  anxiety and depression 82
  help-seeking behaviour 306
  in anxiety disorders 66
  in children 287, 293
  in classification 47–9
  in social phobia 50–2
  influence on treatment modality and therapeutic success 295
  neurotic diagnoses and personality abnormality 92
  patterns of 77
  social phobia and bipolar disorder 98–102
  treatment effectiveness in 112
  with physical illness 338
Composite International Diagnostic Interview (CIDI) 63, 65–7, 81, 98, 350–1
computer-assisted personal interview (CAPI) 350

Computer Automatic Virtual Environment (CAVE) 221
context in classification 47–9
contextual fears 145
contingency management in children 265–6
continuation treatment in children 271
cost effectiveness 334
criterion symptoms 87
crowds 7
cultural factors 83
Culture and Mental Disorders 83
cumulative disability 75

decision making 304
defence systems 150
demographic data 310
dental phobia 130–1
depersonalization–derealization syndrome 19
depression 11, 19, 23, 28–9, 56, 99, 123, 126, 166, 176, 334
  across three generations 343
  comorbid 114
  epidemiological aspects 350
  healthcare service utilization 311
  impact of subthreshold symptoms on outcomes 86–7
  in primary care 342
depressive disorders, epidemiological dissection 81
developmental fears in children 290–1
diagnosis 1–32, 53, 59–60
  commentaries 33–60
  review 1–32
Diagnostic and Statistical Manual *see* DSM
diagnostic classifications 3
diagnostic criteria 35, 50
Diagnostic Interview Schedule (DIS) 63, 81, 98, 110
diagnostic issues in psychotherapeutic interventions 238
diffuse shyness 12, 37
dimensional approach 59–60
direct costs 310–12, 340
direction of causation 94
disability
  attributed to panic and phobias 70–1
  in panic/agoraphobia group of disorders 74–5

INDEX

Disability-Adjusted Life Years (DALYs) 340
Disability Assessment Schedule 53
dizziness 37
DNA, interstitial duplication of stretch of 84
doctor-filtering barriers to treatment 309
dopaminergic neurocircuitry 125
dot probe task 56
drug abuse 318–20
DSM 1–2, 105
DSM-III 39, 63, 67, 303, 319
DSM-III-R 37, 50, 63, 65–6
DSM-IV 34–5, 37, 40, 46–7, 63–4, 67, 73, 86, 246–7, 292, 299, 317, 353
DSM-IV-TR 14, 53–4, 60
DSM-V 60
Duke University Epidemiological Catchment Area Study 86
dynamic context for exposure 241
dysmorphophobia 19, 23, 25–8, 57, 130
    differential diagnosis 26
    onset and discourse 26

Early Developmental Stages of Psychopathology (EDSP) study 66, 308
eating disorders 71
economic aspects of treatment 320–2
economic burden *see* social and economic burden
economic impact, functional impairment 309
educational-supportive group therapy 192
effectiveness vs. efficacy studies 239
efficacy studies vs. effectiveness 239
emergency room (ER) and laboratory visits 346
emotion-focused psychotherapy 241
emotion-focused therapy (EFT) 185, 187
emotional problems 71
empirical findings and clinical theories 94–8
endophenotypes 37
environmental costs 309
environmental influences 254, 281
epidemiological aspects
    of anxiety disorders 337, 350
    of depression 350
Epidemiological Catchment Area (ECA) study 64, 69, 106, 110, 303–5, 329

epidemiological renaissance 89
epidemiology of phobias
    challenges for 89–91
    commentaries 81–115
    early intervention of anxiety disorders 113–15
    in children 247–9
    in clinical settings 304
    old terminology and new relevance 105–8
    review 61–80
epidemiology of social phobia 73–4
epilepsy 27
escitalopram 122
European College of Neuropsychopharmacology 153
European Study of the Epidemiology of Mental Disorders (ESEMeD-MHEDEA 2000) 350
evidence-based treatment guidelines for agoraphobia 168
exposure, dynamic context for 241
exposure *in vivo*
    agoraphobia *see* agoraphobia
    efficacy of 220–3
    social phobia 221
exposure therapy 13, 34, 44, 129, 168, 217–19, 238
    application 218–19
    clinical implications 233–4
    efficacy of 232–4
    feedback manipulations 233
    in children 289
    manipulation of cognitive parameters 233
    manipulation of safety behaviours 233
    phenomenology and process 218
    rationale 218
    research questions 219
exposure/habituation paradigm 168
external context 48–9
extinction 224
Eysenck Personality Questionnaire 83

fainting 6, 12–13, 37
familial aggregation 95
familial loading of social phobias 343
familiality 12
Fear Questionnaire 111, 321
Fear Survey Schedule (FSS) 111

fear(s) 110, 245–7
  acquisition of 253
  and panic disorder 97
  focus of 48
  from same or different syndromes 9
  in adolescence 76
  in children 285–8
  irrational 61–3
  normal 4–5, 246
  of dying 37
  of falling 12–13, 49
  of illness 27
  of lifts 61
  of psychiatric disorder 90
  propensity of 76
  protective 4–5
  symptoms 109
  vs. phobias 246
fluoxetine 42, 122, 192, 270
fluvoxamine 122
flying phobia 175
Food and Drug Administration (FDA) 39
frequency of panic/phobia group of disorders 74
Freud, Sigmund 33
functional disability measures 315
functional impairment, economic impact 309, 315–17

GABA system 144
GABAergic system 127
gabapentin 126
gender distribution across phobias 49
gender factor 12
  in anxiety disorders 295
  in childhood phobias 298
general neurotic syndrome 84, 92
general practitioner 92
generalized anxiety disorder (GAD) 29, 51, 168, 176, 351
genetic epidemiology 81–5
  of anxiety disorders 83
genetic factors 37, 83, 95, 254
genetic influences 257
  in behavioural inhibition 296
genetic isolates 82–3
genetic nosology 37
genetic predisposition 44
genetic studies 46–7
genome scans 84

germ phobia, use of term 166
Global Burden of Disease 305, 340
Great Smoky Mountain Study (GSMS), age of onset 298
group cognitive behavioural therapy (CBT) 118–20, 125

habituation 224
Hamilton Rating Scale for Anxiety 321
Harvard/Brown Anxiety Research Program 243
Head Mounted Display (HMD) 221
health, definition of 330
health-related quality of life
  social phobia 335–7
  use of term 335
  see also quality of life
health service use
  areas still open to research 323
  barriers to treatment 307–9
  consistent evidence 322–3
  determinants of 305–7, 344–8
  incomplete evidence 323
  panic disorders 345
  use in phobias 304–9
height phobias 49
heritability of phobias 253–4
hierarchy rules 64
higher education 333
hippocampally-based implicit memories 145
5-HT_{1A} antagonist 128
5-HT_3 antagonist 126
Hutterites 82–3
hypersensitivity 95
hyperventilation 95
hypervigilance to specific panic- and agoraphobia-related words 55
hypochondriasis 7–8, 25–7, 55, 57, 130
  differential diagnosis 28
  distress and disability in 27
(hypo)mania 101
hypothalmic–pituitary–adrenal axis activation 97

ICD 1, 105, 353
ICD-10 14, 34–5, 40, 46–7, 53–4, 60, 63–4, 66–7, 86
illness fears 27
illness phobia 28, 130

INDEX 361

imipramine 42, 128–9, 147, 149–50, 156, 168
Index of Social Phobia Improvement (ISPI) 321
indirect costs 312–13, 340
inhibition/uninhibition 255–6
internalizing factor 11
International Classification of Diseases *see* ICD
International Classification of Functioning, Disability and Health (ICF) 353
International Personality Disorders Examination 54
International Spectrum Project 87
interoceptive exposure (IE) 225
interpretation biases in social phobia 56
interstitial duplication of stretch of DNA 84
introversion vs. extroversion 254, 296

joint laxity risk 84

"Katharina" 33
kava-kava extract 129

lack of self-assertion 22
lactate infusions 37
late-life anxiety disorders 107
Latin America, psychotherapeutic treatment 242–4
Liebowitz Social Anxiety Scale (LSAS) 53, 123, 155, 171, 312, 316, 321
lifts, fear of 61
limited symptom panic attack 45
lithium 100
Longitudinal Interval Follow-up Evaluation (LIFE) 227

maintenance treatments in children 271
major depressive disorder (MDD) 86–7
Marks, Isaac 33, 36–40, 42–3, 45, 49, 52
Mataix-Cols, David 34–40, 42–3, 49, 52
Medical Outcome Studies (MOS) Short-form (SF-36) 335
medical practitioner consultations 71–2
memory of trauma 84
mental disorders, identifying 62
Meyer, Adolf 35
moclobemide 120–1, 123, 132
modelling techniques in children 262–5

monoamine oxidase B 121
monoamine oxidase inhibitors (MAOIs) 42, 118–19, 128, 144, 146, 149, 161, 163, 170
monoaminergic systems 127
mood disorders 39, 343
mood stabilizers 100
mouse models 96
multiple illness phobias 26–7
Munich EDSP survey 72

National Anxiety Disorders Screening Day 317
National Comorbidity Survey (NCS) 64–5, 158, 297, 303, 305–7, 329, 340
National Institute of Mental Health (NIMH) 329
National Psychiatric Morbidity Surveys of Great Britain 66
nefazodone 124
Netherlands Mental Health Survey 66
neuraesthenia 33
neuropsychology of defence 148–52
neuroscience research 59
neuroscientific theory 148
neurotic disorders, classes of drugs effective in treating 150
neurotic syndromes 149
New York Longitudinal Study 254
nicotine dependence in social phobia 319
non-associative models 95
non-criterion symptoms 87
non-phobia-like syndromes 16
noradrenaline reuptake inhibitors 124
norepinephrine 147
nosology 46–7, 50–2
nosophobia 7

obsessive–compulsive disorder (OCD) 6, 8–9, 19, 23, 25–6, 28, 33, 39, 44, 57, 71, 130, 150, 166, 168, 293
odansetron 126
oedipal crisis 143
one-session therapy 296
outcome measures 321
outpatient services 72
overanxious disorder in children 249

panic
    definition 6

panic (*cont.*)
  experience of 6
  uncued 7
  use of term 45
panic and agoraphobia group of disorders, disability in 74–5
panic and phobia group of disorders, frequency of 74
panic and phobias 68–73
  as major public health problem 76
  chronicity 68–9
  disability attributed to 70–1
  sociodemographic characteristics 68
panic attacks 34, 36–7, 40, 61, 147, 168
  and agoraphobia 171–2
  frequency of 171
  management of 236
  role of spontaneous, unexpected 40–2
  use of term 45
panic control treatment (PCT) 184–5, 187, 199
panic disorder 19, 33–4, 36, 95, 114, 128, 156, 334
  and agoraphobia 16–19, 41–2, 44, 99, 185–6, 199, 243
    differentiation of 42
    in parents 255
    predictors of treatment outcome 186
    prodromes 41
  and fear 97
  and phobias
    phenotype–genotype relationships in 84
    treatments for 75–6
  and social phobia, comorbidity in 51
  antidepressants 128
  areas still open to research 200
  cognitive therapy for 34
  consistent evidence 198
  costs 346
  diagnosis 7
  Harvard/Brown Anxiety Research Program 243
  health service use 345
  in primary care 334
  incomplete evidence 199
  pharmacotherapy 128, 345
  psychotherapeutic interventions 179–80, 183–6
  treatment effectiveness studies 229
  without agoraphobia 225, 243
panic-focused psychodynamic psychotherapy (PFPP) 185–6, 199, 239
paranoid syndromes 19, 23
parenting influences 253
Parkinson's disease and phobic disorders 164
paroxetine 42, 122, 129, 144, 170, 270
patient-filtering barriers to treatment 308–9
personal relationships 309
pervasive developmental disorders (PDD) 286
pharmacological interventions in children 269–70, 297
pharmacotherapeutic agents used in social phobia, behavioural toxicity of 172–4
pharmacotherapy 34, 199
  and psychotherapy 216
  as front-line treatment 301–2
  of agoraphobia 128–9, 159, 167–70
  of miscellaneous phobias 130–1
  of panic disorder 345, 128
  of phobias
    commentaries 143–77
    development of 163
    new neuroscience context 143–5
    review 117–42
    theories and effectiveness 175–7
  of phobic disorders, future directions 156–8
  of social anxiety disorder (SAD) 154–5, 158–60
  of social phobia 117–28
    long–term 170–2
  of specific phobia 129–30
  vs. CBT 191–2, 238
phenelzine 42, 118–19, 125, 129, 170, 192
phenomenology of social phobia 148–9
phenotype–genotype relationships in panic disorder and phobias 84
phobia
  areas still open to research 30
  characterization 245
  clinical picture 246–7
  clinical significance of 108
  consequences of untreated 349–50
  consistent evidence 30
  cues 4

INDEX 363

definitions 246
differential diagnosis 246–7
examples 4
external or internal cues 10
facts or fiction 110–12
handy or handicapping conditions 91–4
history of concept 1–2
incomplete evidence 30
neglected or minor disorders 52–4
occurrence 4
persistence over years 9–10
presence of non-phobic (uncued) symptoms 10–11
prevalence of 303, 338–9
reflections on definitions 108–10
specific or multiple cues 7–10
stigma associated with 352
subjective experience of the cue 5–7
subtypes 37
unanswered questions 352–3
underrecognition 350–1
use of term 43
vs. fears 246
phobia-like syndromes 15
phobic clusters 8–9
phobic disorders
  psychoanalytic treatment of 144
  range of treatment approaches 153
phobic syndromes 15–29
physical illness, comorbidity with 338
physician education, need of 333–4
physiological dependency 161
physiological symptoms 117
pindolol 128
Plan–Do–Study–Act (PDSA) method 353
post-traumatic stress disorder 19, 23, 25, 28–9, 57, 70–1, 168, 242, 351
  differential diagnosis 29
  onset and discourse 28
potential cognitive impairment 125
preferential processing of social-threat-related words 56
pregabalin 127, 132, 144
Present State Examination 110
prevalence of phobias 63–7, 76–7, 303, 338–9
primary care
  collaborative care intervention in 334
  depression in 342

panic disorder in 334
phobias in 342–4
vs. secondary care 92
principal complaint technique 71
proportional impairment ratio (PIR) 173–4
propranolol 127
prototypical mental disorders 60
psychiatric disorder, fear of 90
psychiatric epidemiology 85–8
psychiatric nosology 330
psychoanalytic treatment of phobic disorders 144
psychobiology of phobias 146–8
psychodynamic approaches to phobic disorders 238
psychodynamic group therapy 243
psychodynamic therapy, anxiety disorders 238
psychoeducation 124
psychological reliance 161
psychological treatment
  in agoraphobia 228–9
  in children 290–1
  in phobias 228–32
  in social phobia 229–30
  in specific phobias 230–1
psychopharmacology treatment of phobias and avoidance reactions 160–2
psychosocial interventions
  in adolescence 257–69
  in childhood 257–69, 273, 281–2
psychotherapeutic interventions
  agoraphobia 179–80
  diagnostic issues in 238
  in Latin America 242–4
  panic disorder 179–80, 183–6
  psychoanalytic-attachment perspective 237–41
  review 179–210
  social phobia 187–93
  specific phobia 193–8
psychotherapy 34, 176
  and pharmacotherapy 216
public health perspective, treatment of phobic disorders 235–7
public policy 112

quality of life 172–3, 314–20
  and comorbidity 348

quality of life (cont.)
  burden of phobias on 329
  domains that need to be assessed 321
  dysfunction 330
  generic measures 315
  measures 330
  rating scales measuring 315
  specific phobias 349
  see also health-related quality of life
questionnaire vs. clinical interview 91

randomized controlled trials (RCTs) 117, 119, 121, 123, 126, 133, 262–3
regression strategies 71
relaxation training 188
remission 176
research, areas still open to 77
response to treatment 13–14, 39
reversible inhibitors of monoamine oxidase A (RIMAs) 119–21, 163–4
risk-factor epidemiology 81–5
role impairment 315–17

Schedule of Affective Disorders and Schizophrenia (SADS) 99
Schedule of Assessing Assertive Behaviour 53
schizophrenia 71, 99, 166
school phobia 130
school-refusing children 249
seasonal affective disorders (SAD) 155
selective serotonin-reuptake inhibitors see SSRIs
selegiline 121
self-exposure 192
self-help, cost-saving approach 236
self-report studies 253
sensation-focused therapy (S-FIT) 183, 187
separation anxiety disorder 130
  in children 249
serotonergic antidepressants 161–2
serotonergic drugs 151
serotonin antagonists 124
serotonin-noradrenaline reuptake inhibitor (SNRI) antidepressants 153
serotonin-norepinephrine reuptake inhibitor 159
serotonin reuptake inhibitors (SRIs) 121, 124, 130, 146–7
sertraline 42, 122, 144, 170

service utilization 71–3
sex preponderance 65
sexual dysfunciton 162
sexual functioning in social phobias 317
sexual theories 33
Short Form-12 (SF-12) 71
shyness 22, 51, 152–3
  vs. sociability 254, 296
shyness clinics 153
Signals, Inhibition and Anxiety 143
simple phobia
  age of onset 297
  help seeking and use of medication 305
situational phobia 47
situationally bound panic attack 45
small animal phobias in children 251
snake phobia 175, 251, 253
social and economic burden
  agoraphobia 348
  anxiety disorders 337–9
  commentaries 329–53
  early diagnosis in 348–50
  patient factors 332
  review 303–28
  social anxiety disorder 348
  system issues 332
  treatments needed to reduce 344–8
social anxiety disorder (SAD) 38, 93, 101, 117, 155, 175, 351
  differentiation of generalized and non-generalized 341
  impairments 333
  in children 176
  low professional accomplishment due to 349
  non-response to treatment 157
  pharmacotherapy of 154–5, 158–60
  social and economic burden 348
  unemployment due to 349
  see also social phobias
social avoidance 90
social fears 37
social/occupational impairment 90
social phobia 8–9, 11, 18–23, 25–6, 37, 46–7, 99, 109, 339
  age of onset 297–8
  and bipolar disorder comorbidity 98–102
  and comorbidity, healthcare service utilization 311

and panic disorder comorbidity 51
areas still open to research 132–3,
  200–1
attentional bias in 56
behavioural toxicity of pharmacotherapeutic agents used in 172–4
burden and impairment 340
comorbidity 50–2
consistent evidence 131, 198
cynicism about 153–4
differential diagnosis 23
epidemiology 73–4
exposure *in vivo* 221
familial loading 343
future studies 347
generalized vs. non-generalized
  forms 54, 306–7
healthcare service utilizaion 311
health-related quality of life 335–7
help seeking and use of medication
  305, 307
in childhood 247, 251
in vivo exposure 189–90
inadequacy of treatment 340–1
incomplete evidence 131–2, 199–200
interpretation biases 56
longitudinal study 335
medications 118
misunderstanding 152–4
nicotine dependence 319
onset and discourse 22
pharmacotherapy 117–28
phenomenology 148–9
predictors of treatment outcome
  190–1
psychological treatment 229–30
psychotherapeutic interventions
  187–93
reason of close attention to 340
sexual functioning in 317
symptoms 118
treatment of 144
see also social anxiety disorder
Social Phobia Endstate Improvement
  Functioning Index (SPEFI) 321
social relationships 309
social skills training 188
social-threat-related words, preferential
  processing of 56
Society of Clinical Psychology 190
socioeconomic status 333

space phobia 12–13, 49
specific phobia 28, 44
  age of onset 298
  areas still open to research 201
  behavioural experimentation 225
  combined *in vivo* exposure and
    pharmacotherapy 195
  consistent evidence 198
  criteria of 246
  differential diagnosis 25
  examples 23–5
  external context 48
  future directions 197–8
  in adolescence 252
  in childhood 249, 252, 272–3, 280
    areas still open to research 273–4
  in vivo exposure 193–4
    methods of delivery 195–7
    vs. cognitive therapy 194–5
  incomplete evidence 200
  onset and discourse 24
  pharmacotherapy 129–30
  predictors of treatment outcome 197
  psychological treatment 230–1
  psychotherapeutic interventions 193–8
  quality of life 349
  residual category 48
  technological advances in treatment
    196–7
  traumatic onset 29
sphincteric phobia 19, 23
spider phobia 56–7, 175, 195
SSRIs 39, 42, 122–4, 128–32, 144, 159,
    163–4, 168, 170, 175–6, 269–70, 346
  in adolescent social phobia 124
  in childhood 124, 284
stigma associated with phobias 352
stress–diathesis model 95
Stroop test 56
Structured Clinical Interview of DSM-IV
  (SCID) 99
structured interviews 69, 99
substance abuse 50, 69, 113, 176
subthreshold criteria and non-criterion
  symptoms 87
subthreshold patients 87
suicidality 317–18
symptom substitution 143
symptoms, research on 59
syndromes, use of term 5

systematic desensitization in children 258–62

tachycardia 12
taijin-kyofusho (TKS) 130, 175–6
Task Force on Promotion and Dissemination of Psychological Procedures 190
taxonomy 55
  phobic symptoms 3–5
  potential bases 5–14
temperament 254, 257, 281
  as vulnerability factor 296
time delay between onset of phobia and beginning of treatment 77
transsexualism 26
tranylcypromine 170
trauma, memory of 84
treatment
  economic aspects of 320–2
  effectiveness in comorbidity 112
  effectiveness of 92
  of panic disorder and phobias 75–6
  present state of 92
  public health perspective 235–7
treatment-oriented classifications 42
treatment resisting (type R) 93
treatment responses 13–14, 39
treatment seeking (type S) 93

treatment strategy
  of adolescents 271–2
  of children 271–2
tricyclic antidepressants (TCAs) 42, 97, 121–2, 131, 149, 156, 161, 168, 270
twin studies 37, 46–7, 83

unconditioned stimuli 96
US National Advisory Mental Health Council (NAMHC) 310
US National Comorbidity Survey 50

venlafaxine 124, 144, 159
virtual reality (VR) exposure 220–1
vomiting 6, 21–2
vulnerability to phobias 95

water-phobic children 250
weight gain 162
WHO-DAS-II 53
WHO-Five Well-Being Scale 336
WHO-QoL 53
withdrawal symptoms 125
withdrawal vs. approach 254, 296
work difficulties 313
work impairment 313
World Health Organization International Consortium in Psychiatric Epidemiology (ICPE) 65
World Mental Health Survey 81